STP 1306

Environmental Toxicology and Risk Assessment: Biomarkers and Risk Assessment–Fifth Volume

David A. Bengtson and Diane S. Henshel, Editors

ASTM Publication Code Number (PCN):
04-013060-16

ASTM
100 Barr Harbor Drive
West Conshohocken, PA 19428-2959
Printed in the U.S.A.

ISBN: 0-8031-2031-1
ISSN: 1071-720X
PCN: 04-013060-16

Photocopy Rights

Authorization to photocopy items for internal, personal, or educational classroom use, or the internal, personal, or educational classroom use of specific clients, is granted by the American Society for Testing and Materials (ASTM) provided that the appropriate fee is paid to the Copyright Clearance Center, 222 Rosewood Drive, Danvers, MA 01923; Tel: (508) 750-8400; online: http://www.copyright.com/.

Peer Review Policy

Each paper published in this volume was evaluated by three peer reviewers. The authors addressed all of the reviewers' comments to the satisfaction of both the technical editor(s) and the ASTM Committee on Publications.

To make technical information available as quickly as possible, the peer-reviewed papers in this publication were prepared "camera-ready" as submitted by the authors.

The quality of the papers in this publication reflects not only the obvious efforts of the authors and the technical editor(s), but also the work of these peer reviewers. The ASTM Committee on Publications acknowledges with appreciation their dedication and contribution of time and effort on behalf of ASTM.

Printed in Philadelphia, PA
October 1996

Foreword

This publication, *Environmental Toxicology and Risk Assessment: BioMarkers and Risk Assessment—Fifth Volume*, contains papers present at the symposium of the same name, held on 3-5 April 1995 in Denver, Colorado. The symposium was sponsored by ASTM Committees E-47 on Biological Effects. David A. Bengtson of the University of Rhode Island in Kingston, RI and Diane S. Henshel of Indiana University in Bloomington, IN presided as symposium chairpersons and are editors of the resulting publication.

Contents

Overview

This volume includes papers presented at the ASTM Fifth Symposium on Environmental Toxicology and Risk Assessment, held in April 1995, in Denver, Colorado and sponsored by ASTM Committee E-47 on Biological Effects and Environmental Fate. The theme of the Symposium was Biomarkers and Risk Assessment. From the total of more than 100 oral and poster presentations at the Symposium, this volume represents a select few for which manuscripts were submitted and subjected to a rigorous peer-review process. As with the previous four ASTM Symposia on Environmental Toxicology and Risk Assessment, presentations at the meeting included a mixture of theme-session and non-theme contributions. The contributions to this volume are similarly divided between papers on the biomarker theme and those on general environmental toxicology and risk assessment.

The goals of the plenary session and the several biomarker-focused sessions throughout the Symposium were both to explore the usefulness of established biomarkers and to identify new biomarkers that are under development. A critical question is "How might biomarkers be useful in the future in the environmental and risk assessment processes?"

What is a biomarker? As defined by ASTM, a biomarker is 'a biological measure (within organisms) of exposure to, effects of, or susceptibility to environmental stress using molecular, genetic, biochemical, histological or physiological techniques.'' Thus, biomarkers are generally sublethal changes. Ideally, they should be consistently quantifiable (that is, the measured results should be readily replicable). The quantifiability of different biomarker techniques varies. Histopathological markers tend to be more qualitative, whereas biochemical and physiological markers tend to be very quantitative. Biomarkers are being developed at several levels of biological organization. Those at higher levels (anatomical or physiological) are presumed to integrate changes occurring at lower levels of organization (molecular or cellular). One of the most important challenges of biomarkers research is to understand the mechanisms of change at a given level and to then understand whether and how those changes are integrated at the next higher level.

Why use biomarkers in environmental and risk assessments? Classical endpoints used for risk assessment, for example, mortality or tumor induction, are either too severe or take too long to develop. Using death as the endpoint to establish safe levels of exposure leaves very little margin for the variation in sensitivity between individuals in a species or between species. We now estimate safe levels based on some safe or acceptable exposure level, a no-effect level or an effective dose for 10% of the population (ED10), integrating uncertainty and judgment factors into the equation. If our margin of safety is wrong for some untested population, we have allowed the possibility of a lethal effect in some percentage of a particularly sensitive population. If, on the other hand, safe levels are established based on more subtle, sublethal endpoints, such as biomarkers, behavior, or other biological indicators, then even super-sensitive populations will be better protected from such severe effects as increased mortality. In addition, toxicity testing for exposure and effects should be as cost-effective and time-efficient as possible, because many chemicals and sites must be tested with limited funding. Standard testing for cancer (tumorigenesis) is very costly because it requires a large number of animals to be maintained under test conditions for a large portion of their lifespan. Many short-term, biomarker-based mutagenicity tests have been developed and more are in development. Each such test has its limitations and appropriate uses, but a battery of such tests can be used to screen chemicals that require further testing as potential mutagens or carcinogens to target animal species. Another example of the potential uses of biomarkers is in the relatively new field of endocrine disruption. Until recently, chemicals that disrupt the endocrine system were only identified during testing for reproductive effects, which is also a costly endeavor in terms of time and money. More rapid and less costly screening techniques have recently been developed to assess the potential for chemicals to affect the endocrine system. It is becoming clear that some chemicals disrupt parts of the endocrine system beyond those involved in reproduction. Biomarker-based assays are facilitating the search for other endocrine-disrupting effects of environmental compounds (natural and anthropogenic). In the long term, there will be a need for molecular-level biomarkers that allow determination of "effect" and "no effect" levels for chemicals that will be protective of even sensitive populations.

The three invited speakers in the plenary session, Drs. John Stegeman, John McLachlan and Steven Bartell, discussed biomarkers and their use in the environmental and risk assessment process. Dr. Stegeman discussed many types of biomarkers, especially some of the more well-established biochemical and molecular markers now in use. He pointed out that each marker (measurement) has its own unique utility and pitfalls. Each measurement has a different time course, a different sensitivity and something separate to contribute to our understanding of a process, such that maximum information about an exposure is gained when several measurements are made in concert. Several factors must be considered when developing biomarker-based assays, such as the relative species and chemical specificities of the endpoints being measured; these specificites can often be determined empirically. Understanding the mechanisms controlling the interaction of the chemical with the measured endpoint helps to identify the potential functional significance of changes in that endpoint. Further understanding mechanisms under different physiological conditions (including such natural influences as daily or seasonal homeostatic fluctuations) improves our ability to interpret a given biomarker endpoint. Dr. Stegeman further pointed out that one needs to understand the causes of both increases and decreases in the signal that one measures in order to adequately interpret the measurements. Once the measurements are made, their biological implications for the animal must be understood. The effects measured must be interpreted within the context of the animal or species to respond. Determination of linkages between the measured biomarker effects and biologically significant effects at the organismal and population levels represent a research challenge for the future.

The second plenary speaker, Dr. McLachlan, addressed the need for standardization in biomarker-based assays. Given the important role that standardization generally plays in research, and the fact that we have no real standards as yet in the biomarker arena, it is time to focus on the devlopment of standards. Biomarker assays are based on perturbations in the normal homeostatic mechanisms of the body and are useful specifically because there are interactions between chemicals and cells and chemicals in cells, between cells in tissues, between tissues in organs, between organs in organisms, between organisms in populations, and between populations in communities. Effects or perturbations detected at one level of organization can have and do have effects at other levels of organization. When we understand these interactions, we can better interpret the relevance of perturbations in biomarker assays to the system as a whole. Dr. McLachlan pointed out that, during the last 20 years, there has been considerable research on, and production of standards for, the interaction of the environmental agents with genetic material leading to disease and dysfunction. We know a lot about, and have tests to measure, interactions of chemicals with our genome. We have many assays to look at mutation frequnecy and to try to correlate it with a variety of dysfunctions, especially cancer. Dr. McLachlan identified a currently emerging area of research as the study of environmental agents working through signaling molecules,

not only membrane-related proteins but the whole array of gene regulation, gene express
and signals that enter the cell and result in a variety of adverse effects. He predicted that th
would present a greater challenge both in terms of research and standards development tha
did the previous genetic research because the genetic research had "archival" material in
the structure of DNA. The signaling research will be hampered by the differences in time
scales over which the signaling events may occur and by the transient nature of the signals,
such that they may not be detectable at the time the dysfunction is expressed. The new
challenge presented by this research over the next 20 years will require as much ingenuity as
has been applied to understanding the interactions of environmental agents with the genome
over the last 20 years. The issue of environmental estrogens is one example of signaling
mechanisms and their possible use in biomarker assays. Environmental estrogens are estrogen mimics and can be considered a metaphor for molecules in the environment that mimic
our internal signaling molecules. These environmental mimics work at the interface between
the internal and external environment. Environmental estrogens will be increasingly important as metaphors for understanding signaling changes in a variety of systems and we need
to know more about them and the biological systems they affect.

The third plenary speaker, Dr. Bartell, discussed how the development of biomarkers,
which have allowed us to characterize exposure and effects for some metals, organics and
pesticides, could help us improve the ecological risk assessment process. Ecological risk
assessment recognizes and attempts to identify, quantify and propagate all of the uncertainties inherent in the analysis and to express the results of the assessment as a probabilistic
term based on those uncertainities. Dr. Bartell pointed out that biomarkers could help us
with both exposure assessment and response with regard to the dose-response components
of the ecological risk estimation. Biomarkers can indicate exposure to, or effects of, an
environmental agent, but they cannot by themselves indicate what changes have been
imposed upon the ecosystem as a whole. However, if we could develop relationships
between intensities of different biomarkers and survivorship or reproduction probabilities,
we could extrapolate from the biochemical level up to the population level. By understanding the linkages between cellular, organismal, and population levels, we could use
biomarker results to predict probabilities at the higher levels of organization. The process of
researching and understanding these linkages would very likely enable us to better understand the complexity of ecosystems generally. Thus, biomarkers might provide a catalyst for
a more general understanding of the relationships between different levels of biological
organization through the analysis of the propagation of perturbations through systems. Dr.
Bartell concluded his remarks with the opinion that there is no inherent reason why we
could not ultimately make intelligent decisions on regulation of contaminants directly from
biomarkers, because we don't necessarily have to focus on population, community, or
ecosystem level impacts. If the scientific basis is available, we could decide to use
biomarkers as valid endpoints for decision making. Some biomarkers may be most useful in
ecological risk assessment in the context of evaluation of sites with multiple contaminants.
If biomarkers could be used to conduct an initial screening to help narrow the scope of the
problem, so that attention could be focused on the contaminants posing the greatest risk, that
could be a very beneficial use of biomarkers in risk assessment, in Dr. Bartell's opinion.

The biomarkers section of this volume includes papers on a variety of biomarker responses, including molecular, cellular, genetic, developmental and neurotoxicological, measured in a variety of organisms from bacteria to humans. Some of these biomarkers are well
established and have been tested in a number of species. Others are still being developed.
The first two papers (Palmer & Selcer and Denslow et al.) address the use of vitellogenin as
a biomarker for environmental estrogens and therefore contribute to the growing body of
knowledge on the effects of endocrine disrupting chemicals and potential biological indica-

~s that may be used to assess exposure to these chemicals. Vitellogenin appears to be one ~ch biomarker that will be useful across a variety of submammalian species. The next ~aper (Hewitt et al.) discusses findings that might also be related to reproductive problems in fish. Anderson et al. and Melancon describe the usefulness of assessing the induction of specific cytochromes P450 as biomarkers of exposure to specific classes of chemicals, including many PAH's, as well as laterally substituted chlorinated dioxins and PCB's. The reporter gene system described by Anderson et al. is currently under consideration for inclusion as an ASTM standard. A series of three papers (Lucas & Straume, Law et al., and Donnelly et al.) on genotoxicity follows, describing biomarkers that are being developed as indicators of exposure and effects and providing evidence of genetic damage due to both chemical agents and radiation. This section on cellular- and molecular-level biomarkers closes with a set of papers on smoke exposure in humans (Rees et al.), aromatic hydrocarbon toxicity in plants (Gensemer et al.), identification of proteins (Bradley et al.) and toxic effects in cladocerans (Fort et al.). The Gensemer et al. paper is noteworthy in its correlation of the biomarker endpoint with a population-level effect. Fort et al. demonstrate that subtle changes in membrane potential are clearly biomarkers of functional effect at the cellular level. The next set of three papers (Fort and Stover, Dickerson et al. and Henshel) explore embryological development as an integrator of cellular-level effects of toxicants on organisms. Embryonic development is a very sensitive life stage and there are relatively few well-established biomarkers to assess adverse developmental effects. The FETAX assay, which is extended in the paper by Fort and Stover, is one of the better-tested biomarkers of effects on embryonic development in field situations. The early embryo assay, discussed in the papers by Dickerson et al. and Henshel, is now being developed for future use in field assessments. Finally, the last two papers in the Biomarkers section (Henshel et al. and Eells et al.) examine potential biomarkers of neurotoxicity in birds and mammals. Henshel et al. provide information on a biomarker for developmental neurotoxic effects, for which there is a paucity of biomarker assays at present. The papers by Eells et al. and Henshel discuss the critical question of the use of appropriate animal models in the devlopment of biomarkers; use of an appropriate model may determine whether the biologically relevant effect (retinal degeneration induced by methanol exposure in the case of Eells et al.) will be observed or not. The question is important when one tries to mimic effects seen in a particular species, for example, humans, because biochemical differences among species have been well documented. The Eells et al. paper especially emphasizes the importance of understanding the mechanism underlying the change measured as an effect.

The papers presented in this section thus represent an up-to-date, broad survey of the several classes of biomarkers that are currently being studied and the several classes of vertebrates and invertebrates in which these methods can be evaluated.

The second section of this volume contains papers from the Symposium that do not include biomarkers among the techniques used. The first two papers are in the field of aquatic toxicology. Lussier et al. provide information that can be used to improve an existing ASTM standard on life-cycle tests with saltwater mysids. Lytle and Lytle then present results from toxicity tests with a salt marsh macrophyte, which represents a group of organisms relatively little tested in comparison to their importance in the environment. The next two papers (Pinza et al. and McCauley et al.) deal with problems (ammonia in sediments and porewater extraction, respectively) that have vexed sediment toxicologists for years. The three papers on beahvior (Lipton et al., Nepomnyashchikh et al. and Misra et al.), each of which is interesting in its own right, provide a useful reminder of the connection of biomarker parameters to higher levels of biological factors, such that behavioral changes can be used as an indicator of functional effect; both behavior and biomarkers are most useful when they yield information about sublethal effects of toxicants. Indeed, behavior-based assays are being developed for use in toxicity assessments for application to risk assessment. Harrass and Klemm and Hall provide excellent reviews and valuable advice on quality assurance and toxicity identification, respectively, in the context of laboratory toxicity testing. Peterson and Knowlton then describe a computer-based risk assessment system and Mahoney et al. discuss the difficulties for risk assessors when dealing with different forms of chromium in the environment. Finally, papers by Hsu and Yeung and Li and Yeung provide a mathematical model and a new method of data interpretation, respectively, for engineering problems associated with volatile organic compounds (VOC), although these papers may have more general relevance to those outside the VOC field as well. The papers in this second section thus provide a potpourri of interesting and valuable information ranging over the broad spectrum of the field of environmental toxicology and risk assessment.

We wish to thank both the authors and reviewers of the papers for their considerable efforts, the editorial staff of ASTM (especially Shannon Wainwright) for their constant help, and Kenneth St. John of the ASTM Committee on Publications for continually pushing us to meet deadlines.

Diane S. Henshel

Indiana University, School of Public and Environmental Affairs, Bloomington, IN 47405; Symposium Chairperson and Editor.

David A. Bengtson

University of Rhode Island, Department of Biological Sciences, Kingston, RI 02881; Symposium Chairperson and Editor.

Biomarkers

Brent D. Palmer[1] and Kyle W. Selcer[2]

VITELLOGENIN AS A BIOMARKER FOR XENOBIOTIC ESTROGENS: A REVIEW

REFERENCE: Palmer, B. D. and Selcer, K. W., **"Vitellogenin as a Biomarker for Xenobiotic Estrogens: A Review,"** *Environmental Toxicology and Risk Assessment: Biomarkers and Risk Assessment—Fifth Volume, ASTM STP 1306,* David A. Bengtson and Diane S. Henshel, Eds., American Society for Testing and Materials, 1996.

ABSTRACT: A number of chemical pollutants have physiological effects mimicking those of estrogen. These xenobiotic estrogens pose an insidious risk to wildlife and humans by disrupting reproductive and developmental processes, thereby impairing both the exposed individuals and their offspring. Xenobiotic estrogens are impacting both wildlife and human health, thus it is important to screen chemicals for estrogenic potential, and to monitor environmental levels of estrogenic pollutants. Although most known xenobiotic estrogens show little structural similarity, they do produce predictable physiological responses. This allows the use of functional estrogenicity assays employing specific biomarkers of estrogen action, such as vitellogenin. Vitellogenin is an egg-yolk precursor protein produced by the liver in response to estrogens and estrogen agonists. Vitellogenin is normally found only in the serum of adult female oviparous vertebrates, but it can be induced in males and immature females by estrogen. Vitellogenin induction bioassays can be used to screen chemicals for estrogenic and antiestrogenic activity, to test water for the presence of xenobiotic estrogens, and to screen wildlife populations for exposure to environmental estrogens.

KEYWORDS: Vitellogenin, biomarker, xenobiotic, estrogen

[1]Assistant Professor, Laboratory of Reproductive Ecology, Department of Biological Sciences, Ohio University, Athens, OH 45701

[2] Assistant Professor, Department of Biological Sciences, Duquesne University, Pittsburgh, PA 15282.

3

XENOBIOTIC ESTROGENS

The insidious effects of some environmental contaminants are mediated by their ability to mimic natural hormones in the body. One of the best known and most widespread of these endocrine disrupters are those that mimic the steroid hormone estrogen. Some of these pollutants were designed to be estrogenic and are present in the environment as a result of their widespread use. For example, quantities of oral contraceptives are released via the urine into community waste water systems (Rall and McLachlan 1980). The artificial estrogen diethylstilbestrol (DES) was taken by approximately 5 million pregnant women worldwide from 1941-1971. DES also was released extensively in the United States when it was used for increasing weight gain in livestock (Knight 1980). However, most environmental estrogens were not designed to have endocrine functions and are inadvertently estrogenic. These agents, often termed xenobiotic estrogens, include pesticides and many common industrial chemicals (Table 1). Xenobiotic estrogens are important because they have been implicated in the disruption of reproductive and developmental processes in both wildlife and humans. Particularly, levels of estrogenic compounds that do not induce cancer may have enormous impact on reproductive and developmental systems. This indicates that levels that have been considered "safe" based on cancer studies may actually cause serious health effects. Compounding this is the fact that many xenobiotics, since they are organic, biomagnify in the food web, bioaccumulate in fatty tissues, and are additive in their effects (Soto et al. 1996).

Xenobiotic estrogens have been found to adversely affect reproduction and development of a wide variety of species. Many Xenobiotics both cross the placental barrier (van den Berg et al. 1987) and are transferred to newborns via breast milk (Courtney and Andrews 1985). In wildlife, xenobiotics accumulate in eggs (Bishop et al. 1991). Much of the information on biological effects of environmental estrogens comes from studies of wildlife populations. Effects from exposure to xenobiotic estrogens include: alterations in development of the reproductive tract (Gray et al. 1989), sex changes and feminization (Fry and Toone 1981; Davis and Bortone 1992; Gray 1992; Guillette et al. 1994), altered hormone ratios (Guillette et al. 1994, 1995) and reproductive failure (Fox 1992; Patnode and Curtis, 1994). A large body of correlative evidence suggests that there may be global consequences from contamination of the environment with estrogenic chemicals (Colborn and Clements 1992).

There may be human health effects associated with exposure to xenobiotic estrogens, although these have not been demonstrated unequivocally. Associations have been proposed between increased levels of xenobiotic estrogens in the environment and several human reproductive and developmental anomalies, including: precocious puberty (McLachlan 1985), increased incidence of breast cancer (Wolff et al. 1993), testicular cancer (Brown et al. 1986; Østerlind 1986; Boyle et al. 1987) and prostate cancer (Hoel et al. 1992) and reduced sperm count (Carlsen et al. 1992; Sharpe and Skakkebaek 1993). That there is concern about the possibility of xenobiotic estrogens impacting human health is evidenced by the large amount of attention this topic has received in recent years (e.g., Colborn et al. 1993; McLachlan 1993; Raloff 1993, 1994; Shore et al. 1993; Cotton 1994; Ginsburg 1994).

TABLE 1--Xenobiotic estrogens*.

_____

Pesticides

    DDT and metabolites (*o,p'*-DDT, *p,p'*-DDT, *o,p'*-DDD)
    Methoxychlor metabolites (mono- and didemethylated methoxychlor)
    Chlordecone (Kepone)
    Dieldren
    Alpha and beta-endosulfan
    Gamma-hexachlorocyclohexane (g-HCH: lindane)
    Toxaphene

Industrial Chemicals

    Polychlorinated biphenyls (PCBs)
    Alkylphenol polyethoxylates
    Bisphenol-A
    t-Butylhydroxyanisole (BHA)
    Benzylbutylphthalate
    Diphenylphthalate

_____

*From Soto et al. 1996.

    There are a variety of ways that chemicals can influence estrogenic pathways in the body. Some PCBs and dioxins operate through the Ah receptor to influence steroid levels (by altering their metabolism) or downregulate estrogen receptor levels (Gasiewicz and Rucci 1991; Lin et al. 1991a; Zacharewski et al, 1991, 1992). Activation of the Ah receptor may also cause downregulation of growth factor receptors, which serve to mediate estrogenic responses (Lin et al. 1991b; Abbot et al. 1992; Schrenck et al., 1992). However, most xenobiotic estrogens bind to the endogenous estrogen receptors and elicit either agonistic and/or antagonistic responses. DDT is a xenobiotic estrogen, and probably the best studied example of an exogenous hormone mimic (Bulger and Kupfer 1983a, b; McLachlan 1985). The earliest laboratory account of the estrogenic nature of DDT was the discovery that DDT was uterotropic (increased uterine weight) in rats (Levin et al. 1968; Welch et al. 1969). Further, mice exposed to DDT exhibited prolonged estrous cycles and decreases in ova implantation (Lundberg 1973). It was established that the *o,p'*-isomer of DDT was largely responsible for the uterotropic activity (Welch et al. 1969). DDT binds to the estrogen receptor, and initiates the same sequence of events as natural estrogens (Nelson 1974). This includes an increase in uterine DNA synthesis (Ireland et al. 1980) and induction of protein synthesis and secretion (Stancel et al. 1980). Many of these induced proteins are enzymatic in nature (Singhal et al. 1970; Cohen et al. 1970; Kaye et al. 1971; Bulger et al. 1978a; Bulger and Kupfer 1978 1983b). Particularly notable, one of the proteins induced by *o,p'*-DDT in the rat uterus is the receptor molecule for another sex steroid, progesterone (Mason and Schulte 1980).

Other xenobiotics are also hormone mimics. PCBs are a wide class of compounds and a major industrial pollutant. Many PCB congeners have either estrogenic or antiestrogenic properties (Jansen et al. 1993). PCBs have extensive effects on reproductive systems (Reijnders 1988), including stimulation of uterotropic effects, prolonged estrous cycles, impaired fertility, reduced number of young, and reduced maternal ability to carry young to term (see Swain et al. 1993). In reptiles, 2', 4', 5'-trichloro-4-biphenylol has been shown to be estrogenic and induce complete sex-reversal during embryonic development (Bergeron et al. 1994). These effects are mediated in part by PCBs ability to bind to estrogen receptors (Nelson 1974; Korach et al. 1988). Alkylphenols are another group of widespread industrial pollutants that are estrogenic (Soto et al. 1991). They are used in making plastics, aerosols and surfactants, and are an ingredient in many other products, such as spermicidal foams.

Some xenobiotics mimic endogenous hormones only after being metabolized, or activated, in the body. Methoxychlor (bis-p-methoxy DDT) is a proestrogen, and is metabolized by the hepatic mixed-function oxidase (MFO) system into estrogenic products (Nelson et al. 1976, 1978; Bulger et al. 1978b; Ousterhout et al. 1979, 1981). The estrogenic metabolite of methoxychlor was shown to be about 10 times more active than o,p'-DDT in rodents (Ousterhout et al. 1981).

A variety chemicals known to be estrogenic show little structural similarity (McLachlan 1993). The only structural component shared by most (but not all) of the natural, synthetic and xenobiotic estrogens is a phenyl ring (Daux and Weeks 1980). Otherwise, estrogenic compounds vary dramatically in their structure. However, many xenobiotic estrogens bind agonistically to the estrogen receptor to elicit estrogenic responses. The molecular basis of estrogenicity appears to reside in a compound's ability to bind to the estrogen receptor and elicit biological effects (Daux and Weeks 1980; Katzenellenbogen et al. 1980; McLachlan et al. 1987; Korach et al. 1988). The result of an estrogenic compound binding to the estrogen receptor is usually an alteration in the rate of transcription of estrogen-dependent genes and subsequent changes in synthesis of estrogen-dependent proteins (O'Malley and Tsai 1992). Thus, the definition of an estrogenic compound relies more on function than structure (McLachlan 1993).

FUNCTIONAL ASSAYS FOR XENOBIOTIC ESTROGENS

The lack of structural similarity among xenobiotic estrogens precludes the development of a test method for estrogenicity based on molecular structure. Recently, several researchers have proposed the use of functional assays for the screening of potentially estrogenic compounds. Soto et al. (1992) developed an assay based on growth of estrogen-dependent breast cancer cells. McLachlan (1993) has proposed the use of cells transfected with the estrogen receptor and a specific reporter gene. Vitellogenin induction is another effective means of assessing estrogenicity. These proposed assays differ in the endpoint they use; however, they are all similar in that they measure some aspect of biological activity known to be estrogen specific. It is likely that each will prove to be useful in determining the estrogenicity of various compounds.

Functional assays for xenobiotic estrogens should meet several criteria (Palmer and Palmer 1995). They should measure a physiological response to estrogenic compounds. This response should ideally be through known biochemical pathways that are thoroughly understood. The endpoint of the functional assay must be quantifiable and dose-responsive. The response should also be applicable to a wide variety of vertebrates in order to screen diverse wildlife populations. Finally, the assay should preferably utilize samples that can be readily obtained in the laboratory or field without causing undo stress or harm to the animal.

VITELLOGENIN AS A BIOMARKER

Vitellogenin is a serum protein occurring naturally in adult female nonmammalian vertebrates (Ho 1987; Lazier and MacKay 1993). Vitellogenin is the precursor molecule for egg yolk, which is essential as the source of metabolic energy for the developing embryo. The liver synthesizes and secretes vitellogenin, which is carried in the bloodstream to the oocytes. The developing oocytes take up vitellogenin and cleave it into the egg yolk proteins lipovitellin and phosvitins (Lazier and MacKay 1993).

Vitellogenin is a phospholipoglycoprotein that usually circulates as a dimer of 400-500 kilodaltons (kDa)(Callard and Ho 1987). The vitellogenin polypeptides of various species are commonly about 200-250 kDa. There are multiple vitellogenin forms present in the plasma of several species, including chicken, several fish and *Xenopus* (Ho 1987; Lazier and MacKay 1993). The basic organization of the vitellogenin polypeptide is similar among various species of vertebrates. The vitellogenin polypeptide consists of lipid-rich and phosphate-rich regions. These regions are separated by enzymatic cleavage in the oocyte into the yolk proteins lipovitellin and phosvitin, respectively. Vitellogenin is glycosylated and contains about 1.4 % carbohydrate by weight. The lipovitellin region of the molecule is lipidated and contains as much as 20 % lipid by weight. The phosvitin region of the molecule consists of a large percentage (up to 50 %) of serine residues, most of which are phosphorylated, resulting in as much as 10 % phosphorus by weight for this region of the molecule.

Estrogen is the primary stimulus for vitellogenin production. Estrogen promotes vitellogenesis in members of all nonmammalian vertebrate classes (Ho 1987; Lazier and MacKay 1993). In each of these groups, the time of vitellogenin production in adult females corresponds to the period of elevated estrogen levels. Furthermore, vitellogenin production can be induced in males and in nonvitellogenic females by administration of estrogen (Ding et al. 1989; Kishida et al. 1992). The production of vitellogenin in response to estrogenic compounds is rapid, sensitive, and dose-dependent (Ho et al. 1981; Lazier and MacKay, 1993). The strength of the vitellogenic response indicates the relative ability of xenobiotic compounds to stimulate estrogenic pathways. Estrogen is the primary inducer of vitellogenin (Tata and Smith 1979), although other factors have a role in modulating the vitellogenic response (Ho et al. 1981; Wangh 1982; Carnevali and Mosconi 1992; Carnevali et al. 1992; Carnevali et al, 1993). A recent study found that cortisol may have a transient effect on inducing vitellogenin mRNAs in fish by an unknown mechanism, although these are rapidly cleared and do not result in production of vitellogenin protein (Ding et al. 1994).

The utility of vitellogenin as a biomarker for estrogenic compounds is based on several facts. Vitellogenin induction is a physiological response to the presence of estrogen or estrogenic chemicals. The mechanism of vitellogenin production has been extensively studied as a model for steroid action. Vitellogenin is universally produced by all nonmammalian vertebrates in a dose-dependent manner. Vitellogenin is normally female-specific, but vitellogenin is inducible in male animals by estrogen and estrogenic compounds. Male oviparous vertebrates normally will not have vitellogenin in their blood unless they are exposed to estrogen or an estrogenic compound. Therefore, the presence of vitellogenin in the blood of male oviparous animals can serve as an indicator of exposure to xenobiotic estrogens. Finally, vitellogenin is readily quantified. These characteristics make vitellogenin uniquely qualified to serve as a functional biomarker for exposure to estrogenic compounds.

UTILITY OF VITELLOGENIN ASSAYS

Recent information on the abundance and potential health hazards of xenobiotic contamination of the environment has brought attention to the need for assays to screen chemicals for estrogenic activity (Colborn et al. 1993; McLachlan 1993). Vitellogenin induction assays can be employed in various ways to investigate different aspects of environmental estrogens. Potential uses include screening compounds for estrogenicity and antiestrogenicity, testing waters for the presence of xenobiotic estrogens, and evaluating exposure of wildlife populations to estrogenic compounds. In fact, vitellogenin induction is unique in that this same estrogen-dependent response can be employed for screening compounds both *in vitro* and *in vivo*.

The *in vitro* vitellogenin induction assay involves the use of primary cultures of hepatocytes. Pelissero et al.(1993) first proposed the use of cultured rainbow trout hepatocytes as a test for estrogenic chemicals. They demonstrated the relative estrogenicity of several natural and artificial estrogens (e.g., ethinylestradiol and diethylstilbestrol) as well as six phytoestrogens. The various chemicals showed dose-responsive induction of vitellogenin. This induction was blocked by the antiestrogen tamoxifen, confirming that the mechanism of vitellogenin induction was via the estrogen receptor. Trout hepatocytes have subsequently been used to identify alkylphenolic and phthalate compounds that are estrogenic *in vitro* (Jobling and Sumpter 1993; White et al. 1994). Other sources of hepatocytes should also prove useful for vitellogenin induction assays.

Primary hepatocyte cultures have certain advantages for estrogenicity screening, including ready availability of tissues and the ability to rapidly screen large numbers of chemicals. However, there are also limitations associated with the use of primary cultures. Primary cultures are subject to variation in response due to the use of livers from different individuals. Furthermore, the responsiveness of hepatocytes generally diminishes with time. This limits the screening to relatively short-term exposures. Flouriot et al. (1993), using estrogen receptor and vitellogenin as markers of estrogen responsiveness, reported that monolayers of trout hepatocytes became unresponsive to estrogens within 5-10 days. However, they found that aggregates of hepatocytes in defined medium remained responsive to estrogens for up to 30 days. Perhaps the major limitation of *in vitro* screening assays is the potentially limited metabolism of the test compounds compared with the whole animal. Some known xenobiotic compounds are estrogenic only after metabolic conversion. While hepatocytes have an array of metabolic enzymes, it is unlikely they possess the full complement found in the whole animal. Furthermore, cell culture systems lack other important factors that may influence estrogenicity, such as serum transport proteins, which influence effective exposure levels.

While *in vitro* systems are advantageous for screening large numbers of compounds for estrogenic effects, *in vivo* studies can provide a more precise measure of potential effects in living organisms. *In vivo* systems allow evaluation of uptake, transport, metabolism, and excretion of test compounds. Furthermore, *in vivo* systems lend themselves to long-term studies of exposure to xenobiotic estrogens. The classic method of assessing estrogenicity *in vivo* is the ovariectomized rodent uterotropic assay, which has proven to be a sensitive and reliable indicator of estrogenicity. However, the vitellogenin induction assay has several advantages over the uterotropic assay, not the least of which is that it employs nonmammalian model systems. Another advantage of the vitellogenin induction assay is that it can be employed to assess the effects of exposure to xenobiotic estrogens in aquatic systems. To date, vitellogenin induction assays have been applied to fish (Pelissero et al. 1991a, b; Purdom et al. 1994) as well as to aquatic reptiles and amphibians (Palmer and Palmer 1995). Palmer and Palmer (1995) reported that DES and the persistent pesticide *o,p'*-DDT cause dose-dependent induction of vitellogenin in the red-eared turtle and in *Xenopus*, demonstrating the potential utility of vitellogenin induction as a screen for xenobiotic estrogens. Chakravorty et al. (1992) used the suppression of vitellogenin levels in determining the antiestrogenic effects of endosulfan in catfish.

The *in vivo* vitellogenin induction assay can be adapted to test waters for the presence of estrogenic contaminants. This involves placing caged aquatic animals, known to lack vitellogenin, into waters suspected of containing xenobiotic estrogens, then regularly sampling their serum for vitellogenin. Although the causative compound is not identified by this method, it serves as a rapid and inexpensive test of water quality. Positive results can be followed up with chemical analyses to identify the causative agents and their concentrations. Purdom et al. (1994) used this approach to test sewage effluent for estrogenicity, using caged trout and carp as model organisms. They found induction of vitellogenin in the plasma of males in the mg/ml range, which is comparable to levels reached in vitellogenic females.

Vitellogenin assays can also be used to screen wildlife population for exposure to xenobiotic estrogens (Palmer and Selcer 1994; Palmer et al. 1994). Many wildlife species have experienced unexplained declines in population size over the past few decades. It has been suggested that environmental endocrine disrupters may be one causative factor (Colborn et al. 1993). Thus, population biologists are increasingly interested in determining if particular populations are being affected by xenobiotic estrogens. This can be accomplished by testing plasma samples of males or juvenile females for the presence of vitellogenin. If vitellogenin is found, there is a high probability that the local environment contains estrogenic agents. However, for these types of studies to be meaningful, several considerations must be taken into account. The normal levels of vitellogenin (from a reference population) for males and juveniles of the species in question must be determined. For example, there have been several reports of low levels of vitellogenin in male fish (So et al. 1985; Copeland et al. 1986; Copeland and Thomas 1988; Pelissero et al. 1989; Goodwin et al. 1992; Kishida and Specker 1993). It is important to assay for endogenous estrogens, which may be artificially elevated for due to other causes. Also, the vitellogenin of the species in question should be characterized with regard to number of vitellogenin forms, molecular weight, and cross-reactivity with any antibodies used in the assay.

METHODS FOR MEASURING VITELLOGENIN

Use of vitellogenin induction as a biomarker of estrogenicity requires a method for measuring vitellogenin levels in cell culture medium or plasma. A number of techniques have been employed to quantify vitellogenin. Because vitellogenin is a calcium-binding phospholipoprotein, indirect estimates of vitellogenin have been made based on changes in plasma phosphoprotein, calcium or lipid (e.g., Dessauer and Fox 1959; Redshaw et al. 1969; Craik 1978; Elliott et al. 1979). Some techniques require separation of vitellogenin, which is then measured colorimetrically. Vitellogenin can be purified by precipitation or chromatography, followed by protein assay. Alternately, vitellogenin can be separated from other plasma proteins by polyacrylamide gel electrophoresis and quantified by computerized densitometry (Palmer and Palmer 1995). Most commonly, vitellogenin is measured using immunological approaches. The most widely employed of these are radioimmunoassays (e.g., Redshaw and Follett 1976; Gapp et al. 1979; Idler et al. 1979; Sumpter 1985; So et al. 1985; Norberg and Haux 1988; Tyler and Sumpter 1990) and enzyme-linked immunosorbent assays (Rodriguez et al. 1989; Carnevali et al. 1991; Goodwin et al. 1992; Kishida et al. 1992; Specker and Anderson 1994; Palmer and Palmer 1995). Both methods are highly specific, sensitive and accurate when used for detection of homologous vitellogenins. For large scale applications, the enzyme-linked immunosorbent assays may be preferable since they do not require radioactivity. Furthermore, the labeled vitellogenin used in the radioimmunoassays may be unstable in some species (Idler et al. 1979; Sumpter 1985).

Regardless of the type of immunoassay used, a specific vitellogenin antibody is required. The antibody is typically generated from semipurified or purified vitellogenin. Vitellogenin is relatively simple to purify in most species using dimethylformamide precipitation (Hori et al. 1979; Goodwin et al. 1992), EDTA/Mg precipitation (Wiley et al. 1979; Bradley and Grizzle 1989; Selcer and Palmer 1995; Palmer and Palmer 1995) or DEAE chromatography (Wiley et al. 1979; Kashida et al. 1992; Selcer and Palmer 1995). However, purified fish vitellogenin appears to be unstable and more difficult to purify (Tyler and Sumpter 1990). Most studies have utilized polyclonal antibodies, but recently monoclonal antibodies have proven effective in vitellogenin immunoassays (Goodwin et al. 1992). Monoclonal antibodies will be particularly valuable for large-scale screening of chemicals for estrogenicity using the vitellogenin induction assays.

Ideally, a homologous antibody should be used in a vitellogenin immunoassay. However, with the recent interest in evaluation of vitellogenin in diverse wildlife populations, some of which may be threatened, it may be necessary to develop antibodies that demonstrate significant cross-reactivity among species. This would obviate purifying vitellogenin and generating specific antibodies for each species to be examined. Unfortunately, the vitellogenin polypeptides do not show a high degree of homology among species, resulting in fairly low cross-reactivity for most antibodies. However, there are homologous regions of the vitellogenin proteins that may allow development of broadly cross-reactive antibodies. This approach has been attempted for fish vitellogenins. Folmar et al. (1995) generated antibodies against a peptide representing the most homologous portion of the n-terminal amino acid regions of six fish species.

It is likely that a broadly cross-reactive antibody can be developed for vitellogenin. We used the program Clustal to perform a multiple alignment on the five full vitellogenin sequences currently available in the protein databases. These sequences (*Gallus, Ichthyomyzon, Xenopus, Acipenser, and Fundulus*) represent individuals from four classes of vertebrates. After alignment, there were six regions of 10 amino acids or longer that showed reasonably high homology, 60-73 % (Palmer et al. 1994). Antibodies generated against peptides based on these regions may prove to be broadly cross-reactive, even among species in different classes.

Most assays used to measure vitellogenin induction by estrogenic compounds are based on detection of the vitellogenin protein in plasma or culture medium. However, molecular approaches can also be used to measure stimulation of vitellogenin. Estrogen regulation of vitellogenin gene transcription represents one of the classic model systems used to study the molecular mechanisms of steroid hormone action (Tata and Smith 1979; Shapiro et al. 1989). Consequently, methods to measure vitellogenin gene expression are well established. Induction of vitellogenin mRNA is a sensitive and rapid response to the presence of estrogenic agents. Vitellogenin mRNA can be readily measured by Northern blotting and by slot and dot hybridization assays. A more sensitive assay, especially for small samples, can be developed using rt-PCR. Vitellogenin mRNA assays can be employed *in vitro*, using cultured hepatocytes, or *in vivo*. Assays for induction of vitellogenin mRNA may prove to be the best methods for screening large numbers of chemicals for estrogenicity.

CONCLUSIONS AND FUTURE DIRECTIONS

Vitellogenin is a versatile biomarker for exposure to xenobiotic estrogens. It is applicable for screening chemicals for estrogenicity and antiestrogenicity both *in vitro* and *in vivo*, testing water for the presence of estrogenic agents, and assessing the effects of environmental estrogens on wildlife populations. Advancements in techniques will enhance the speed, sensitivity and utility of vitellogenin assay systems. The diversity of species suitable for vitellogenin induction studies should be examined to develop more sensitive models and determine cross-species variation. For *in vitro* systems, the development of immortalized hepatocyte cell lines will reduce interassay variation, increase the potential duration of treatment regimens, and provide uniformity among investigators. New molecular methods, such as rt-PCR, will enhance the sensitivity of vitellogenin assays. In the field, the screening of diverse wildlife species necessitates the development of broad spectrum antibodies that will provide reliable, specific and sensitive cross-reactivities with multiple vertebrate vitellogenins. Lastly, standardization of laboratory and field methodologies will facilitate increased use of vitellogenin assays, replication of studies, and direct comparison of data from multiple investigators. Clearly, the usefulness of vitellogenin as a biomarker for xenobiotic estrogens and antiestrogens is well established. New advancements in the methodologies will only serve to increase its utility.

LITERATURE CITED

Abbot, B. D., Harris, M. W., and Birnbaum, L. S., 1992, "Comparisons of the effects of TCDD and hydrocortisone on growth factor expression provide insight into their interaction in the embryonic mouse palate," Teratology, Vol. 45, pp. 35-53

Bergeron, J. M., Crews, D., McLachlan, J.A., 1994, "PCBs as environmental estrogens; turtle sex determination as a biomarker of environmental contamination," Environmental Health Perspectives Vol. 102, pp. 780-781

Boyle, P., Kaye, S. N., Robertson, A. G., 1987, "Changes in testicular cancer in Scotland," European Journal of Cancer and Clinical Oncology, Vol. 23, pp. 827-830.

Bradley, J. T., and Grizzle, J. M., 1989, "Vitellogenin induction by estradiol in channel catfish, *Ictalurus punctatus*," General and Comparative Endocrinology, Vol. 73, pp. 28-39

Brown, L. M., Pottern, L. M., Hoover, R. N., Devesa, S. S., Aselton, P., Flannery, J. T., 1986, "Testicular cancer in the United States: trends in incidence and mortality," International Journal of Epidemiology, Vol. 15, pp. 164-179

Bulger, W. H., and Kupfer, D., 1978, "Studies on the induction of rat uterine ornithine decarboxylase by DDT analogs. I. Comparison with estradiol-17β activity," Pesticide Biochemistry and Physiology, Vol. 8, pp. 165-177

Bulger, W. H., Muccitelli, R. M., Kupfer, D., 1978a, "Studies on the induction of rat uterine ornithine decarboxylase by DDT analogs. II. Kinetic characteristics of ornithine decarboxylase induced by DDT analogs and estradiol," Pesticide Biochemistry and Physiology, Vol. 8, pp. 263-270

Bulger, W. H., Muccitelli, R. M., Kupfer, D., 1978b, "Studies on the *in vivo* and *in vitro* estrogenic activities of methoxychlor and its metabolites: Role of hepatic mono-oxygenase in methoxychlor activation," Biochemical Pharmacology, Vol. 27, pp. 2417-2423

Bulger, W. H., and Kupfer, D., 1983a, "Estrogenic action of DDT analogs," American Journal of Industrial Medicine, Vol. 4, pp. 163-173

Bulger, W. H., and Kupfer, D., 1983b, "Effect of xenobiotic estrogens and structurally related compounds on 2-hydroxylation of estradiol and on other monooxygenase activities in rat liver," Biochemical Pharmacology, Vol. 32, No. 6, pp. 1005-1010

Callard, I. P., and Ho, S.-M., 1987, "Vitellogenesis and viviparity," In Fundamentals of comparative endocrinology, Chester-Jones, I., Ingleton, P. M., and Phillips, J. G., eds., Plenum Press, New York, pp. 257-282

Carlsen, E., Giwereman, A., Keiding, N., and Skakkebaek, N. E., 1992, "Evidence for decreasing quality of semen during the past 50 years," British Medical Journal, Vol. 305, pp. 609-613

Carnevali, O., and Mosconi, G., 1992, "In vitro induction of vitellogenin synthesis in Rana esculenta: role of the pituitary," General and Comparative Endocrinology, Vol. 86, pp. 352-358

Carnevali, O., Mosconi, G., Angelini, F., Limatola, E., Ciarcia, G., and Polzonetti-Magni, A., 1991, "Plasma vitellogenin and 17β-estradiol levels during the annual reproductive cycle of Podacris s. sicula Raf," General and Comparative Endocrinology, Vol. 84, pp. 337-343

Carnevali, O., Mosconi, G., Yamamoto, K., Kobayashi, T., Kikuyama, S., and Polzonette-Magni, A. M., 1992, "Hormonal control of in vitro vitellogenin synthesis in Rana esculenta liver: effects of mammalian and amphibians growth hormone," General and Comparative Endocrinology, Vol. 88, pp. 406-414

Carnevali, O., Mosconi, G., Yamamoto, K., Kobayashi, T., Kikuyama, S., and Polzonette-Magni, A. M., 1993, "In vitro effects of mammalian and amphibian prolactins on hepatic vitellogenin synthesis in Rana esculenta," Journal of Endocrinology, Vol. 137, pp. 383-389

Chakravorty S., Lal, B., and Singh, T. P., 1992, "Effect of endosulfan (thiodan) on vitellogenesis and its modulation by different hormones in the vitellogenic catfish Clarias batrachus," Toxicology, Vol. 75, pp. 191-198

Cohen, S., O'Malley, B. W., Stastny, M., 1970, "Estrogenic induction of ornithine decarboxylase in vivo and in vitro," Science, Vol. 170, pp. 336-338

Colborn, T., and Clements, C., 1992, Chemically induced alterations in sexual and functional development: the wildlife/human connection, Princeton Scientific Publications, Princeton, New Jersey

Colborn, T., vom Saal, F. S., and Soto, A. M., 1993, "Developmental effects of endocrine-disrupting chemicals in wildlife and humans," Environmental Health Perspectives, Vol. 101, pp. 378-384

Copeland, P. A., Sumpter, J. P., Walker, T. K., and Croft, M., 1986, "Vitellogenin levels in male and female rainbow trout (*Salmo gairdneri* Richardson) at various stages of the reproductive cycle," Comparative Biochemistry and Physiology, Vol. 83B, pp. 487-493

Copeland, P. A., and Thomas, P., 1988, "The measurement of plasma vitellogenin levels in a marine teleost, the spotted seatrout (*Cynoscion nebulosus*) by homologous radioimmunoassay," Comparative Biochemistry and Physiology, Vol. 91B, pp. 17-23

Cotton, P., 1994, "Environmental estrogenic agents area of concern," Journal of the American Medical Association, Vol. 271, pp. 414-416

Courtney, K., and Andrews, J., 1985, "Neonatal and maternal blood burdens of hexachlorobenzene (HCB) in mice: gestational exposure and lactational transfer," Fundamental and Applied Toxicology, Vol. 5, No, 2, pp. 265-277

Craik, J. C. A., 1978, "The effects of oestrogen treatment on certain plasma constituents associated with vitellogenesis in the elasmobranch *Scyliorhinus canicula* L.," General and Comparative Endocrinology, Vol. 35, pp. 455-464

Daux, W. L., and Weeks, C. M., 1980, "Molecular basis of estrogenicity: X-ray crystallographic studies," In Estrogens in the Environment, J. A. McLachlan, ed., Elsevier, New York, pp. 11-31

Davis, W. P., and Bortone, S. A., 1992, "Effects of kraft mill effluent on the sexuality of fishes: an environmental early warning?," In Chemically induced alterations in sexual and functional development: the wildlife/human connection, Colborn, T., and Clement, C., eds., Princeton Scientific Publ., Princeton, New Jersey, pp. 113-127

Dessauer, H. C., and Fox, W., 1959, "Changes in ovarian follicle composition with plasma levels of snakes during oestrus," American Journal of Physiology, Vol. 197, pp. 360-366

Ding, J. L., Lee, P. L., and Lam, T. J., 1989, "Two forms of vitellogenin in the plasma and gonads of male *Oreochromis aureus*," Comparative Biochemistry and Physiology, Vol. 93B, pp. 363-370

Ding, J. L., Lim, E. H., and Lam, T. J., 1994, "Cortisol-induced hepatic vitellogenin mRNA in *Oreochromis aureus* (Steindachner)," General and Comparative Endocrinology, Vol. 96, pp. 276-287

Elliott, J. A. K., Bromage, N. R., and Whitehead, C., 1979, "Effects of estradiol-17β on serum calcium and vitellogenin levels in rainbow trout," Journal of Endocrinology, Vol. 83, pp. 54P-55P

Flouriot, G., Vaillant, C., Salbert, G., Pelissero, C., Guiraud, J. M., Valotaire Y., 1993, "Monolayer and aggregate cultures of rainbow trout hepatocytes: long-term and stable liver-specific expression in aggregates," Journal of Cell Science, Vol. 105, pp. 407-416

Folmar, L. C., Denslow, N. D., Wallace, R. A., LaFleur, G., Gross, T. S., Bonomelli, S., and Sullivan, C. V., 1995, "A highly conserved n-terminal sequence for teleost vitellogenin with potential value to the biochemistry, molecular biology and pathology of vitellogenins," Journal of Fish Biology, Vol. 46, pp. 255-263

Fox, G., 1992, "Epidemiological and pathological evidence of contaminant-induced alterations in sexual development of free-living wildlife," In Chemically induced alterations in sexual and functional development: the wildlife/human connection, Colborn, T., and Clement, C., eds., Princeton Scientific Publ., New Jersey, pp. 147-158

Fry, D. M., and Toone, C. K., 1981, "DDT-induced feminization of gull embryos," Science, Vol. 231, pp. 919-924

Gapp, D. A., Ho, S. M., and Callard, I. P., 1979, "Plasma levels of vitellogenin in Chrysemys picta during the annual gonadal cycle: Measurement by specific radioimmunoassay," Endocrinology, Vol. 104, pp. 784-790

Gasiewicz, T. A., and Rucci, G., 1991, "Alpha-naphthoflavone acts as an antagonist of 2,3,7,8-thtrachlorodibenzo-p-dioxin by forming an inactive complex with the Ah recpetor," Molecular Pharmacology, Vol. 49, pp. 607-612

Ginsburg, J., 1994, "Environmental estrogens," Lancet, Vol. 343, pp. 284 285

Goodwin, A. E., Grizzle, J. M., Bradley J. T., and Estridge, B. H., 1992, "Monoclonal antibody-based immunoassay of vitellogenin in the blood of male channel catfish (Ictalurus punctatus)," Comparative Biochemistry and Physiology, Vol. 101B, pp. 441-446

Gray, L. E., Ostby, J., Ferrell, J., Rehnberg, G., Linder, R., Cooper, R., Goldman, J., Slott, V., and Laskey, J., 1989, "A dose-response analysis of methoxychlor-induced alterations of reproductive development and function in the rat," Fundamental Applied Toxicology, Vol. 12, pp. 92-108

Gray, L. E., 1992, "Chemically-induced alterations of sexual differentiation: a review of effects in humans and rodents," In Chemically induced alterations in sexual and functional development: the wildlife/human connection, Colborn, T., and Clement, C., eds., Princeton Scientific Publ., New Jersey, pp. 203-230

Guillette, L. J., T. S., Gross, G. R., Masson, J. M., Matter, H. F., Percival, and A. R., Woodward, 1994, "Developmental abnormalities of the gonad and abnormal sex hormone concentrations in juvenile alligators from contaminated and control lakes in Florida," Environmental Health Perspectives, Vol. 102, pp. 680-688

Guillette Jr., L. J., Gross, T. S., Gross, D. A., Rooney, A. A., and Percival, H. F., 1995, "Gonadal steroidogenesis in vitro from juvenile alligators obtained from contaminated or control lakes," Environmental Health Perspectives, Vol. 103(supplement 4), pp. 31-36

Ho, S.-M., Dankso, D., and Callard, I. P., 1981, "Effect of exogenous estradiol-17β on plasma vitellogenin levels in male and female Chrysemys and its modulation by testosterone and progesterone," General and Comparative Endocrinology, Vol. 43, pp. 413-421

Ho, S.-M., 1987, "Endocrinology of vitellogenesis,". In Hormones and Reproduction in Fishes, Amphibians, and Reptiles, Norris, D. O., and Jones, R. T., eds., Plenum Press, New York, pp. 145-169

Hoel, D. G., Davis, D. L., Miller, A. B., Sondik, E. J., Swerdlow, A. J. 1992, "Trends in cancer mortality in 15 industrialized countries, 1969-1986," Journal of the National Cancer Institute, Vol. 84, pp. 313-320

Hori, S. H., Kodama, T., and Tanahashi, K., 1979, "Induction of vitellogenin synthesis in goldfish by massive doses of androgens," General and Comparative Endocrinology, Vol. 37, pp. 306-320

Idler, D. R. , Hwang, S. J., and Crim, L. W., 1979, "Quantification of vitellogenin in Atlantic salmon (Salmo salar) plasma by radioimmunoassay," Journal of Fish Research Canada, Vol. 36, pp. 574-578

Ireland, J. S. Mukku, V. R., Robison, A. K. Stancel, G. M., 1980, "Stimulation of uterine deoxyribonucleic acid synthesis by 1,1,1-trichloro-2-(p-chlorophenyl)-2(o-chlorophenyl)ethane (o,p'DDT)," Biochemical Pharmacology, Vol. 29, pp. 1469-1479

Jansen, H. T., Cooke, P. S., Porcelli, J., Liu, T-C., and Hansen, L. G., 1993, "Estrogenic and antiestrogenic actions of PCBs in the female rat: in vitro and in vivo studies," Reproductive Toxicology, Vol. 7, pp. 237-248

Jobling, S., and Sumpter, J. P., 1993, "Detergent components in sewage effluent are weakly oestrogenic to fish: an in vitro study using rainbow trout (Onchohynchus mykiss) hepatocytes", Aquatic Toxicology, Vol. 27, pp. 361-372

Kaye, A. M., Icekson, I., Lindner, H. R., 1971, "Stimulation by estrogens of ornithine and S-adenosylmethionine decarboxylases in the immature rat uterus," Biochimica et Biophysica Acta, Vol. 252, pp. 150-159

Kishida, M., Anderson, T. R., and Specker, J. L., 1992, "Induction by β-estradiol of vitellogenin in striped bass (*Morone saxatilis*): Characterization and quantification in plasma and mucus," General and Comparative Endocrinology, Vol. 88, pp. 29-39

Kishida, M., and Specker, J. L., 1993, "Vitellogenin in tilapia (*Oreochromis mossambicus*): Induction of two forms by estradiol, quantification in plasma and characterization in oocyte extract. Fish Physiology and Biochemistry, Vol. 12, pp. 171-182

Korach, K. S., Sarver, P., Chae, K., McLachlan, J. A., and McKinney, J.D., 1988, "Estrogen receptor-binding activity of polychlorinated hydroxybiphenyls: conformationally restricted structural probes," Molecular Pharmacology, Vol. 33, No. 1, pp. 120-126

Katzenellenbogen, J. A., Katzenellenbogen, B. S., Tatee, T., Robertson, D. W., and Landvatter, S. W., 1980, "The chemistry of estrogens and antiestrogens: Relationships between structure, receptor binding, and biological activity," In Estrogens in the Environment, McLachlan, J. A., ed., Elsevier, New York, pp. 33-51

Knight, W. M., 1980, "Estrogens administered to food-producing animals: Environmental considerations," In Estrogens in the Environment, McLachlan, J. A., ed., Elsevier, New York, pp. 391-402

Lazier, C.C., MacKay, M.E., 1993, "Vitellogenin gene expression in teleost fish," In Biochemistry and Molecular Biology of Fishes, Vol. 2, Hochachka, P. W., and Mommsen, T. P., eds., Elsevier, Amsterdam, pp. 391-405

Levin, W., Welch, R. M., Conney, A. H., 1968, "Estrogenic action of DDT and its analogs," Federation Proceedings, Vol. 27, pp. 649

Lin, F. J., Stohs, S. J., Birnbaum, L. S., Clark, G., Lucier, G. W., and Goldstein, J. A., 1991a, "The effects of 2,3,7,8-tetrachlorodibenzo-p-dioxin (TCDD) on the hepatic estrogen and glucocorticoid receptors in congenic strains of Ah responsive and Ah nonresponsive C57BL/6J mice," Toxicology and Applied Pharmacology, Vol. 108, pp. 129-139

Lin, F. J., Clark, G., Birnbaum, L. S., Lucier, G. W., and Goldstein, J. A., 1991b, "Influence of the Ah locus on the effects on 2,3,7,8-tetrachlorodibenzo-p-dioxin (TCDD) on the hepatic epidermal growth factor receptor," Molecular Pharmacology, Vol. 39, pp. 307-313

Lundberg, C., 1973, "Effects of long-term exposure to DDT on the oestru frequency of implanted ova in the mouse," Environmental Physiol Biochemistry, Vol. 3, pp. 127-131

Mason, R. R., Schulte, G. L., 1980, "Estrogen-like effects of o,p'DDT on progesterone receptor of rat uterine cytosol," Research Communic Chemical Pathology and Pharmacology, Vol. 29, pp. 281-290

McLachlan, J. A., 1985, Estrogens in the Environment. II. Influences on Elsevier Science Publishing Company, New York

McLachlan, J. A., Newbold, R. R., Korach, K. S., and Hogan, M., 1987 assessment considerations for reproductive and developmental to oestrogenic xenobiotics," In Human risk assessment: The roles selection and extrapolation, Roloff, M. V., and Wilson, A. W., e Francis, London, pp. 187-193

McLachlan, J. A., 1993, "Functional toxicology: a new approach to det active xenobiotics," Environmental Health Perspectives, Vol. 1

Nelson, J. A., 1974, "Effects of dichlorodiphenyltrichloroethane (DDT polychlorinated biphenyl (PCB) mixtures on 17β-[^{3}H] estradio uterine receptor," Biochemical Pharmacology, Vol. 23, pp. 44

Nelson, J. A., Stuck, R. F., and James, R., 1976, "Estrogenically activ and methoxychlor," Pharmacologist, Vol. 18, pp. 247

Nelson, J. A., Stuck, R. F., and James, R., 1978, "Estrogenic activitie hydrocarbons," Journal of Toxicology and Environmental He 325-340

Norberg, B., and Haux, C., 1988, "An homologous radioimmunoass (Salmo trutta) vitellogenin," Fish Physiology and Biochemis

O'Malley, B. W., and Tsai, M. J., 1992, "Molecular pathways of ste Biology of Reproduction, Vol. 46, pp. 163-167

Østerlind, A., 1986, "Diverging trends in incidence and mortality o Denmark, 1943-1982," British Journal of Cancer, Vol. 53,

Ousterhout, J. M., Struck, R. F., and Nelson, J. A., 1979, "Estroge methoxychlor metabolites," Federation Proceedings, Vol.

Ousterhout, J. M., Struck, R. F., and Nelson, J. A., 1981, "Estroge methoxychlor metabolites," Biochemical Pharmacology,

Palmer, B. D., Palmer, S. K., and Selcer, K. W., 1994, "Effects of environmental endocrine disruptors on reptiles and amphibians," American Zoologist, Vol. 35, No. 4, pp. 13A

Palmer, B. D., and Selcer, K. W., 1994, "Serum proteins as biomarkers for xenobiotic estrogens in wildlife," Biology of Reproduction, Vol. 50, (Supplement 1), pp. 100

Palmer, B. D. , and Palmer, S.K., 1995, "Vitellogenin induction by xenobiotic estrogens in the red-eared turtle and African frog," Environmental Health Perspectives, Vol. 103, Supplement 4, pp. 19-25

Patnode, D. A., Curtis, L. R., 1994, "2,2',4,4',5,5'- and 3,3',4,4',5,5'-Hexachlorobiphenyl alteration of uterine progesterone and estrogen receptors coincides with embryotoxicity in mink (Mustela vison)," Toxicology and Applied Pharmacology, 127:9-18

Pelissero, C., Le Menn, F., and Burzawa-Gerard, F., 1989, "Vitellogenesis and steroid levels in the Siberian sturgeon Acipenser baeri bred in fish farms," General and Comparative Endocrinology, Vol. 74, pp. 253

Pelissero, C., Bennetau, B., Babin, P., Le Menn, F., and Dunogues, J., 1991a, "The estrogenic activity of certain phytoestrogens in the Siberian sturgeon Acipenser baeri," Journal of Steroid Biochemistry and Molecular Biology, Vol. 38, pp. 293-299

Pelissero, C., Le Menn, F., and Kaushick, S., 1991b, "Estrogenic effect of dietary soya bean meal on vitellogenesis in cultured Siberian sturgeon Acipenser baeri," General and Comparative Endocrinology, Vol. 83, pp. 447-457

Pelissero, C., Flouriot, G., Foucher, J. L., Bennetau, B., Dunogues, J., LeGac, F., and Sumpter, J. P., 1993, "Vitellogenin synthesis in cultured hepatocytes: An in vitro test for the estrogenic potency of chemicals," Journal of Steroid Biochemistry and Molecular Biology, Vol, 44, pp. 263-272

Purdom, C. E., Hardiman, P. A., Bye, V. J., Eno, N. C., Tyler, C. R., Sumpter, J. P., 1994, "Estrogenic effects of effluents from sewage treatment works," Chemistry and Ecology, Vol. 8, pp. 275-285

Rall, D. P., and McLachlan, J. A., 1980, "Potential for exposure to estrogens in the environment," In Estrogens in the Environment, McLachlan, J. A., ed., Elsevier, New York, pp. 199-202

Raloff, J., 1993, "EcoCancers: Do environmental factors underlie a breast cancer epidemic ?," Science News, Vol. 144, pp. 10-13

Raloff, J., 1994, "The Gender Benders: Are environmental "hormones" emasculating wildlife ?," Science News, Vol. 145, pp. 24-27

Redshaw, M. R., Follett, B. K., and Nicholls, T. J., 1969, "Comparative effects of the oestrogens and other steroid hormones on serum lipids and proteins in *Xenopus laevis* Daudin," Journal of Endocrinology, Vol. 43, pp. 47-53

Redshaw, M. R., and Follett, B. K., 1976, "Physiology of egg yolk production in the fowl: The measurement of circulating levels of vitellogenin employing a specific radioimmunoassay," Comparative Biochemistry and Physiology, Vol. 55A, pp. 399-405

Reijnders, P., 1988, "Environmental impact of PCBs in the marine environment," In Environmental Protection of the North Sea, Newman, P. J., and Agg, A. R., eds., Heineman Professional Publishing, Oxford, England, pp. 86-98

Rodriguez, J. N., Kah, O., Geffard, M., and LeMenn, F., 1989, "Enzyme-linked immunosorbent assay (ELISA) for sole (*Solea vulgaris*) vitellogenin," Comparative Biochemistry and Physiology, Vol. 92B, pp. 741-746

Schrenk, D., Karger, A., Lipp, H. P., and Bock, K.W., 1992, "2,3,7,8-Tetrachlorodibenzo-p-dioxin and ethinylestradiol as co-mitogens in cultured rat hepatoytes," Carcinogenesis, Vol. 13, pp, 453-456

Selcer, K. W., and Palmer, B. D., 1995, "Estrogen downregulation of albumin and a 170-kDa serum protein in the turtle, *Trachemys script*," General and Comparative Endocrinology, Vol. 97, pp. 340-352

Shapiro, D. J., Barton, M. C., McKearin, D. M., Chang, T.-C., Lew, D., Blume, J., Nielsen, D. A., and Gould, L., 1989, "Estrogen regulation of gene transcription and mRNA stability," Recent Progress in Hormone Research, Vol. 45, pp. 29-64.

Sharpe, R. M. and Skakkebaek, N. E., 1993, "Are oestrogens involved in falling sperm counts and disorders of the male reproductive tract?," Lancet, Vol. 341, pp. 1392-1395

Shore, L. S., Gurevitz, M., and Shemesh, M., 1993, "Estrogen as an environmental pollutant," Bulletin of Environmental Contaminants and Toxicology, Vol. 51, pp. 361-366

Singhal, R. L. Valadares, J. R. E., Schwark, W. S., 1970, "Metabolic control mechanism in mammalian systems. IX. Estrogen-like stimulation of uterine enzymes by *o,p'*-1,1,1,-trichloro-2-2-bis(p-chlorophenyl)ethane," Biochemical Pharmacology, Vol. 19, pp. 21245-21255

So, Y. P., Idler, D. R., and Hwang, S. J., 1985, "Plasma vitellogenin in landlocked Atlantic salmon (*Salmo salar* Ouananiche); isolation homologous radioimmunoassay and immunological cross-reactivity with vitellogenin from other teleosts," Comparative Biochemical Physiology, Vol. 81B, pp. 63-71

Soto, A. M., Justicia, J., Wray, J. W., and Sonnenschein, C., 1991, "p-nonyl-phenol: an estrogenic xenobiotic released from "modified" polystyrene," Environmental Health Perspectives, Vol. 92, pp. 167-173

Soto, A. M., Lin, T., Justicia, H., Silvia, R., and Sonnenschein, C., 1992, "An "in culture" bioassay to assess the estrogenicity of xenobiotics (E-SCREEN)," In Chemically induced alterations in sexual and functional development: the wildlife/human connection, Colborn, T., and Clement, C., eds., Princeton Scientific Publ., New Jersey, pp. 295-309

Soto, A. M., Sonnenschein, C., Chung, K. L., Fernandez, M. F., Olea, N., and Serrano, F. O., 1996, "The E-screen assay as a tool to identify estrogens: an update on estrogenic environmental pollutants," Environmental Health Perspectives, in press

Specker, J. L., and Anderson, T. R., 1994, "Developing an ELISA for a model protein - Vitellogenin," In Biochemistry and Molecular Biology of Fishes, Vol. 3, Hochachka, P. W., and Mommsen, T. P., eds., Elsevier Science Publishers, Amsterdam, pp. 567-578

Sumpter, J. P., 1985, "The purification, radioimmunoassay and plasma levels of vitellogenin from the rainbow trout, *Salmo gairdneri*," Current Trends in Comparative Endocrinology, Lofts, B., ed., Hong Kong University Press, Hong Kong, pp. 355-357

Stancel, G. M., Ireland, J. S., Mukku, V. R., and Robison, A. K., 1980, "The estrogenic activity of DDT: *in vivo* and *in vitro* induction of a specific estrogen inducible uterine protein by *o,p'*DDT," Life Science, Vol. 27, pp. 1111-1117

Swain, W., Colborn, T., Bason, C., Howarth, R., Lamey, L., Palmer, B. D., and Swackhamer, D., 1993, "Great Waters Report. Vol. 2. Exposure and effects of airborne contaminants," U.S. Environmental Protection Agency, Research Triangle Park, North Carolina.

Tata, J. R., and Smith, D. F., 1979, "Vitellogenesis: A versatile model for hormonal regulation of gene expression," Recent Progress in Hormone Research, Vol. 35, pp. 47-95

Tyler, C. R., and Sumpter, J. P., 1990, "The development of a radioimmunoassay for carp, *Cyprinus carpio*, vitellogenin," Fish Physiology and Biochemistry, Vol. 8, pp. 129-140

van den Berg, M., Heeremans, C., Veenhoven, E., and Olie, K., 1987, "Transfer of polychlorinated dibenzo-p-dioxins and dibenzofurans to fetal and neonatal rats," Fundamental and Applied Toxicology, Vol. 9, pp. 635-644

Wangh, L. J., 1982, "Glucocorticoids act together with estrogens and thyroid hormones in regulating the synthesis and secretion of Xenopus vitellogenin, serum albumin, and fibrinogen," Developmental Biology, Vol. 89, pp. 294-298

Welch, R. M., Levin, W., Conney, A. H., 1969, "Estrogenic action of DDT and its analogs," Toxicology and Applied Pharmacology, Vol. 14, pp. 358-367

White, R., Jobling, S., Hoare, S. A., Sumpter, J. P., and Parker, M. G., 1994, "Environmentally persistent alkylphenolic compounds are estrogenic," Endocrinology, Vol. 135, pp. 175-182

Wiley, H. S., Opresko, L., and Wallace, R. A., 1979, "New methods for the purification of vertebrate vitellogenin," Analytical Biochemistry, Vol. 97, pp. 145-152

Wolff, M. S., Toniolo, P., Lee, E., Rivera, M., and Dubin, N., 1993, "Blood levels of organochlorine residues and the risk of breast cancer," Journal of the National Cancer Institute, Vol. 85, pp. 648-652

Zacharewski, T., Harris, M., and Safe, S, 1991, "Evidence for the mechanism of action of the 2,3,7,8-tetrachlorodibenzo-p-dioxin-mediated decrease of nuclear estrogen receptor levels in wild-type and mutant mouse Hepa 1c1c7 cells," Biochemical Pharmacology, Vol. 41, pp. 1931-1939

Zacharewski, T., Harris, M., biege, L., Morrison, V., Merchant, M., and Safe, S, 1992, "6-Methyl-1,3,8-trichlorodibenzofuran (MCDF) as an antiestrogen in human and rodent cancer cell lines: evidence for the role of the Ah receptor," Toxicology and Applied Pharmacology, Vol. 11, pp. 311-318.

Nancy D. Denslow[1], Ming M. Chow[2], Leroy C. Folmar[3], Sherman L. Bonomelli[4], Scott A. Heppell[5], and Craig V. Sullivan[6]

DEVELOPMENT OF ANTIBODIES TO TELEOST VITELLOGENINS: POTENTIAL BIOMARKERS FOR ENVIRONMENTAL ESTROGENS

REFERENCE: Denslow, N. D., Chow, M. M., Folmar, L. C., Bonomelli, S., Heppell, S. A., and Sullivan, C.V., "**Development of Antibodies to Teleost Vitellogenins: Potential Biomarkers for Environmental Estrogens**", *Environmental Toxicology and Risk Assessment: Biomarkers and Risk Assessment—Fifth Volume, ASTM STP 1306,* David A. Bengtson and Diane S. Henshel, Eds., American Society for Testing and Materials, 1996.

ABSTRACT: We describe 2 IgG class and an IgM class monoclonal antibodies and a polyclonal antiserum which recognize a wide variety of teleost vitellogenins. Based on these and previous results we discuss the potential for developing a "universal" ELISA to recognize all vertebrate vitellogenins.

[1] Director, Program in Biotechnologies for the Ecological, Evolutionary and Conservation Sciences (BEECS), Interdisciplinary Center for Biotechnology Research, University of Florida, Gainesville, FL 32610.

[2] Technical Assistant, Department of Biochemistry and Molecular Biology, University of Florida, Gainesville, FL 32610.

[3] Senior Research Physiologist, U.S. Environmental Protection Agency, Sabine Island, Gulf Breeze, FL 32561.

[4] Research Associate, Interdisciplinary Center for Biotechnology Research, University of Florida, Gainesville, FL 32610.

[5] Research Asistant, Department of Zoology, North Carolina State University, Raleigh, NC 27695-7617.

[6] Associate Professor, Department of Zoology, North Carolina State University, Raleigh, NC 27695-7617.

KEYWORDS: Environmental Estrogens, Vitellogenin, Biomarkers

INTRODUCTION

There have been numerous recent reports on how estrogenic chemicals in the environment affect a variety of aquatic species (Pelissero et al. 1991, Colborn et al. 1993, Jobling and Sumpter 1993, Hileman 1994, Purdom et al. 1994, Sumpter 1995). These chemicals include detergents, plasticizers and a wide variety of chlorinated hydrocarbons. An initial review of those chemicals known to be estrogenic shows little structural similarity, making a *priori* identification of estrogenic chemicals potentially difficult (McLachlan 1993).

Vitellogenin (VTG), the estrogen-inducible egg yolk precursor protein found in all oviparous vertebrates (Wallace 1985, Specker and Sullivan 1994), is a promising biomarker to verify exposure of animals to environmental contaminants that mimic estrogen. VTG is normally synthesized in the liver of maturing females with growing oocytes. Males of some species (Ding et al. 1989, Kishida and Specker 1993) are also capable of producing measurable quantities of VTG, but most males only produce VTG when exposed to exogenous estrogens or estrogen mimics. Here we discuss development of polyclonal antisera and monoclonal antibodies to VTGs of teleost fishes, their cross reactivities within and among teleost families and their potential use in bioassays of estrogenic activity.

MATERIALS AND METHODS

Purification of Vitellogenin:

Striped bass (*Morone saxatilis*) and rainbow trout (*Oncorhynchus mykiss*) VTGs used to make monoclonal antibodies were purified from fish treated with estradiol-17β (E$_2$) as described previously (Tao et al. 1993, Hara et al. 1993).

Preparation of Antibodies:

Anti-VTG peptide antisera were raised in rabbits against a peptide fifteen amino acids long. This peptide was derived from a consensus sequence to the N-terminal portion of several vertebrate vitellogenins (Folmar et al. 1995), including striped bass, pinfish (*Lagodon rhomboides*), brown bullhead (*Ameiurus nebulosus*), yellow perch (*Perca flavescens*), and medaka (*Oryzias latipes*) (Heppell et al. 1995).

Monoclonal antibody 2D8 was raised against rainbow trout in Balb/C mice and tested against striped bass and rainbow trout VTGs as described previously (Heppell et al. 1995, Heppell 1994). Monoclonal antibodies HL1081-1C8 and HL1082-3H1 were raised against purified striped bass VTG in Balb/C mice. Specifically, mice were immunized by intraperitoneal injection with 100 ug of striped bass VTG mixed 1:2 with Freund's complete adjuvant. Mice were boosted two times at three week intervals with 50 ug antigen in incomplete adjuvant. Mouse serum was collected from the tail vein to check for antibody production before sacrificing the mice. Hybridoma's were produced by standard methods (Harlow and Lane 1988), and each colony was screened for VTG cross-reactivity by direct ELISA using both striped bass and rainbow trout VTGs. Colonies which showed immunoreactivity with both rainbow trout and striped bass VTGs were selected for cloning. Monoclonal antibodies (mabs) were harvested by collecting tissue culture supernatant and were used in Western blots as described below.

Western Blots:

Serum samples from eel (*Anguilla rostrata*), carp (*Cyprinus carpio*), brown bullhead, hardhead catfish (*Arius felis*), rainbow trout, striped bass, largemouth bass (*Micropterus salmonides*), bluegill sunfish (*Lepomis macrochirus*), pinfish and white mullet (*Mugil curema*) were diluted ten-fold with Laemmli sample buffer (Laemmli 1970) for naturally vitellogenic fish and fifty-fold for E_2-induced fish and run in 7 1/2% polyacrylamide tris-tricine SDS gels (Schagger and von Jagow 1987). For each species, samples presumably devoid of VTG (untreated males) were used as controls. Each sample represents a single animal. These results, however, are representative of hundreds of analyses, although the exact number varies from species to species.

For Western blot analysis, the gels were electroblotted to PVDF membranes (Millipore, Immobilon P). Membranes were blocked with 5% non-fat dry milk (Johnson et al. 1984) in TBST (10 mM Tris, pH 7, 150 mM NaCl, 0.5% Tween) overnight, incubated with primary antibody (1:3,000 dilution for the anti-VTG peptide antibody in 5% milk or directly with the tissue culture supernatant for monoclonal antibodies) for two hours at room temperature, washed with TBST and then probed with goat anti-rabbit or anti-mouse alkaline-phosphatase conjugated secondary antibody (dilution 1:5,000) for 1 hr. The blots were developed by incubating with bromochloroindolyl phosphate/nitro blue tetrazolium substrate which marks cross-reactive VTGs in purple.

RESULTS

Previously we reported on the preparation of a monospecific anti-VTG peptide antiserum and an IgM class monoclonal VTG antibody (Heppell et al. 1995). In this report we further characterize their specificities and compare them with new IgG class monoclonal antibodies prepared in balb/C mice immunized with striped bass VTG.

The consensus peptide used to immunize rabbits for the monospecific antiserum was based on N-terminal sequences for VTGs from 6 teleost fish: striped bass, mummichog, pinfish, brown bullhead, yellow perch and medaka (Folmar et al. 1995; Heppell et al. 1995). Sequences at this end of the molecule were not identical among all of these species, but they were highly conserved (87-100%).

This polyclonal antiserum cross-reacts well with all species in this group, reacting with VTG from striped bass, pinfish, brown bullhead, and hardhead catfish (Fig. 1). However, the antiserum does not cross-react with VTG from more primitive fishes, such as common carp and rainbow trout, and it appears to have some cross-reactivity with other serum proteins in some of the fish tested. For example, it does not react with VTG from rainbow trout, but does react with a 76 kDa serum protein present in serum from both female and male trout (Fig. 1).

The monoclonal antibody, 2D8 (IgM class), raised against rainbow trout VTG was identified for its strong cross-reactivity with striped bass and trout VTGs, the initial selection criterion used for screening (Heppell et al. 1995). These two fish are widely separated in evolutionary time, increasing the likelihood that any epitope the monoclonal antibody recognized in both species would be a very conserved region. Western blot tests of that antibody indicated that it did not cross-react with normal male plasma from either species, suggesting that the epitope is unique to VTG (Heppell et al. 1995).

In this study, we tested the 2D8 antibody by Western blot against a panel of VTGs obtained from different fish species, including pinfish, striped bass, rainbow trout, hardhead catfish, brown bullhead, and carp (Fig. 2). Normal male (control) serum from each species was also tested for non-specific binding to the antibody. Antibody 2D8 reacted with all VTGs tested (Fig. 2).

Additional monoclonal antibodies were developed in mice using an experiment reciprocal to the one employed for the production of monoclonal 2D8, i.e., the mice were initially immunized with purified striped bass VTG. We obtained 25 hybridomas specific for striped bass VTG of which only two (HL1081-1C8 and HL1082-3H1) cross-reacted with rainbow trout

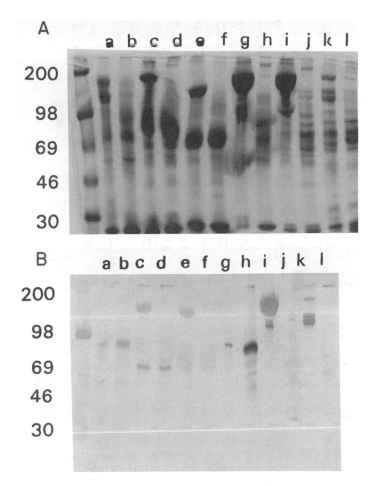

FIG. 1.   SDS-PAGE and Western blot analysis of six different
fish sera probed with the anti-VTG peptide antibody.   Lanes
a-b, E2-stimulated carp serum and male control; lanes c-d,
serum from a vitellogenic female brown bullhead and male
control; lanes e-f, serum from a vitellogenic female
hardhead catfish and male control; lanes g-h, E2-induced
plasma from rainbow trout and male control; lanes i-j, E2-
induced serum from striped bass and male control; lanes k-l,
E2-induced serum from pinfish and male control.   (A) 7.5%
acrylamide tris-tricine gels stained with Coomassie blue,
(B) Corresponding Western blots probed with the anti-VTG
peptide antibody.   Molecular mass standards, rainbow
molecular weight markers from Amersham (first lane) are
Myosin, 200 kDa; Phosphorylase b, 97 kDa; Bovine Serum
Albumin, 69 kDa; Ovalbumin, 46 kDa; Carbonic anhydrase, 30
kDa and Trypsin inhibitor, 21.5 kDA.

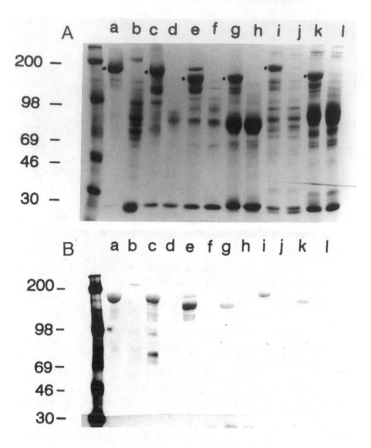

FIG. 2.   SDS-PAGE and Western blot analysis of ten
different fish sera using the monoclonal 2D8.   Lanes a-b,
E2-stimulated striped bass serum and male control; lanes c-
d, E2-stimulated rainbow trout plasma and male control;
lanes e-f, E2-induced carp serum and male control; lanes g-
h, female vitellogenic hardhead catfish serum and male
control; lanes i-j, E2-induced pinfish serum and male
control; lanes k-l, female vitellogenic brown bullhead
serum and male control.   (A) 7.5% acrylamide tris-tricine
gels stained with Coomassie blue, (B) Corresponding Western
blots probed with the monoclonal 2D8 (IgM) antibody.   MW
markers are as described for Fig. 1.

VTG. Both appear to react specifically with VTG since neither cross-reacted with serum proteins from control males (Figs. 3 and 4). The two antibodies appear to recognize different epitopes as judged by the different pattern of recognition obtained with slightly degraded vitellogenin. For example, antibody HL1082-3H1 recognized a high MW VTG band (>180 kDa) and a number of smaller MW bands, presumably degradation products of the 180 kDa band. This is especially evident with the bluegill VTG sample in which the 180 kDa band is totally missing, but a number of smaller bands are present. Antibody HL1081-1C8 recognizes both the 180 kDa band and a ca. 120 kDa band   when both are present in the sample. Antibody HL1081-1C8 reacts with VTG from white mullet, pinfish, largemouth bass, bluegill sunfish, striped bass and rainbow trout, but not with hardhead catfish, brown bullhead, carp or eel. Antibody HL1082-3H1 reacts with the same VTGs and also with VTG from eel, but not with VTG from carp, brown bullhead or hardhead catfish.

DISCUSSION

Considering the nutritional role of VTG in developing embryos of invertebrates and four classes of vertebrates, it seems likely that there would be few evolutionary constraints imposed on the primary structure of VTG. The few sequences of VTGs found in the protein databases confirm that, at the amino acid level, VTGs from fishes vary extensively (Specker and Sullivan 1994). This variation probably accounts for the poor cross-reactivity of polyclonal antibodies from one species to another (Campbell and Idler 1980, So et al. 1985). VTGs, however, do share spotty but significant stretches of similarity (Carnevali and Belvedere 1991). This raises the possibility that we could prepare monospecific or monoclonal antibodies to these regions, reagents that could be used across all classes of oviparous vertebrates for VTG immunoassays.

The four VTG antibody preparations we have used apparently recognize different epitopes conserved to differing degrees. The first antibody preparation we developed was a polyclonal, monospecific antiserum made against a peptide representing the N-terminal sequence of VTG from several teleost fish. This antiserum has the narrowest range of phylogenetic cross-reactivity, possibly because the N-terminal sequence of VTG has changed during vertebrate evolution. It also is a low affinity antibody, with an association constant in the order of 10^6 mol^{-1} (the lowest measurable affinity by Western blot analysis, Harlow and Lane 1988).

Monoclonal 2D8 appears to be the most "universal" of the antibodies we have made to date. In addition to cross-

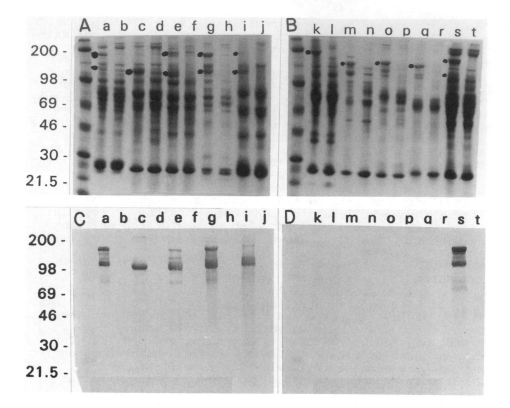

FIG. 3.   SDS-PAGE and Western blot analysis of ten different
fish sera probed with the monoclonal antibody HC1081-1C8.
Serum samples from vitellogenic females and male controls.
Lanes a-b, striped bass; lanes c-d, bluegill sunfish; lanes
e-f, largemouth bass; lanes g-h, pinfish; lanes i-j, white
mullet; lanes k-l, eel; lanes m-n, carp; lanes o-p, brown
bullhead; lanes q-r, hardhead catfish; lanes s-t, rainbow
trout.   (A and B) 7.5% poly acrylamide tris-tricine gels
stained with Coomassie blue.   (C and D) Western blots probed
with the HL1081-1C8 (IgG class) antibody.   Molecular mass
standards are as described for Fig. 1 (● = VTG band).

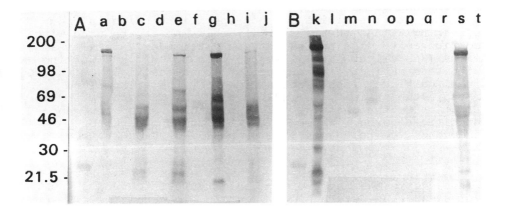

FIG. 4. Western blot analysis of the ten different fish
sera used in Figure 3 probed with the monoclonal antibody
HL1083-3H1. Serum samples from vitellogenic females and
male controls. Molecular mass standards are as described
for Fig. 1.

reacting with all the species of fish we tested in this
study, antibody 2D8 recognizes gag grouper (<u>Mycteroperca
microlepis</u>) and fathead minnow (<u>Pimephales</u> <u>promelas</u>)
(Sullivan and Heppell, unpublished) and also cross-reacts
with VTGs from bullfrogs (*Rana catesbeiana*), chickens
(*Gallus domestica*), and black rat snakes (*Elaphe obsoleta*)
(Heppell 1994), suggesting that the relevant epitope is
highly conserved among vertebrate animals. This antibody is
in the IgM class, which is a group that is notoriously
sticky and of low affinity. Non-specific binding to other
serum proteins (Fig. 2) is a characteristic of IgM class
antibodies.. Under optimal conditions, this non-specific
binding can be diluted out in Western blots.   Although this
antibody still exhibits low non-specific binding in
screening ELISAs (Heppell 1994), this mAb can be used with
confidence to distinguish between vitellogenic females and
males (Heppell et al. 1995). We plan to continue working
with this antibody, determine its cross-reactivity with VTG
from additional fish species, identify the epitope and
measure the affinity to individual VTGs. We also intend to
fractionate the antibody into FAb fragments to reduce no-
specific binding. These tests will be important for
choosing a corresponding "universal" VTG standard for
bioassay development.

    The antibodies with the highest affinities for
vitellogenin are the IgG antibodies HL1081-1C8 and
HL1082-3H1, as determined by Western blot analysis. These
antibodies cross-react only with serum or plasma from
vitellogenic females or males that have been induced with E_2.
Each of these antibodies recognizes a different VTG epitope
as suggested by their pattern of recognition on the Western
blot. In the vitellogenins that are recognized, both
antibodies bind to the larger VTG band (>180 kDa). The
binding site for HL1081-1C8 is also present in the smaller
VTG band (ca. 120 kDa) as demonstrated in Fig. 3 C and D. It
appears that the 180 kDa band is more easily degraded,
giving rise to a number of smaller fragments that are still
recognized by antibody HL1082-3H1. These smaller fragments
do not appear to be normal serum proteins, since they are
not present in the serum from untreated males (Fig. 4 A and
B). This is most apparent when looking at the serum sample
for bluegill sunfish in which the 180 kDa band for VTG is
missing from the sample. In this case, HL1082-3H1 binds
only to the lower molecular weight bands in the female and
not in the male, while HL1081-1C8 binds only to the ca. 120
kDa band in the female. We plan to do further experiments
to determine whether the 180 KDa and 120 kDa proteins are
different gene products or whether the 120 kDa band
originates from the 180 kDa band.

    The epitopes for HL1081-1C8 and HL1082-3H1 appear to
differ from the one recognized by antibody 2D8, described

above.   Neither of these IgG-class antibodies has the full
cross-reactivity with other VTGs observed with antibody 2D8,
implying that their corresponding epitopes are not as highly
conserved. We are producing additional monoclonal
antibodies, using other fish VTGs as immunogens in order to
develop an extensive panel of antibodies that can be used
individually or in combination for VTG detection and
quantitation.

There are over 27,000 chemicals on the Toxic Substances
Act (TOSCA) inventory, of which several hundred are
considered estrogenic or estrogen receptor agonists.   We
have recently developed a quantitative VTG ELISA which
enhances our ability to screen large numbers of samples.
This ELISA will be essential to develop Quantitative
Structure Activity Relationships (QSARs) to determine the
relative estrogenicity for this vast array of chemicals;
however, the presence of VTG does not differentiate between
direct activation of the estrogen receptor and
hyperproduction of the natural ligand.

REFERENCES

Benfey, T.J., Donaldson, E.M., and Owen, T.G. 1989. An Homologous Radioimmunoassay for Coho Salmon (*Oncorhynchus kisutch*) Vitellogenin, with General Applicability to other Pacific Salmonids. General and Comparative Endocrinology **75**:78-82.

Campbell, CM. and Idler, D.R. 1980. Characterization of an estradiol-induced protein from Rainbow Trout Serum as Vitellogenin by the Composition and Radioimmunological Cross Reactivity to Ovarian Yolk Fractions. Biology of Reproduction **22**:605-617.

Carnevali, O. and Belvedere, P. 1991. Comparative Studies of Fish, Amphibian, and Reptilian Vitellogenins. Journal of Experimental Zoology 259:18-25.

Colborn, T., vom Saal, F.S. and Soto, A.M. 1993. Developmental Effects of Endocrine-Disrupting Chemicals in Wildlife and Humans. Environmental Health Perspectives **101**:378-384.

Ding, J.L., Hee, P.L. and Lam, T.J. 1989. Two Forms of Vitellogenin in the Plasma and Gonads of Male Oreochromis aureus. Comparative Biochemistry and Physiology. 93B:363-370.

Folmar, L.C., Denslow, N.D., Wallace, R.A., LaFleur, G., Gross, T.S., Bonomelli, S. and Sullivan, C.V. 1995. A Highly Conserved N-terminal Sequence for Teleost Vitellogenin with Potential Value to the Biochemistry, Molecular Biology and Pathology of Vitellogenesis. Journal of Fish Biology **46**:255-263.

Hara, A., Sullivan, C.V. and Dickhoff, W.W. 1993. Isolation and some Characterization of Vitellogenin and its Related Egg Yolk Proteins from Coho Salmon (Oncorhynchus kisutch). Zoological Science **10**:245-256.

Harlow, E. and Lane, D., 1988, Antibodies, A Laboratory Manual, Cold Spring Harbor Laboratory, Cold Spring   Harbor, New York, pp. 28-29.

Heppell, S.A. 1994. Development of Universal Vertebrate Vitellogenin Antibodies M.Sc. Thesis. Department of Zoology, North Carolina State University.

Heppell, S.A., Denslow, N.D., Folmar, L.C. and Sullivan, C.V. 1995. 'Universal' Assay of Vitellogenin as a Biomarker for Environmental Estrogens. Environmental Health Perspectives (In press).

Hileman, B. 1994. Environmental Estrogens Linked to Reproductive Abnormalities, Cancer. Chemistry and Engineering News 72:19-23.

Jobling S. and Sumpter, J.P. 1993. Detergent Components in Sewage Effluent are Weakly Oestrogenic to Fish: an In Vitro Study using Rainbow Trout (Oncorhynchus mykiss) Hepatocytes. Aquatic Toxicology 27:361-372.

Johnson, D.A., Gautsch, J.W., Sportsman, J.R. and Elder, J.H. 1984. Improved Technique Utilizing Non-fat Dry Milk for Analysis of Proteins and Nucleic Acids Transferred to Nitrocellulose. Gene Analytical Techniques 1:3-8.

Kishida, M. and Specker, J.I. 1993. Vitellogenin in Tilapia (Oreochromis mossambicus): Induction of Two Forms by Estradiol, Quantification in Plasma and Characterization in Oocyte Extract. Fish Physiology and Biochemistry 12:171-182.

Laemmli, U.K. 1970. Cleavage of structural proteins during the assembly of the head of bacteriophage T4. Nature 227:680-685.

McLachlan, J.A. 1993. Functional Toxicology: A New Approach to Detect Biologically Active Xenobiotics. Environmental Health Perspectives 101:386-387.

Pelissero, C., Le Menn, F. and Kaushick, F. 1991. Estrogenic Effect of Dietary Soya Bean Meal on Vitellogenisis in Cultured Siberian Sturgeon Acipenser baeri. General and Comparative Endocrinology 83:447-457.

Purdom C.E., Hardiman, P.A., Bye, V.J., Eno N.C., Tyler, C.R. and Sumpter, J.P. 1994. Estrogenic Effects of Effluents from Sewage Treatment Works. Chemical Ecology 8:275-285.

Schagger, H. and von Jagow, G. 1987. Tricine-Sodium Dodecyl Sulfate Polyacrylamide Gel Electrophoresis for the Separation of Proteins in the Range from 1 to 100 kDa. Analytical Biochemistry 166:368-379.

So, Y.P., Idler, D.R. and Hwang, S.J. 1985. Plasma Vitellogenin in Landlocked Atlantic Salmon (Salmo salar Oaunaniche): Isolation, Homologous Radioimmunoassay and Immunological Cross-reactivity with Vitellogenin from other Teleosts. Comparative Biochemistry and Physiology 81B:63-71.

Specker, J. and Sullivan, C. V. 1994. "Vitellogenesis in
        Fishes: Status and Perspectives," Perspectives in
        Comparative Endocrinology, K. G. Davey, R. G.
        Peter, and S. S. Tobe, eds. National Research
        Council of Canada Ottawa pp 304-315.

Sumpter, J.P. 1995. Estrogenic Surfactant-Derived
        Chemicals in the Aquatic Environment. Environmental
        Health Perspectives (In press).

Tao, Y., Hara, A., Hodson, R.G., Woods, L.C. III and
        Sullivan C.V. 1993. Purification,
        Characterization and Immunoassay of Striped Bass
        (Morone saxatilis) vitellogenin. Fish Physiology
        and Biochemistry 12:31-46.

Wallace, R. 1985. "Vitellogenesis and Oocyte Growth in
        Non-mammalian Vertebrates," Developmental Biology
        Vol. 1. L. W. Browder ed. Plenum Press, New York
        pp. 127-177.

L. Mark Hewitt[1,2], Ian M. Scott[2], Glen J. Van Der Kraak[3], Kelly R. Munkittrick[2], Keith R. Solomon[1], and Mark R. Servos[2],

DEVELOPMENT OF TIE PROCEDURES FOR COMPLEX MIXTURES USING PHYSIOLOGICAL RESPONSES IN FISH

REFERENCE: Hewitt, L. M., Scott, I. M., Van Der Kraak, G. J., Munkittrick, K. R., Solomon, K. R., and Servos, M. R., "**Development of TIE Procedures for Complex Mixtures Using Physiological Responses in Fish,**" *Environmental Toxicology and Risk Assessment: Biomarkers and Risk Assessment—Fifth Volume, ASTM STP 1306,* David A. Bengtson and Diane S. Henshel, Eds., American Society for Testing and Materials, 1996.

ABSTRACT: Methodology was developed for the isolation and recovery of compounds from a commercial lampricide formulation associated with hepatic mixed function oxygenase (MFO) enzyme induction in fish. MFO induction in laboratory bioassays was characterized and optimized prior to fractionation experiments. Recovery and isolation of MFO activity directed the chemical fractionations. Fractionation techniques were developed on a preparative scale so that fish exposures could be conducted directly. Formulation impurities associated with MFO induction were separated from the active lampricide using solid phase extraction. Subsequent HPLC fractionations isolated activity in distinct fractions, indicating that multiple formulation impurities are associated with the observed MFO induction. Activity was recovered from each fraction using toluene extraction and the extracts were characterized by GC-MS. No activity was associated with several compounds confirmed in the bioactive fractions and other structures are proposed. A preliminary application of these techniques to potential reproductive dysfunctions in fish is discussed.

KEYWORDS: TIE, MFO induction, Lampricide, TFM, Method Development

[1]Department of Environmental Biology, University of Guelph, Guelph Ontario N1G 2W1 Canada
[2]GLLFAS, Department of Fisheries and Oceans, Burlington Ontario L7R 4A6 Canada
[3]Department of Zoology, University of Guelph, Guelph Ontario N1G 2W1 Canada

37

Induction of the P450IA1 isosyme of hepatic mixed function oxygenase (MFO) enzymes from aquatic exposure to anthropogenic pollutants is well documented for several fish species. The mechanism of induction of this enzymatic system has been intensively studied and characterized. Induction, and in some cases, subsequent toxicity, is mediated by binding of the chemical within the cell to the aryl hydrocarbon (Ah) receptor (Poland et al. 1976; Safe et al. 1985, 1986; Safe 1986). Several classes of compounds which demonstrate a high affinity for the Ah receptor are persistent, bioaccumulative and toxic substances. These compound classes are planar aromatic hydrocarbons such as polychlorinated biphenyls (PCBs) (Safe et al. 1985) and selected polyaromatic hydrocarbons (PAHs) (Klotz et al. 1983). 2,3,7,8-tetrachlorodibenzo-*p*-dioxin (TCDD) has one of the highest affinities for the receptor and the potencies of other compounds are frequently expressed relative to TCDD (North Atlantic Treaty Organization 1986, Parrott et al. 1995). Induction of P450IA1 in aquatic species is considered as a biomarker for the presence of these types of compounds and an indication of potential toxicity (Payne et al. 1987). However, in environmental situations induction is often a result of the presence of multiple inducers, known and unknown. It is desirable to identify the responsible chemicals in these cases because of the potential toxicity associated with materials which are known to cause MFO induction. Existing protocols on toxicity identification/evaluations (TIE) for bioactive substances from environmental matrices deal with compounds associated with acute and chronic toxicity (U.S. Environmental Protection Agency, 1991, 1992, 1993a, 1993b) and have not been applied to fractionations directed by indicators of potential toxicity such as MFO induction.

The objective of this research was to develop toxicity identification/evaluation (TIE) fractionation techniques to consistently recover and isolate compounds from complex matrices associated with MFO induction in fish. Methodologies have been developed using a field formulation of the lampricide containing 3-trifluoromethyl-4-nitrophenol (TFM). Periodic TFM treatments of nursery streams have been the primary means of controlling sea lamprey (*Petromyzon marinus*) populations in the Great Lakes Basin since the late 1950s. MFO induction at remote, non-industrialized sites was recently associated with lampricides (Munkittrick et al. 1994). Detailed experiments showed that induction was not associated with TFM itself and was presumably a contaminant in the field formulation. Using the lampricide formulation, this paper describes an approach to isolate and identify the compounds associated with MFO induction from complex matrices.

TIE METHOD DEVELOPMENT

Optimization and Standardization of Fish Exposures

Rainbow trout exposure conditions were modified from the previous study. The objective of the optimization was to generate consistent, maximal MFO induction for tracking during TIE experiments, while minimizing acute toxicity. The acute toxicity of TFM to salmonid species is well documented and is highly dependent on pH (Bills et al. 1988) and dissolved oxygen (Seelye and Scholefield 1990). All TIE method development experiments were performed on the formulation batch (Hoescht 1990-2; Sea Lamprey Control Centre, Sault Ste Marie ON) used in the previous study (Munkittrick et al. 1994). Exposures were conducted using juvenile rainbow trout (3-5 g; Rainbow Springs Hatchery, Thamesford, ON) in darkness and glass aquaria containing 12 L of dechlorinated Burlington city tap water (pH 7.5 - 8.0, hardness 128 - 133 mg/L $CaCO_3$), at a loading density of 2.5 g/L (n = 6). Fish were acclimated to 13°C and fed (Martin's Feed Mill, Elmira ON) *ad libitum* until 6 d prior to exposures and were not fed during exposures.

Data was checked for normality and equal variances using SYSTAT software. One-way analyses of variance (ANOVA, p<0.001) were conducted for individual experiments using log transformed data. Tukey's HSD pairwise comparisons and Post Hoc contrasts were used to compare differences between treatments. Bars on all graphs depict ±1 standard error of the mean.

The first experiment determined the optimal concentration of the field formulation for exposures. Dose response exposures showed high levels of MFO induction at 150µL field formulation/12 L water or 4.6 mg/L TFM (Fig. 1) after 72 h static exposures (Fig. 1). High levels of mortality were encountered above this concentration (data not shown). Steep toxicity curves are associated with fish exposure to TFM itself (National Research Council of Canada 1985). This concentration is within the range of treatment concentrations (1.0 - 14.0 mg/L (National Research Council of Canada 1985)) used in the Great Lakes basin.

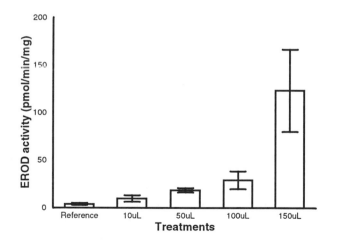

Figure 1.   Relationship between rainbow trout hepatic EROD activity and concentration of the TFM field formulation. Formulation aliquots were diluted in 12 L holding water for exposures. EROD activities have been normalized for protein content.

Due to the high throughput of fractions anticipated from the TIE, it was desirable to utilize exposure conditions which minimized labour intensity. Static conditions would be suited for these experiments. Although these conditions do not exactly match field situations (12-18 h continuous, followed by depuration) potentially higher levels of MFO may be necessary for charting induction during detailed TIE experiments. Once identified and obtained in pure form, candidate compounds would then be tested under treatment conditions as part of the confirmation process. Using 4.6 mg/L of the active ingredient, static exposures showed an apparent induction maximum in fish exposed for 72 h (Fig. 2) without acute toxicity.

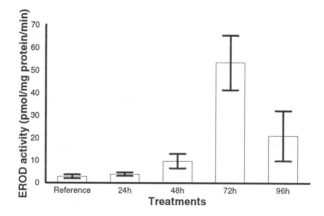

Figure 2.   Rainbow trout hepatic EROD activity for static exposures to 4.6 mg/L (active ingredient) TFM formulation after 24, 48, 72 and 96 h.

For each experiment, positive and negative references were conducted concurrently. Positive references consisted of one exposure to a known inducing fraction corresponding to a previous fractionation experiment as well as one exposure to whole filtered (<1 μm) formulation; filtering had previously shown no effect on MFO induction (Munkittrick et al. 1994). Negative reference fish were exposed to the maximum amount of solvents and/or buffer associated with the exposed fractions. Duplicate negative references were performed for each experiment. The development of these exposure conditions enabled the comparative assessment of the potential to induce fish MFO activity of batches from two manufacturers. The batch used for TIE method development (1990-2) was utilized as a positive reference for formulation batch testing (Fig. 3).

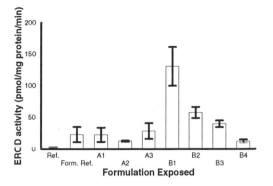

Figure 3.   Rainbow trout hepatic EROD activity associated with TFM field formulation batches from two manufacturers. Fish were exposed under conditions developed for TIE experiments. (Form. Ref.) refers to fish exposed to the batch used for TIE method development and as a positive reference for batch testing.

Rainbow Trout Hepatic MFO Activity

The measurement of hepatic MFO activity as ethoxyresorufin-O-deethylase (EROD) induction followed the methods of McMaster et al. (1991) but was optimized for TIE exposures by utilizing liver homogenates rather than traditional post mitochondrial supernatants (PMS) containing microsomes. This provided greater sensitivity for detecting MFO induction and reduced analysis time. EROD activities are reported in fluorescence units (FU), corresponding to the amount of substrate produced during the enzymatic assay. A high correlation (FU = 0.569(pmol/mg/min) + 1.28; $r^2 - 0.89$) between homogenate and post mitochondrial supernatant (PMS) activities normalized for protein was shown for fish exposed to a range of formulation concentrations (Fig. 4).

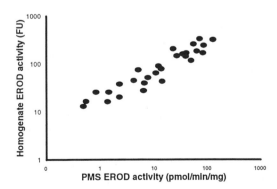

Figure 4.   Relationship between EROD activities derived from whole liver homogenates (FU) and post mitochondrial supernatants normalized for protein (pmol/min/mg protein). Both values were derived from the same individual fish.

Under the exposure conditions developed, the relative induction of filtered formulation over negative reference activity was 31 ±6.2 (SE) fold for over 50 separate experiments.

Isolation of Bioactive Formulation Impurities

There are several approaches to the isolation of bioactive compounds, which depend on matrix characteristics as well as the bioassay method. Standard protocols (U.S. Environmental Protection Agency 1991, 1992, 1993a, 1993b) begin with some form of bulk fractionation where separations are based on compound class properties, for example, purgeables. Once isolated, separations can then be initiated within a compound class. A similar approach was adopted for the lampricide formulation but for a different objective. The first objective in the isolation procedure was to separate bioactive impurities from the primary formulation ingredient, TFM. The TFM field formulation is a mixture of TFM (37% w/v), isopropanol and aqueous sodium hydroxide; the pH of the formulation is approximately 9.5. It was desirable to separate bioactive components from TFM because it was demonstrated that TFM was not associated with MFO induction (Munkittrick et al. 1994) and it was suspected that the bioactive compounds are present at low levels in the formulation. In order to isolate trace amounts of bioactive impurities from the mixture of contaminants presumably present, it is necessary to concentrate the mixture. Exposures to higher concentrations of the contaminants would not be possible with TFM present because of the acute toxicity encountered above 4.6 mg/L.. Chromatographic separations would also be facilitated once the large TFM interference was removed.

Solid phase extraction experiments

Previous HPLC separations using C_{18} columns demonstrated that TFM could be separated from bioactive components using this stationary phase (Munkittrick et al. 1994). However, formulation characteristics (namely pH) caused a rapid deterioration in column efficiency. It was hypothesized that the same separations could be achieved using solid phase extraction (SPE) C_{18} cartridges. It was speculated that the inducing contaminants were less polar than TFM, and following the methods of Burkhard et al. (1991) it should be possible to selectively elute TFM from the cartridge, leaving bioactive formulation impurities adsorbed to the packing. Bioactive impurities could then be recovered in a separate, less polar solvent elution. All fractionations were performed on a preparative scale using 150 uL formulation so that the fractions generated were exposed directly using the standardized bioassay. The presence of TFM in each fraction was monitored visually and at its absorbance maximum, 290 nm. The first experiment used a 100 mg C_{18} cartridge and employed solvent conditions similar to those used previously for HPLC separations (Munkittrick et al. 1994). Fig. 5 shows the EROD activity associated with these fractions.

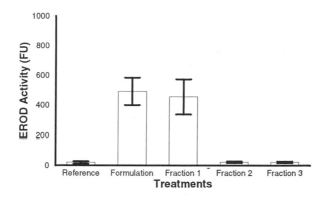

Figure 5.   Rainbow trout hepatic EROD activity associated with fractions
generated from solid phase extraction of the TFM formulation using 100 mg C_{18}
cartridges.

Fraction 1 was collected with 1 mL 25:75 methanol:pH 4 0.2M acetate buffer,
fraction 2 with a subsequent 2 mL 85:15 methanol:buffer and fraction 3 with 2 mL
100% methanol. Formulation TFM was distributed between fractions 1 and 2 and
separation from induction was unsuccessful. A slightly improved separation was seen
when the polarity of the first solvent/ buffer mixture was increased to 10:90
methanol:buffer (Fig. 6).

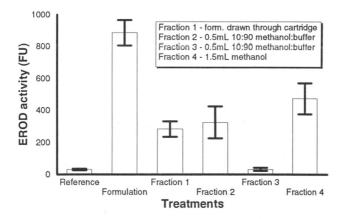

Figure 6.   Rainbow trout hepatic EROD activity associated with fractions
generated from solid phase extraction of the TFM formulation using 100 mg C_{18}
cartridges and a more polar initial elution solvent mixture.

It was hypothesized that the incomplete separation of TFM from inducing contaminants may be due to insufficient chromatographic capacity of the 100 mg SPE cartridges. Under slightly modified elution conditions, a larger cartridge size (500 mg) showed an enhanced separation of TFM from induction (Fig. 7).

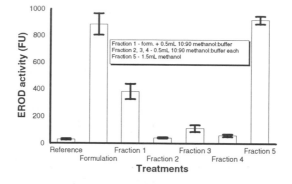

Figure 7.   Rainbow trout hepatic EROD activity associated with fractions generated from solid phase extraction of the TFM formulation using 500 mg C_{18} cartridges.

Elution volumes were slightly modified because of the larger packing. Fraction 1 was eluted with the formulation volume plus 0.5 mL of 10:90 methanol:acetate buffer; fractions 2,3 and 4 were eluted with 0.5 mL 10:90 methanol:acetate buffer, and fraction 5 was eluted with 1.5 mL methanol. TFM was absent from fractions 4 and 5. These observations suggested that the capacity of the smaller cartridges may have been exceeded. Further experiments utilized 500 mg SPE cartridges.

Methanol fractions after 500 mg SPE fractionations were profiled by HPLC and showed a significant amount of residual TFM. It was hypothesized that protonation of TFM was occurring during elution with the methanol:pH 4 acetate buffer mixture; the pK_a of TFM is approximately 6.1 (National Research Council of Canada 1985). A buffer with a pH above the pK_a of TFM should maintain TFM dissociation and facilitate its complete elution. Trials using a pH 8 0.2M (trihydroxymethyl)amine buffer with low proportions of methanol demonstrated removal of TFM only after relatively large elution volumes (>10 mL). Increasing the proportion of methanol to 40:60 methanol:tris buffer showed >99.99% removal of TFM after 9 mL (SPE-1). Formulation impurities were visibly removed in a post 1.5 mL methanol elution (SPE-2). Fish exposures to both fractions showed no induction was associated with SPE-1 and that formulation activity was recovered in the methanol fraction (SPE-2) (p<0.001) (Hewitt et al. 1996). SPE-2 fractions could now be fractionated directly using preparative HPLC.

HPLC separations

The objective of HPLC fractionation experiments was to isolate activity in a narrow chromatographic window to facilitate chemical characterizations on a minimum number of candidates. HPLC separations were conducted on a preparative scale so that SPE-2 fractions could be fractionated without volume adjustment. The fractions generated from the HPLC could then be directly exposed to fish. HPLC fractionations were carried out using a Waters (Millipore Corp., Milford, MA) system consisting of a 717 autosampler, a 600E system controller, a 610 valve station and a 481 spectrophotometer UV detector set at 254 nm (Millipore Corp.). UV detection at 254 nm provided a crude means of detecting materials containing one or more aromatic rings, a characteristic common to known inducers. It should be emphasized however, that experiments were directed by MFO induction; this detection method provided consistent reference locations within chromatograms for fractionation purposes.

Separations were achieved with a 500 mm x 9.4 mm i.d. reverse phase Partisil 10 ODS 2 column (Watman Inc., Clifton, NJ). Methanol and a pH 4 0.2M acetate buffer were used for HPLC separations as they were previously successful in eluting inducing formulation impurities (Munkittrick et al. 1994). Solvent programming was optimized to achieve maximal resolution of components visible at 254 nm: flow rate 4 mL/min, column preconditioning and an initial 2 min hold of 10:90 (%) methanol:0.2 M pH 4 acetate (Caledon Laboratories) buffer, linear gradient to 100% methanol at 34 min and hold for 21 min..

To ensure recovery of activity from the HPLC system, fish were exposed to the entire run from an injection of SPE-1 (Fig. 8). EROD activity was recovered in the region showing visible peaks at 254nm. Fractions from this region were initially collected during the elution of three main segments. Further collections corresponded to the location of large peaks for reproducibility. Activity was eventually isolated in two distinct narrow regions which demonstrated that a minimum of two formulation impurities were associated with MFO induction (Fig. 8). For complete resolution of activity at the chromatographic limit of the HPLC method, the final collections were exposed at 5 formulation equivalents.

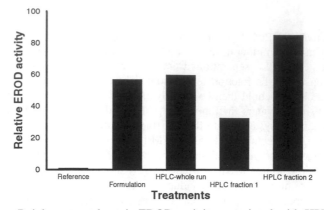

Figure 8.   Rainbow trout hepatic EROD activity associated with HPLC fractions generated after solid phase extraction of the TFM formulation. Activities are expressed relative to reference because exposures were performed separately. Both final active fractions were exposed at 5 formulation equivalents.

Chemical Characterizations of Bioactive Fractions

The bioactive fractions generated by HPLC fractionation of SPE-2 were characterized by GC-MS. GC-MS analyses were performed using a Hewlett Packard 5890 GC equipped with a retention gap consisting of 1 m x 0.53 mm i.d. deactivated fused silica gel connected to a 2.5 m x 0.25 mm i.d. section of deactivated fused silica. The retention gap was fitted to a 60 m x 0.25 mm i.d. DB-5 (J&W Scientific, Folsom, CA) column bonded to 0.25 µm phase thickness. The GC was interfaced at 280°C to a VG Autospec-Q mass spectrometer (Fisons, VG Analytical, Manchester, UK). Injections were 2 µL on-column with a helium (ultra high purity carrier grade, CANOX) carrier. GC injections were cold on-column to ensure complete delivery of bioactive extracts onto the GC column and to reduce the risk of decomposition of thermally labile compounds. Injector temperatures were programmed to follow oven conditions. GC oven temperatures were gradually increased over a wide temperature range to resolve compounds covering a broad range of polarities. Oven and injector temperatures were initially held at 80°C for 0.1 min then programmed at 4°C/min to 280°C, held for 2 min, programmed at 4°C/min to 290°C and held for 10 min. Positive ion electron impact mass spectra were obtained using both full scan and selection ion monitoring techniques. Full scan mass spectra of unknowns are necessary for structure determination. The identifications assigned to components detected by GC-MS in the bioactive fractions should follow published guidelines concerning identification of unknowns (Christman 1984). Tentative identifications are assigned when the postulated structure of an unknown is based solely on interpretation of its mass spectrum. Identifications are noted as confident when there is no authentic standard available but either the spectral or chromatographic data matches closely published data, including mass spectral data bases and retention indices. Compounds are described as confirmed when retention times and mass spectra match those for authentic standards analyzed under identical conditions.

The bioactive fractions were a mixture of methanol and acetate buffer and required solvent exchange prior to characterization. To determine the recovery of bioactive compounds, each fraction was solvent extracted, the extracts reduced in volume to just dryness and then redissolved in methanol for fish exposures. MFO induction in the resuspended extracts were compared to separate original bioactive fractions. Fish exposures to ethyl ether extracts of both fractions showed partial recovery of activity (71% and 43% respectively) while toluene extractions showed complete recovery of activity in both fractions ($p<0.001$) (Fig 9). This also indicated that the responsible compounds were relatively nonvolatile.

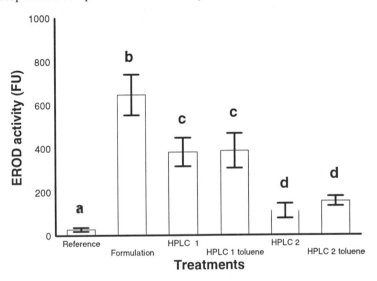

Figure 9.   Rainbow trout hepatic EROD activity associated with inducing HPLC fractions and their respective toluene extracts. The fractions and extracts were each exposed at 3 formulation equivalents. Letters above bars correspond to groups which were statistically independent of each other.

The chromatograms of the bioactive fractions were compared in detail with analysis blanks for the determination of unique constituents. The major components of the bioactive fractions were confirmed by synthesis as nitro-, trifluoromethyl-, and/or chloro diphenyl ethers. Fish exposures to the pure materials at a range of formulation equivalent concentrations showed no MFO induction was associated with these compounds (Hewitt et al. 1996). Although the identities of the compounds responsible for induction remained unknown at this juncture in the TIE, it could be concluded that these impurities were not associated with induction. These findings are significant because low levels of MFO induction have been associated with diphenyl ethers (Chui et al. 1986) and relatively high levels of these materials were present in the formulation (Hewitt et al. 1996). It should be emphasized that even if the TIE is ultimately unsuccessful in that the responsible compounds are not fully characterized, the elimination of materials identified during the course of the TIE that are not associated with the endpoint can yield useful information (Hewitt et al. 1995). Further, properties of the responsible compounds which become evident during the TIE (polarity, volatility) will augment characterizations. Ideally, as in this case, the materials were obtained in pure form from custom synthesis and were exposed in known, accurate concentrations to assess their bioactivity potential.

Further separations were necessary to isolate the responsible compounds. Although not employed here, other techniques such as normal phase HPLC could be applied. For the lampricide formulation being investigated further separations were realized by reinjection onto the reverse phase column under modified elution conditions.

HPLC Subfractionations

The bioactive fractions were concentrated three-fold prior to reinjection to facilitate the resolution of trace materials. Solvent conditions were optimized for each fraction to achieve the greatest resolution of components visible at 254nm. Recovery of activity after passage through the HPLC system was verified for both new elution conditions prior to fractionation experiments ($p < 0.001$). Activity from both reinjections were eventually recovered in a total of three new fractions. A trisubstituted dibenzo-p-dioxin possessing chloro-, nitro-, and trifluoromethyl substituents was confidently identified in two of these fractions by GC-MS (Hewitt et al. 1996).

Application to Other Physiological Responses

The goal of the development of the TIE techniques described is their application to a variety of physiological responses. In addition to elevated levels of MFO activity, altered levels of circulating sex steroid hormones in both male and female goldfish were associated with waterborne exposures to the lampricide formulation (Munkittrick et al. 1994). The TIE methodology developed using MFO induction was tested using circulating levels of sex steroids in fish as an endpoint. Preliminary experiments were conducted using the SPE-2 fraction of the TFM formulation. Male goldfish were dosed by intraperitoneal injection and basal levels of circulating steroids were measuresed after 4 days using the methods described in Munkittrick et al. (1994). Significantly decreased levels of both testosterone and 11-ketotestosterone were associated with exposure to the SPE-2 fraction (Fig. 10). Using this endpoint, the TIE methodology can be applied to determine the identity of the chemicals responsible for this response. Each step of the TIE must be validated for recovery of the biological activity as was documented here for MFO induction.

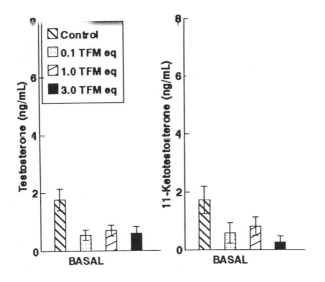

Figure 10.   Circulating levels of testosterone and 11-ketotestosterone in male goldfish exposed by intraperitoneal injection to 0.1, 1 and 3 lampricide formulation equivalents of the SPE-2 fraction containing formulation impurities.

SUMMARY

A TFM lampricide formulation was utilized to develop TIE techniques directed by hepatic MFO induction in fish. Prior to fractionation experiments, bioassay conditions were optimized to consistently obtain the highest response while maintaining low toxicity. Hepatic MFO determinations were modified from traditional assays to increase sensitivity and reduce analysis time. Solid phase extraction was successful in separating bioactive formulation impurities from the primary formulation ingredient, TFM. Induction was recovered after solid phase extraction which enabled direct fractionation by preparative HPLC. Activity was not compromised after passage through the HPLC system and was eventually isolated in two distinct fractions. Further fractionations were eventually achieved by reinjection of each fraction onto the HPLC under modified conditions. Bioassays verified that activity was recovered from each fraction by toluene extraction preceding chemical characterizations. Toluene extracts were characterized by cold on-column GC-MS. Characterization of bioactive fractions by GC-MS resulted in the elimination of three nitro-, trifluoromethyl- and/or chloro- diphenyl ethers as inducers. A chloro-, nitro-, trifluoromethyl dibenzo-p-dioxin has also been confidently identified in two active fractions. These techniques have also been initiated for the identification of compounds associated with potential reproductive abnormalities in fish.

ACKNOWLEDGEMENTS

The authors wish to acknowledge the assistance of Susan Huestis, Beth Chisholm, Bev Blunt, Vic Gillman, Larry Schleen and John Carey. This project was funded by the Canadian Department of Fisheries and Oceans, the Great Lakes Fishery Commission and the Reproductive Endorcrine Toxicology program of the Canadian Network of Toxicology Centres.

REFERENCES

Bills, T.D., Marking, L.L., Howe, G.E. and Rach, J.J., 1988, "Relation of pH to toxicity of lampricide TFM in the laboratory", Great Lakes Fishery Commission, Technical Report. no. 53, Ann Arbor, MI, pp. 6-13

Burkhard L.P., Durhan, E.J. and Lukasewycz, M.T., 1991, "Identification of nonpolar toxicants in effluents using toxicity-based fractionation with gas chromatography/mass spectrometry", Analytical Chemistry, Vol. 63, pp. 277-283

Christman, R.F., 1985, "Editorial policy changes", Environmental Science and Technology, Vol. 18, p. 203A

Chui, Y.C., Hansell, M.M., Addison, R.F. and Law, F.C.P., 1986, "Effects of chlorinated diphenyl ethers on the mixed-function-oxidases and ultrastructure of rat and trout liver", Toxicology and Applied Pharmacology, Vol. 81, pp. 287-294

Hewitt, L.M. Carey, J.H., Dixon, D.G. and Munkittrick, K.R. , 1995, "Examination of bleached kraft mill effluent fractions for potential inducers of mixed function oxygenase activity in rainbow trout ", In Environmental Fate and Effects of Bleached Pulp Mill Effluents, M.R. Servos, J.H. Carey, K.R. Munkittrick and G.J. Van Der Kraak eds., St. Lucie Press, Delray Beach, FL, in press

Hewitt, L.M., Munkittrick, K.R., Scott, I.M., Carey, J.H., Solomon, K.R. and Servos, M.R., 1996, "Use of a MFO-directed toxicity identification evaluation to isolate and characterize bioactive impurities from a lampricide formulation", Environmental Toxicology and Chemistry, in press

Klotz, A.V., Stegeman, J.J. and Walsh, C., 1983, "An aryl hydrocarbon hydroxylating hepatic cytochrome P-450 from the marine fish Stenotomus chrysops", Archives of Biochemistry and Biophysics, Vol. 226, pp. 578-592

McMaster, M.E., Van Der Kraak, G.J., Portt, C.B., Munkittrick, K.R., Sibley, P.K., Smith, I.R. and Dixon, D.G., 1991, "Changes in the hepatic mixed function oxygenase (MFO) activity, plasma steroid levels and age to maturity of white sucker (Catostomas commersoni) population exposed to bleached pulp mill effluent", Aquatic Toxicology, Vol. 21, pp. 199-218

Munkittrick, K.R., Servos, M.R., Parrott, J.L., Martin, V., Carey, J.H., Flett, P. and Van Der Kraak, G.J., 1994, "Identification of lampricide formulations as a potent inducer of MFO activity in fish", Journal of Great Lakes Research, Vol. 20, pp. 355-365

National Research Council of Canada., 1985, "TFM and Bayer 73: Lampricides in the aquatic environment", NRCC No. 22488, Environmental Secretariat, Ottawa, ON, 184p

North Atlantic Treaty Organization, 1986, "Pilot study on the international information exchange on dioxins and related compounds: International toxic equivalency factor method of risk assessment for complex mixtures of dioxin and related compounds." Report 176, U.S. Government Printing Office, Washington, DC, pp. 1-26

Parrott, J.L., Hodson, P.V., Servos, M.R., Huestis, S.Y. and Dixon, D.G., 1995, "Relative potency of polychlorinated dibenzo-p-dioxins and dibenzofurans for inducing mixed function oxygenase activity in rainbow trout", Environmental Toxicology and Chemistry, Vol.14, pp.1041-1050

Payne, J.F., Fancey, L.L., Rahimtula, A.D. and Porter, E.L., 1987, "Review and perspective on the use of mixed-function oxygenase enzymes in biological monitoring", Comprehensive Biochemistry and Physiology, Vol. 86C, No. 2, pp. 233-245

Poland A., Glover, E. and Kende A.S., 1976, "Stereospecific, high affinity binding of 2,3,7,8-tetrachlorodibenzo-p-dioxin by hepatic cytosol", The Journal of Biological Chemistry, Vol. 251, No. 16, pp. 4936-4946

Safe, S.H., 1986, "Comparative toxicology and mechanism of action of polychlorinated dibenzo-p-dioxins and dibenzofurans", Annual Reviews of Pharmacology and Toxicology, Vol. 26, pp. 371-399

Safe, S., Bandiera, S., Sawyer, T., Zmudzka, B., Mason, G., Romkes, M., Demomme M.A., Sparling, J., Okey, A.B. and Fujita, T., 1985, "Effects of structure on binding to the 2,3,7,8-TCDD receptor protein and AHH induction - Halogenated biphenyls", Environmental Health Perspectives, Vol. 61, pp. 21-33

Safe, S., Fujita, T., Romkes, M., Piskorska-Pliszczynska, J., Homonko, K. and
    Denomme M.A., 1986, "Properties of the 2,3,7,8-TCDD receptor - A QSAR
    approach", Chemosphere, Vol.15, pp. 1657-1663

Seelye, J.G. and Scholefield, R.J., 1990, "Effects of changes in dissolved oxygen on
    the toxicity of 3-trifluoromethyl-4-nitrophenol (TFM) to sea lamprey and
    rainbow trout", Great Lakes Fishery Commission, Technical Report no. 56,
    Ann Arbor, MI, pp. 6-13

U.S. Environmental Protection Agency, 1991, "Methods for aquatic toxicity
    identification evaluations: Phase I toxicity characterization procedures", 2nd
    Edition, EPA/600/6-91/003, Environmental Research Laboratory, Duluth, MN

U.S. Environmental Protection Agency, 1992, "Characterization of chronically toxic
    effluents, phase I", EPA/6-91/005F, Environmental Research Laboratory,
    Duluth, MN

U.S. Environmental Protection Agency, 1993a, "Methods for aquatic toxicity
    identification evaluations: Phase II toxicity identification procedures for
    samples exhibiting acute and chronic toxicity", EPA/600/R-92/080,
    Environmental Research Laboratory, Duluth, MN

U.S. Environmental Protection Agency, 1993b, "Methods for aquatic toxicity
    identification evaluations: Phase III toxicity identification procedures for
    samples exhibiting acute and chronic toxicity", EPA/600/R-92/081,
    Environmental Research Laboratory, Duluth, MN

Jack W. Anderson[1], F. C. Newton[2], John Hardin[2], Robert H. Tukey[3] and Keneth E. Richter[4]

CHEMISTRY AND TOXICITY OF SEDIMENTS FROM SAN DIEGO BAY, INCLUDING A BIOMARKER (P450 RGS) RESPONSE

REFERENCE: Anderson, J. W., Newton, F. C., Hardin, J., Tukey, R. H., and Richter, K. E., **"Chemistry and Toxicity of Sediments from San Diego Bay, Including a Biomarker (P450 RGS) Response,"** *Environmental Toxicology and Risk Assessment: Biomarkers and Risk Assessment—Fifth Volume, ASTM STP 1306,* David A. Bengtson and Diane S. Henshel, Eds., American Society for Testing and Materials, 1996.

ABSTRACT: Thirty sediment samples were collected from the vicinity of the Naval Docking Facility in San Diego Bay and used to conduct bioassays with amphipods (solid-phase), oyster larvae (elutriate), Microtox, and a new rapid screening test called the cytochrome P450 Reporter Gene System (RGS). This RGS cell line, from a human liver cancer cell, has been engineered to produce luciferase, when the CYP1A1 gene on the chromosome is induced by toxic and carcinogenic organics (dioxin, coplanar PCBs, PAHs). Elutriates were tested with both Microtox and oyster larvae, and organic extracts of sediments were tested with Microtox and the P450 RGS assay. Chemical analyses included total organic carbon (TOC), and acid volatile sulfides (AVS) along with a wide range of metals and organic chemicals. The simultaneously extracted metals (SEM) to AVS ratio was compared to the toxic response of oyster larvae and amphipods. Along each of the piers sampled, contaminant concentrations decreased with distance from shore. A correlation matrix analysis of all biological and chemical data was conducted. The strongest correlation (0.78, $r^2=0.61$) between a chemical measurement and a biological response was that of total PAH versus the P450 RGS response. The use of P450 RGS as a screening tool to assess the relative risk of contaminants on sediments is biologically meaningful, and is a rapid and inexpensive means of determining which samples require complete chemical characterization.

KEYWORDS: San Diego Bay, Cytochrome P450, PAHs, Sediment, Toxicity, Contamination

1 Columbia Analytical Services, Carlsbad, CA
2 MEC Analytical Systems, Carlsbad, CA
3 Department of Pharmacology, University of California, San Diego, CA
4 NRaD, U.S. Navy, San Diego, CA

Location

San Diego Bay is the southern-most embayment on the west coast of the United States. Located approximately 16 km north of the U.S.-Mexican Border, the Bay is about 24 km in length and varies in width from 0.4 km to 4 km. Depths vary from approximately 12 m in the ship channel, to about 1 m in many areas in the South Bay. The Bay has a deep entrance to the harbor and an extensive area for sheltered anchorage.

While the Bay is classified as an estuarine system, freshwater input has been greatly reduced over the years as a result of dam construction, the extensive use of ground waters, and diversion of the San Diego River. Freshwater input is now limited to that from periodic surface drainage of the metropolitan area and intermittent flow from several streams during periods of rainfall.

Objectives

This study was conducted to determine if sediments in and around the Naval facilities in San Diego Bay posed an ecological risk to the biota inhabiting the Bay, or possibly to humans consuming fish or shellfish from the Bay. Sediments were collected from 25 stations in the vicinity of the Naval Station (near National City) and 5 stations off the Naval Amphibious Base to determine contaminant concentrations and toxicity (Figure 1). Five sample stations along each of the transect lines (A-E) were located to reveal sediment contaminant concentration gradients perpendicular to the shoreline. Contaminant concentrations were also examined for longshore gradients, particularly near the mouth of Chollas (station A-1) and Paleta (station C-1) Creeks. The five stations off the Amphibious Base were randomly chosen in locations that were presumed to be reference stations.

The basic design for toxicity evaluations was to conduct testing that would subject the organisms or test systems to contaminants that were either water-soluble, or required extraction with an organic solvent. Tests were selected which ranged in duration from a few minutes to 10 days. Two separate tests were used to evaluate the toxicity of a water extract and two additional tests evaluated the toxicity of organic extracts. Dilutions of the seawater extract (elutriate) of a sediment sample were first tested with Microtox (luminescent bacteria) and oyster (*Crassostrea gigas*) embryos. Dilutions of the dichloromethane (DCM) extract of a sediment were tested again with Microtox and with the new P450 Reporter Gene System (RGS). A longer term test was the 10-day solid phase amphipod test, using *Rhepoxynius abronius*. Reference toxicants were included in each test to determine the relative sensitivities of the organisms, in relation to previous testing, and in relation to each other.

Methods

Sampling Design

The aerial distribution of sampling stations can be described as a simple grid (Figure 1) with station designations containing two characters, a letter (A-F) and a number (1-5). Stations with the same letter (A-E) were associated with transects orthogonal to shore. Orthogonal transects were ordered from A in the North to E in the South. Reference stations

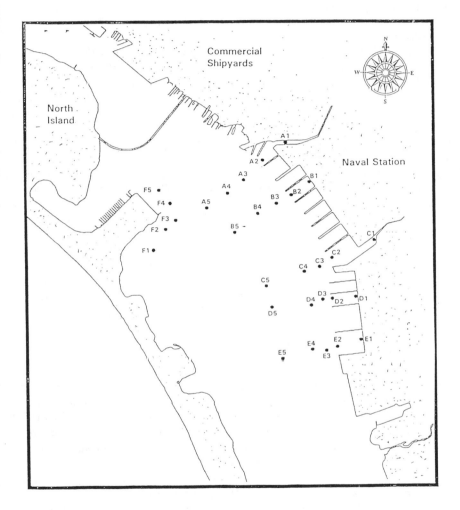

FIG. 1 — *Location of Sediment Sampling Stations in San Diego Bay. Transects A to E, in the Naval docks, are on the East side of the Bay, numbered from shore (1 stations) to the ship channel (5 stations). Reference stations are located on the West side of the Bay, near the Naval Amphibious Base.*

(F), across the Bay in an area presumed to be relatively uncontaminated, were numerically ordered from South (F1) to North (F5). Other stations (A-E) with the same number (e.g., 1) were associated with transects parallel to shore. Parallel transects were ascendingly ordered from shore (1 stations) to the ship channel (5 stations).

Field Collection Methods

Sediments for this program were collected from the Navy research Vessel *ECOS* on two occasions. Samples for chemistry, Microtox, P450 RGS and amphipod toxicity tests were collected on July 1 and 2, 1993. Samples for the bivalve elutriate test were obtained on September 2, 1993. Station locations were pre-plotted and entered into a differential geographic positioning system (GPS) which was utilized for navigation. Sediments were collected with a modified chain-rigged Van Veen sampler. Upon retrieval to the vessel, excess water was carefully poured off, with minimal loss of the surface layer of fine sediment. The grab was inspected and if any indication of incomplete collection was observed, such as visible washing out of the sample or incomplete closure of the grab, the sample was rejected. Sediment was collected from the top 6 centimeters with a Teflon spatula, taking care not to touch the sides of the grab. Samples were placed into pre-cleaned, labeled containers, using glass jars for organic constituents and toxicity tests and polyethylene containers for evaluation of metals and particle size. Sediments were stored in ice chests with blue ice and kept at 4° C while being transported to the Carlsbad, CA laboratory of Columbia Analytical Services (CAS). Samples for chemical analysis were carefully packaged to prevent breakage and shipped at 4° C with full chain of custody documentation to the CAS laboratory in Kelso, Washington for chemical analyses. At the Carlsbad laboratory, sediments to be used in toxicity testing were stored at 4° C for less than two weeks before test initiation.

Analytical Chemical and Biological Methods

Table 2 lists the methods used in both chemical and biological testing. The majority of the procedures are standard EPA or ASTM methods, so they will not be described in detail here. As discussed under objectives, the biological testing was designed to detect both water-soluble and solvent extractable contaminants. As described in the U.S. Army Corps of Engineers "Greenbook" (COE 1991), sediment elutriates were prepared, using 1:4 (by weight) slurries of sediment to seawater. These slurries were agitated for one hour in a rotary mixer and the water (elutriate) was then filtered through 0.45 micron filters to remove fine particles and bacteria. The elutriates were maintained at 4° C for 2 days until toxicity testing was initiated. Biological tests used with these elutriates were Microtox (luminescent bacteria) and the oyster larval bioassay (normal development). Dilutions of 0, 12.5, 25, 50 and 100% elutriate were used to determine the potential toxicity of the sediment samples. After testing dilutions of several samples with Microtox, it was observed that even the 100% elutriate of several samples failed to significantly reduce light emission. Therefore, the 100% elutriates of the remaining samples were tested first, to determine if there was any significant toxicity.

Organic extracts of the sediment samples were first prepared by the standard EPA 3540 method using 40 g of wet sediment and dichloromethane (DCM). The volume of DCM was reduced to 1 mL by evaporation, and then 1 mL of additional DCM was added back before dividing this volume to two 1 mL portions. One of the vials with 1 mL of DCM was used in testing with the P450 Reporter Gene System (RGS), while the DCM in the second vial was exchanged with non-denatured ethanol to be used in the Microtox assay. For Microtox, dilutions of 0, 12.5, 25, 50 and 100% were prepared. As described in the Microtox protocol, ethanol extracts were tested to determine the extent of luminescent reduction. The calculated dilution that produced a 50% light reduction (EC_{50}) was determined with a statistical program supplied with the instrument. The P450 RGS induction was determined by applying 2 µL of the DCM extract to 2 mL of media covering approximately one million 101L cells in individual wells. The induction response from DCM alone was used as control and set equal to unity. Responses from sediment extracts were expressed as fold induction, after dividing by the control response.

The chemical analyses listed in Table 1 include some of the most recent approaches, such as total organic carbon (% TOC) normalization of the concentrations of organic compounds and acid volatile sulfide (AVS) normalization of the simultaneously extracted metals (SEM).

TABLE 1 — *Methods used to Measure Study Parameters*

MEASUREMENT	METHOD
Grain Size	Plumb 1981
% Solids	EPA 160.3
Total Organic Carbon	ASTM D4129-82 Modified
Total Sediment Metals	EPA 6010 Most Metals EPA 7060 Arsenic EPA 7471 Mercury EPA 7740 Selenium EPA 7841 Thalium
Acid Volatile Sulfide	EPA 1991 Draft, Allen et al. 1993
Simultaneously Extracted Metals	EPA 1991 Draft , Allen et al. 1993
PCBs and Pesticides	EPA 3540/8080
Polycyclic Aromatic Hydrocarbons	EPA 3540/GC/MS SIM
Organic Extraction	EPA 3540, with and without modifications described by Microbics, Inc. for Microtox
Biological Analyses	
Elutriate Preparation	COE Greenbook 1991
Microtox with Elutriate	Battelle 1992
Oyster larval test with Elutriate	ASTM 1993
Microtox with Organic Extract	Battelle 1992
P450 with Organic Extract	Anderson et al. 1995
Solid Phase test with Amphipods	ASTM 1993

Data Evaluation

Several numerical techniques were employed in the analysis of the project data including descriptive, quantal, and hypothesis tests. Descriptive statistics were used to provide a summary of gathered information and included arithmetic mean, standard deviation, coefficient of variation (Sokal and Rohlf 1969), Pearson's correlation (SAS 1982) and histograms.

Due to the quantal nature of the data collected during the conduct of the bivalve bioassays, probit analyses (Hewlett and Plackett 1979), a parametric procedure and the spearman-Karber Method (Finney 1978), a non-parametric procedure, were used to evaluate effects. Quantal procedures were used to estimate the amount of test substance (sediment elutriate) needed to affect 50 % of the developing bivalve embryos in a 48-hour period; or more commonly stated the 48-hour EC_{50} value. Other toxicological parameters, including the no effects concentration (NOEC) were processed using ToxCalc software.

The One-Way analysis of Variance (ANOVA) was used for testing two null hypotheses on transects A to E; 1) transects parallel to shore do not differ significantly (p< or =0.05) from each other with respect to parameters tested, and 2) transects orthogonal to shore do not differ significantly (p< or =0.05) from each other with respect to the parameters tested. The reference stations (group F) were not selected in the same manner as A to E stations, and these were not included in the ANOVA. Additionally, the Student-Newman-Kuels multiple range test (Steel and Torrie 1980) was used to separate transects that were found to differ significantly (p< or =0.05). Forty-three biological and chemical parameters were reviewed using ANOVA.

Results

Sediment Analyses

The sediments were composed of mixtures of sand, silt and clay, with little if any gravel present (Fig. 2). Station E3 contained 27% gravel, but all others were 0 to 7% gravel and

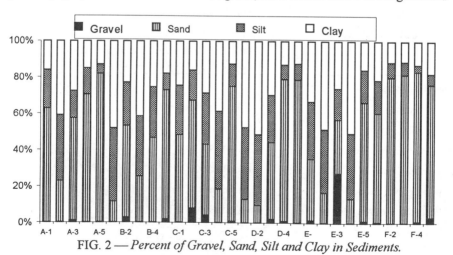

FIG. 2 — *Percent of Gravel, Sand, Silt and Clay in Sediments.*

most contained zero. Sand varied from a low of 9% at D2 to 82% at station F4. The average sand content of F stations was greater than that of other station groups. While there were exceptions, the stations that were most distant from land tended to contain the higher proportion of sand. In Figure 3, the percentage of solids in the sediment samples is plotted against the percentage of silt and clay combined. As the amount of fine material increased, the percent solids decreased. The percentage of total organic carbon increased with the increase in percentage of fine-grained material (Fig. 4).

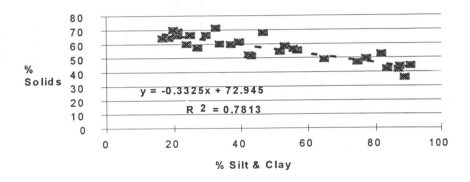

FIG. 3 — *Relationship between % Solids and Fine Grain Material in Sediments.*

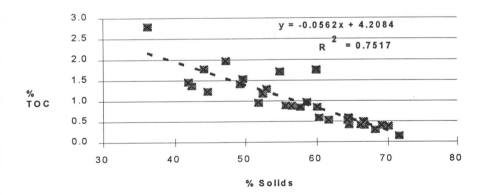

FIG. 4 — *Relationship between % Total Organic Carbon and % Solids in Sediment Samples.*

TABLE 2— *Total Metals Concentrations (mg/kg) in Sediments*

Station	Barium	Chromium	Copper	Lead	Mercury	Nickel	Tin	Vanadium	Zinc
A1	85	22	30	64	0	0	0	56	134
A2	110	45	117	197	0.5	12	0	64	206
A3	62	38	90	35	0.4	0	0	48	135
A4	39	26	51	25	0.4	0	0	30	97
A5	16	15	30	0	0	0	0	15	60
B1	139	99	486	120	1.5	25	19	91	444
B2	69	24	41	0	0	0	0	45	69
B3	123	118	162	82	2	24	22	82	313
B4	82	47	98	42	0.5	11	0	56	162
B5	28	22	44	20	0.2	0	0	25	91
C1	116	49	156	102	0.4	12	0	58	516
C2	164	20	30	0	0	0	0	48	58
C3	93	38	87	26	0.3	11	0	62	124
C4	124	70	161	57	0.7	16	0	87	227
C5	28	21	46	0	0.2	0	0	24	91
D1	137	84	358	68	1.5	19	10	93	330
D2	133	99	89	41	1.2	19	11	96	191
D3	95	46	129	34	0.5	11	0	66	161
D4	36	24	60	0	0	0	0	31	94
D5	25	18	36	21	0	0	0	20	74
E1	117	63	371	74	1	16	11	72	313
E2	108	60	400	42	0.4	17	0	88	244
E3	96	53	188	36	0.4	14	0	78	189
E4	101	59	185	42	0.5	17	11	81	222
E5	56	36	73	26	0.3	0	0	46	137
F1	41	29	50	24	0.3	0	0	36	106
F2	27	22	42	25	0.2	0	0	25	99
F3	40	28	56	22	0.3	0	0	34	112
F4	17	17	33	0	0	0	0	19	80
F5	24	22	46	0	0.2	0	0	26	106

TABLE 3 — *Acid Volatile Sulfide and Simultaneously Extracted Metals (mg/kg) in Sediments*

Station	AVS	Arsenic	Beryllium	Cadmium	Chromium	Copper	Lead	Mercury	Nickel	Selenium	Silver	Zinc
A1	550.15	1	0	0	7	20	64	0	5	0	0	11
A2	27.89	3	0	0.7	19	92	118	0	6	0	0	19
A3	159.98	2	0	17.8	18	61	31	0.3	0	0	0	11
A4	39.11	2	0	0	16	43	26	0	0	0	0	9
A5	50.98	0	0	6.1	9	22	15	0	0	0	0	6
B1	820.09	4	0	1.3	67	401	133	0.3	10	0	3	49
B2	11.86	0	0	0	5	17	11	0	0	0	0	2
B3	9.94	3	0.6	5	64	108	93	0.3	11	0	3	3
B4	33.98	4	0	0	25	80	47	0.3	0	0	0	14
B5	42.00	2	0	0	12	34	20	0	0	0	0	7
C1	749.88	3	0	1.1	25	129	102	0	6	0	0	42
C2	0.00	0	0	0	4	15	0	0	0	0	0	2
C3	10.90	1	0	0	16	59	27	0	0	0	0	9
C4	92.97	3	0	0	33	116	59	0.3	6	0	1	15
C5	45.85	1	0	6.1	13	36	22	0.2	0	0	0	8
D1	389.85	4	0	0	42	260	65	0.2	8	0	2	25
D2	66.04	0	0	4.2	36	22	27	0	0	0	0	1
D3	59.95	2	0	0	22	83	33	0	5	0	1	1
D4	140.10	1	0	0	13	43	20	0	0	0	0	8
D5	53.86	1	0	0	11	28	16	0	0	0	0	6
E1	240.13	4	0	0.6	32	181	68	0.3	6	0	1	25
E2	86.88	3	0.5	0	30	161	48	0.2	6	0	0	15
E3	109.97	2	0	0	22	91	37	0	0	0	0	14
E4	209.99	2	0	0	28	105	45	0	0	0	1	12
E5	159.98	2	0	0	18	50	25	0	0	0	0	13
F1	21.16	1	0	0	14	30	22	0	0	0	0	8
F2	5.77	2	0	0	13	35	24	0	0	0	0	9
F3	550.15	2	0	33	16	42	26	0	0	3	0	106
F4	74.06	0	0	0	9	20	14	0	0	0	0	6
F5	200.05	1	0	0	14	33	20	0	0	0	0	9

Table 2 shows the total metals composition of the 30 sediment samples, including non-toxic elements such as Al, Ca, Fe, Mg, K, and Na. Metals that may be problems in bays and estuaries (Long and Morgan 1990) are copper, chromium, lead and zinc (Fig. 5). Values between 50 and 100 mg/kg (ppm) for these metals were quite common. Copper and zinc reached high concentrations (300 ppm) at stations B1, C1, D1, and E1. This was the first indication that stations in the inner most (1 stations, nearshore) portion of each sampling group (A-E) may contain the highest contamination level of that specific group of stations.

The highest values for acid volatile sulfide (moles of AVS) were in most cases found in the first sample (1 stations) within each group (A-E). For example, the highest values were A1(=17), B1 (=26), C1 (=23), D1 (=12), and E1 (=8). An exception was within the high-sand F group, where the highest value was 17 moles of sulfide for station F3. As noted above, sediments from stations near the shoreline were also the samples that contained the highest levels of total Cu, Cr and Zn. The mild acid extractions used to measure the sulfide content of sediments were also used to measure the Simultaneously Extracted Metals (SEM). Significant concentrations were measured for Cr, Cu, Pb, and Zn in most samples (Table 3). As in the case of total metals, the SEM values were quite high in samples B1, C1, D1 and E1. Sample B1 had the highest concentrations for Cr, Cu, Pb and Zn. Those stations, which we expected would serve as reference stations (F), were the lowest in concentrations of these metals.

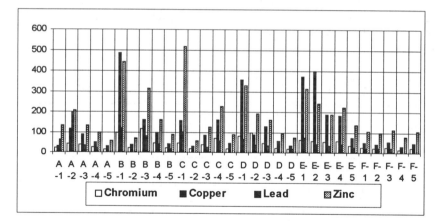

FIG. 5 — *Concentrations (mg/kg) of Total Chromium, Copper, Lead,and Zinc in Sediment Samples.*

Figure 6 compares the levels of potentially toxic metals (Cu. Cr, Pb, and Zn) from the total metals analyses to those from SEM analyses. As would be expected, there was a close relationship between the two sets of data. Because the presence of sulfides in sediments generally decreases the bioavailability of metals (Allen et al. 1993), the molar ratios of SEM to AVS are shown in Fig 7. Values greater than one are considered to show the potential for toxicity and bioavailability, while those with ratios less than one would not likely be toxic. Samples A2, B3, C3, and F2 showed the highest ratios, and would be expected to produce the most significant biological effects from metals.

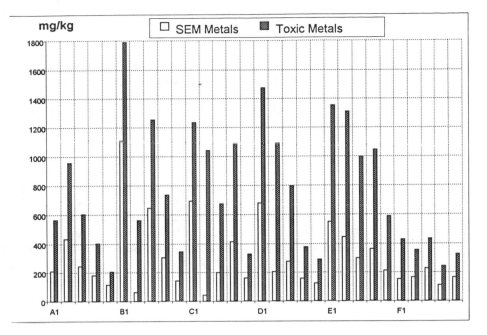

FIG. 6 — *Distribution of Total Potentially Toxic Metals (Cr, Cu, Pb, Zn) in Sediments and the Same Simultaneously Extracted Metals (SEM) in the Sediment Extracts.*

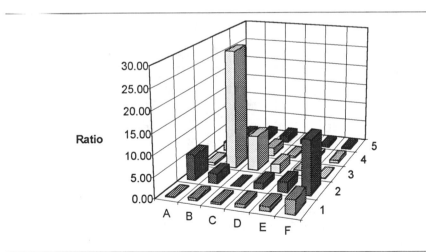

FIG. 7 —*Ratio of the combined moles of chromium, copper, lead, and zinc in the SEM extract to moles of sulfur in the AVS. Ratios of 1 or less are presumed to indicate low potential metal toxicity and bioavailibility.*

Because of the high water content of the sediments, and the methods used to quantify the PCBs and chlorinated pesticides, the detection limits for PCBs were either 100 or 200 µg/kg (ppb). PCBs were not found in any of the sediment samples at concentrations above these detection limits. At the lower detection limit of 20 ppb for most of the pesticides, none of those listed on the EPA Priority Pollutant List were found at concentrations above the detection level in any of the sediment samples.

The PAH characteristics of the sediments were measured by quantification of 36 compounds, or groups of compounds (i.e. C1-Naphthalenes = methylnaphthalenes) at individual detection limits of 20 ppb. Table 4 shows the composition of individual PAHs in sediment samples, and the total PAH content. In most cases the PAH components found were in the intermediate to high molecular weight range (phenanthrene to benzo[g,h,i]perylene). The first station in each transect, however, also contained significant contamination from some of the lower molecular weight compounds (A1, B1, C1, D1, and E1), except for the F group. As shown in Figure 8, these nearshore stations contained the highest levels of total PAH (from 7 to 20 ppm). Table 4 lists the total organic carbon (TOC) in the sediments so that the individual PAH concentrations can be normalized to ng of PAH/ g TOC. This may be useful in order to compared the data to Draft EPA Sediment Criteria, and Washington State Sediment Criteria, as will be done in the Discussion section.

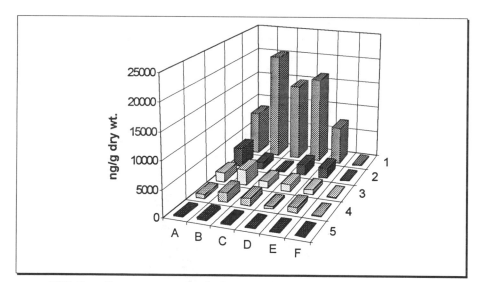

FIG. 8 — *Concentrations (ng/g dry weight) of Total Polycyclic Aromatic Hydrocarbons (PAHs) in Sediments.*

TABLE 4 — PAH Concentrations (ng/g sediment dry weight).

Analyte	A1	A2	A3	A4	A5	B1	B2	B3	B4	B5	C1	C2	C3	C4	C5
Naphthalene	ND	ND	ND	ND	ND	25	ND	21	ND	ND	ND	ND	ND	ND	ND
C1-Naphthalenes	ND	ND	ND	ND	ND	ND	ND	ND	ND	ND	ND	ND	ND	ND	ND
C2-Naphthalenes	52	ND	ND	ND	ND	34	ND	ND	ND	ND	32	ND	ND	ND	ND
C3-Naphthalenes	75	ND	ND	ND	ND	22	ND	ND	ND	ND	39	ND	ND	ND	ND
C4-Naphthalenes	70	ND	ND	ND	ND	31	ND	ND	ND	ND	290	ND	ND	ND	ND
Acenaphthylene	22	36	20	ND	ND	190	ND	29	ND	ND	62	ND	ND	ND	ND
Acenaphthene	110	ND	ND	ND	ND	ND	ND	ND	ND	ND	ND	ND	ND	ND	ND
Fluorene	110	ND	ND	ND	ND	32	ND	ND	ND	ND	ND	ND	ND	ND	ND
C1-Fluorenes	51	ND	ND	ND	ND	ND	ND	ND	ND	ND	140	ND	ND	ND	ND
C2-Fluorenes	66	ND	ND	ND	ND	59	ND	ND	ND	ND	550	ND	ND	ND	ND
C3-Fluorenes	140	ND	ND	ND	ND	ND	ND	ND	ND	ND	840	ND	ND	ND	ND
Phenanthrene	500	91	41	23	ND	310	24	50	37	ND	130	ND	20	24	ND
Anthracene	310	42	35	ND	ND	420	32	28	26	ND	210	ND	24	23	ND
C1-Phenanthrenes/Anthracenes	290	87	48	26	ND	380	25	56	34	26	330	ND	25	31	ND
C2-Phenanthrenes/Anthracenes	270	50	29	ND	ND	250	20	38	23	ND	550	ND	ND	ND	ND
C3-Phenanthrenes/Anthracenes	37	32	33	ND	ND	300	ND	53	25	ND	840	ND	ND	ND	ND
C4-Phenanthrenes/Anthracenes	83	38	28	ND	ND	360	ND	56	ND	ND	640	ND	ND	ND	ND
Dibenzothiophene	ND	ND	ND	ND	ND	ND	ND	ND	ND	ND	ND	ND	ND	ND	ND
C1-Dibenzothiophenes	ND	ND	ND	ND	ND	ND	ND	ND	ND	ND	ND	ND	ND	ND	ND
C2-Dibenzothiophenes	34	ND	ND	ND	ND	ND	ND	ND	ND	ND	ND	ND	ND	ND	ND
C3-Dibenzothiophenes	110	ND	ND	ND	ND	ND	ND	90	ND	ND	600	ND	ND	ND	ND
Fluoranthene	1,700	170	100	55	30	720	130	260	130	47	900	20	48	62	20
Pyrene	890	280	130	80	30	1,700	99	180	180	41	1,400	ND	64	88	ND
C1-Fluoranthenes/Pyrenes	500	190	110	55	21	1,600	120	120	110	27	1,200	23	57	69	ND
Benzo(a)anthracene	550	140	92	49	ND	950	93	120	100	29	630	ND	60	72	20
Chrysene	520	170	140	52	24	1,400	130	130	150	36	780	25	83	94	ND
C1-Chrysenes	190	134	66	28	ND	850	54	97	58	ND	520	ND	51	50	22
C2-Chrysenes	95	94	52	27	ND	300	ND	46	50	ND	230	ND	25	28	25
C3-Chrysenes	71	60	ND	ND	ND	230	ND	ND	ND	ND	120	ND	ND	ND	ND
C4-Chrysenes	49	48	25	ND	ND	97	62	ND	ND	ND	47	ND	ND	ND	24
Benzo(b)fluoranthene	370	560	200	85	40	3,600	140	330	190	66	1,170	57	230	200	45
Benzo(k)fluoranthene	230	280	150	62	27	1,300	120	170	130	31	760	52	100	110	ND
Benzo(a)pyrene	250	410	160	78	29	2,900	97	330	140	41	750	39	160	140	22
Indeno(1,2,3-cd)pyrene	140	320	140	60	30	1,100	69	270	140	41	460	35	130	130	25
Dibenzo(a,h)anthracene	54	ND	ND	20	ND	170	24	62	42	ND	160	ND	50	48	ND
Benzo(g,h,i)perylene	150	310	140	64	31	860	62	300	150	41	380	29	120	130	24
Total PAH	8089	3542	1739	764	262	20190	1239	2836	1715	426	14550	280	1247	1299	156
TOC (% dry weight)	1.76	1.54	1.19	0.5	0.59	2.8	0.3	1.98	0.98	0.85	1.72	0.15	0.89	1.3	0.4

TABLE 4 (Continued)

Analyte	D1	D2	D3	D4	D5	E1	E2	E3	E4	E5	F1	F2	F3	F4	F5
Naphthalene	ND	ND	ND	ND	ND	23	ND	ND	ND	ND	ND	ND	ND	ND	ND
C1-Naphthalenes	ND	ND	ND	ND	ND	ND	ND	ND	ND	ND	ND	ND	ND	ND	ND
C2-Naphthalenes	ND	ND	ND	ND	ND	ND	ND	ND	ND	ND	ND	ND	ND	ND	ND
C3-Naphthalenes	ND	ND	ND	ND	ND	ND	ND	ND	ND	ND	ND	ND	ND	ND	ND
C4-Naphthalenes	27	ND	ND	ND	ND	ND	ND	ND	ND	ND	ND	ND	ND	ND	ND
Acenaphthylene	180	ND	ND	ND	ND	42	24	ND	ND	ND	ND	ND	ND	ND	ND
Acenaphthene	ND	ND	ND	ND	ND	ND	ND	ND	ND	ND	ND	ND	ND	ND	ND
Fluorene	34	ND	ND	ND	ND	ND	ND	ND	ND	ND	ND	ND	ND	ND	ND
C1-Fluorenes	21	ND	ND	ND	ND	20	ND	ND	ND	ND	ND	ND	ND	ND	ND
C2-Fluorenes	ND	ND	ND	ND	ND	ND	ND	ND	ND	ND	ND	ND	ND	ND	ND
C3-Fluorenes	ND	ND	ND	ND	ND	ND	ND	ND	ND	ND	ND	ND	ND	ND	ND
Phenanthrene	160	88	27	ND	ND	160	31	20	24	ND	ND	ND	ND	ND	ND
Anthracene	310	35	26	ND	ND	140	41	26	20	ND	ND	ND	ND	ND	ND
C1-Phenanthrenes/Anthracenes	220	50	26	ND	ND	140	40	23	22	ND	ND	ND	ND	ND	ND
C2-Phenanthrenes/Anthracenes	150	32	26	ND	ND	140	29	ND	ND	ND	ND	ND	ND	ND	ND
C3-Phenanthrenes/Anthracenes	170	24	ND	ND	ND	220	20	ND	ND	ND	ND	ND	ND	ND	ND
C4-Phenanthrenes/Anthracenes	120	ND	ND	ND	ND	320	ND	ND	ND	ND	ND	ND	ND	ND	ND
Dibenzothiophene	ND	ND	ND	ND	ND	ND	ND	ND	ND	ND	ND	ND	ND	ND	ND
C1-Dibenzothiophenes	ND	ND	ND	ND	ND	ND	ND	ND	ND	ND	ND	ND	ND	ND	ND
C2-Dibenzothiophenes	ND	ND	ND	ND	ND	ND	ND	ND	ND	ND	ND	ND	ND	ND	ND
C3-Dibenzothiophenes	53	ND	ND	ND	ND	78	ND	ND	ND	ND	ND	ND	ND	ND	ND
Fluoranthene	590	170	54	31	21	420	79	64	49	22	23	ND	ND	ND	ND
Pyrene	1,200	170	69	38	21	590	150	65	72	22	26	ND	ND	ND	ND
C1-Fluoranthenes/Pyrenes	1,100	160	70	33	ND	590	120	63	50	ND	ND	ND	ND	ND	ND
Benzo(a)anthracene	780	110	51	26	ND	330	81	58	41	ND	ND	ND	ND	ND	ND
Chrysene	1,800	120	79	39	ND	640	140	86	55	ND	ND	ND	ND	ND	ND
C1-Chrysenes	750	59	49	ND	ND	290	78	37	32	ND	ND	ND	ND	ND	ND
C2-Chrysenes	260	34	24	ND	ND	130	37	ND	ND	ND	ND	ND	ND	ND	ND
C3-Chrysenes	110	ND	ND	ND	ND	55	ND	ND	ND	ND	ND	ND	ND	ND	ND
C4-Chrysenes	25	ND	ND	ND	ND	22	ND	ND	ND	ND	ND	ND	ND	ND	ND
Benzo(b)fluoranthene	2,500	250	220	93	37	740	250	120	160	37	46	33	30	30	30
Benzo(k)fluoranthene	1,900	100	87	36	ND	560	190	86	61	ND	ND	ND	ND	ND	ND
Benzo(a)pyrene	2,000	190	130	48	21	550	180	85	110	27	27	ND	ND	ND	ND
Indeno(1,2,3-cd)pyrene	910	160	130	51	27	420	160	72	110	ND	37	28	25	24	26
Dibenzo(a,h)anthracene	370	ND	42	ND	ND	66	24	ND	ND	ND	ND	ND	ND	ND	ND
Benzo(g,h,i)perylene	680	180	140	51	27	360	150	68	110	28	41	29	27	26	29
Total PAH	16420	1932	1250	446	154	7046	1824	873	916	136	200	90	82	80	85
TOC (% dry weight)	1.78	1.24	0.88	0.42	0.4	1.42	1.37	0.96	1.46	0.59	0.54	0.38	0.42	0.53	0.85

Biological Analyses

Elutriates.   None of the 100% elutriate samples were found to reduce the light emission of Microtox. In most cases the light emission actually increased, which was likely the result of added nutrients.

A 50 % reduction in normal oyster larval development (EC$_{50}$), after 48 hours of exposure, was not produced by 100 % elutriates of most sediments. An EC$_{50}$ was observed in a few of the elutriates (A5, B5, C1, E2, F4, F5) at concentrations of 34 to 86%. A more sensitive evaluation of the data was to use the no effects concentrations (NOEC) for each sediment and convert these values to chronic toxicity units (TUc) by dividing them into 100. These TUc values are shown for each sediment site in Figure 9. Sediment elutriates producing the greatest effects on the oyster larvae were from stations A4, 5; B1; E2, 5; and F2, 4.

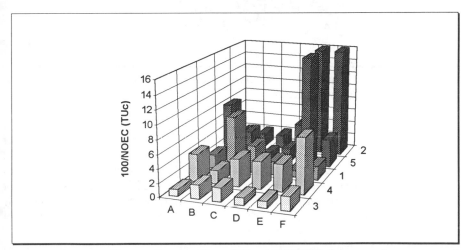

FIG. 9 — *Chronic Toxicity Units (TUc; 100/NOEC) for oyster larvae exposed to sediment elutriates.*

Organic Extracts of Sediments.   The baseline response for the Microtox test was illustrated by sample B2 with an EC$_{50}$ of >100% (Fig. 10). The EC$_{50}$ values for Microtox from an exposure to the organic extracts of sediment become smaller (greater dilution) as the toxicity of the extract increases. To provide an illustration that is easier to understand, and relate to the P450 RGS data, in Fig. 10 the EC$_{50}$ values were divided into 100, producing acute toxicity units (TUa). The greatest effects on the luminescence of Microtox was from sediments extracts of stations A1, 4, 5; B1, 5; C3; D1; E4; and F3, 4. Three of these stations were nearest the shore in their transect (1 stations).

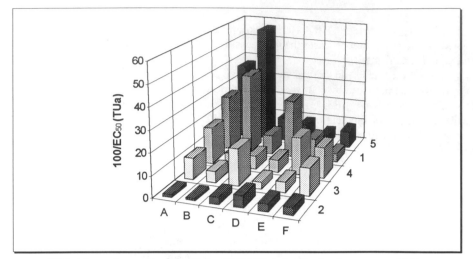

FIG. 10 — Acute Toxicity Units ($100/EC_{50}$) for the luminescence of Microtox exposed to organic extracts of sediments.

Background P450 RGS induction from both biogenic and anthropogenic compounds in these samples was approximately 20 fold, based on the induction produced by the extract of sediment from station F4, which contained relatively low amounts of toxic organic compounds. Studies on marine sediments from other regions have shown the background P450 response is as low as 4 fold (Anderson et al. 1995). Within sample groups A-E, RGS induction was the greatest in the first sample, closest to the shore. In the reference group (F series), F2 produced a slightly higher level of P450 induction. Figure 11 shows the comparison between the responses of Microtox and RGS from exposure to sediment extracts. In Figure 11, the TUa values for Microtox (Fig. 10) were multiplied by a factor of 2 to make the range of values comparable. Increases in the heights of both bars represent increasing toxicity. The trend for RGS responses was a stepwise decrease in induction from the first sample in a group to the last (moving from shore outward). It was difficult to observe any consistent pattern from observation of the Microtox data.

Solid Phase Testing.   The amphipod, *Rhepoxynius abronius*, was used in 10-day sediment tests to determine the toxicity of the 30 samples. No sediments produced 50% or greater mortality for the amphipods (Fig. 12). Only three samples (A2, B1 and D5) produced 40% or greater mortality. Samples D2, D4, F1, and F4 produced between 30 and 40% mortality after 10 days of exposure. Considering the relative sensitivity of this species, and the rather high contamination levels in many of the samples, greater mortality was anticipated. Reference toxicant data gathered during the testing, indicated that these animals were responding as expected to copper (LC_{50} = 230 ppb).

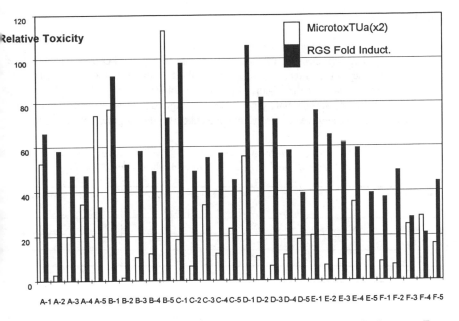

FIG. 11— *Pattern of Responses of the two Tests Used with Organic Extracts of Sediment. The TUa of Microtox was multiplied by 2 to bring the values in the appropriate range.*

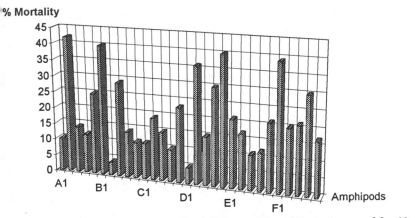

FIG. 12 — *Percent Mortality of Rhepoxynius abronius exposed for 10-days to the Sediment Samples.*

Discussion and Conclusions

Comparative Sensitivities of Biological Tests
    Table 5 summarizes the results of reference toxicant testing with copper and the three species used in this study. It is interesting to note that the 5- and 15-minute EC_{50} values for Microtox are in the same range as the 96-hour LC_{50} values for *R. abronius*. The 48-hour EC_{50} values for oyster larvae are approximately one order of magnitude lower than the other two tests. While the oyster larvae were quite sensitive, the effects on development observed were

TABLE 5 — *Comparison of Copper Toxicity (µg/L) for Microtox, Oyster Larvae (Crassostrea gigas), and Amphipods (Rhepoxynius abronius).*

Measurement	Microtox	Oyster Larvae	Amphipods
5-min. EC_{50}	320; 710		
15-min. EC_{50}	120; 290		
48-hour EC_{50}		17.0; 17.8; 19.0	
96-hour EC_{50}			230; 470; 410

less than anticipated. If there was strong binding of the contaminants identified in this investigation to the sediments, the levels in the elutriates used in the larval exposure could have been very low.
    The first station in each group (A-E), except in the reference series (F), produced the greatest response in the P450 RGS induction, and the Microtox (organic extract) response indicated high toxicity at the nearshore station on three of the transects (A1, B1, D1). The amphipods showed the highest mortality at stations A2, B1, D2, D5, and F1. The greatest impacts on development of bivalve larvae (Fig. 9.) were from elutriates prepared from samples at stations A5, B1, E2, E5, and F2. Station B1 was the only station where all four indicators showed a strong adverse response (Figs. 9,11,12). The responses at the reference stations indicated there was some level of contamination to which the test systems were responding. Each test may be responding to different classes or phases (soluble versus bound) of contaminants. The most specific biological response was the P450 RGS, which likely reacted to low levels of high molecular weight PAHs from petroleum or combustion sources.

Comparison of Toxicity to Other Studies

    The Southern California Coastal Water Research Project (SCCWRP) conducted an investigation of sediments at sites between Santa Monica Bay and San Diego Bay in 1987 (Anderson et al. 1988, 1989). Only three stations were sampled and tested from San Diego Bay, but these were the most likely to produce effects. Two of the stations in this present investigation for NRaD (approximately A1 and C1) were sampled and analyzed by SCCWRP (Chollas Creek and Paleta Creek = 7th Street). SCCWRP found that interstitial water from the sediments of Chollas Creek, Paleta Creek and the NASSCO dock station produced significant reduction in luminescence in the Microtox test. Sediments from these same three stations significantly reduced the survival of the amphipod, *Grandidierella*

TABLE 6 —*Comparative Results of Two Recent Surveys.*

STATION		TOC (% dry wt.)		Mercury (ppm)		Rhepoxynius % Mortality	Grandidierella % Mortality over Reference
CAS	SAIC	CAS	SAIC	CAS	SAIC	CAS	SAIC
A-1/Chollas Crk.	1	1.76	0.306	0	0.04	10	0
A-2	2	1.54	2.27	0.5	0.59	42	0
A-3		1.19		0.4		14	
A-4		0.5		0.4		12	
A-5		0.59		0		25	
B-1	12	2.8	2.7	1.5	1.31	40	39
B-2	15	0.3	2.8	0	1.76	4	25
B-3		1.98		2		29	
B-4		0.98		0.5		14	
B-5		0.85		0.2		11	
C-1/Paleta Crk.		1.72		0.4		11	
C-2	44	0.15	1.29	0	0.69	19	43
C-3		0.89		0.3		15	
C-4		1.3		0.7		10	
C-5		0.4		0.2		23	
D-1	62	1.78	1.76	1.5	0.86	5	39
D-2	58	1.24	1.69	1.2	0.63	36	5
D-3		0.88		0.5		15	
D-4		0.42		0		30	
D-5		0.4		0		40	
E-1	80	1.42	0.93	1	0.38	21	8
E-2	76	1.37	1.75	0.4	0.53	17	7
E-3		0.96		0.4		11	
E-4		1.46		0.5		12	
E-5		0.59		0.3		21	
F-1		0.54		0.3		39	
F-2		0.38		0.2		20	
F-3		0.42		0.3		21	
F-4		0.53		0		30	
F-5		0.85		0.2		17	

japonica, particularly at the two creek stations (60-65% mortality). The growth of sea urchins, *Lytechinus pictus*, was suppressed when held on Paleta Creek sediments for 35 days. This was one of the few studies comparing the sensitivities of two amphipods (*G. japonica* and *R. abronius*) frequently used in sediment toxicity testing. Dilutions of Paleta Creek sediment were tested with both species, and the findings showed them to respond in a very similar manner. At 20, 50, 75 and 100% Paleta Creek sediment, the ranges of percent survival for both species were 60-77, 40-45, 20-40, and 38-43, respectively.

A very recent survey was conducted in the naval docks for the Navy by Science Applications International, Corp. (SAIC). This preliminary investigation included sediment grain size, total organic carbon, mercury, and toxicity for *Grandidierella*. Table 6 compares those findings with the present NRaD study. Nine stations were selected that are close to those used in this study. It is interesting that station B1 produced 40% mortality for *R. abronius* and 39% mortality for *G. japonica*. The agreement at other stations in biological and chemical measurements was not as good. Frequently, the TOC or mercury values were quite similar, but in other cases there was an order of magnitude difference. This comparison suffers from the lack of split-sample intercomparison, as the characteristics of sediments collected only a few meters apart might be quite different.

Relationship Between Levels of Contamination and Station Location

Table 7 demonstrated statistically that there were several contaminants, as well as biological tests, that showed a significant relationship to distance from shore. It was evident that the nearshore (1 and 2) stations, within each group (A-E) along the piers, contained sediments that were higher in contamination and produced greater biological effects. Acid volatile sulfides and total PAHs produced the most significant relationships with distance from shore (p=0.000). Values down the right column of Table 7 to Arsenic (p=.0665) are significantly related to the distance from shore. P450 RGS was the biological measure that was most strongly related to the distance from shore, likely because of the distribution pattern of total PAHs.

Correlations Between Toxicity and Chemical Analyses

All chemical and biological data were first tested for the level of correlation in a massive Pearson correlation matrix. Those combinations of parameters showing a correlation of 0.6 or greater were then selected and evaluated (Table 8). The only biological parameter that correlated significantly with any of the chemical measures, was the P450 RGS. The correlation of 0.779 (r^2= 0.607) for RGS versus total PAH concentrations, was the highest value observed in this investigation. Since there was a considerable amount of co-occurence of high values for multiple pollutants, the correlations of RGS with several other toxicants (individual PAHs and metals) were also high. Figure 13 shows that the responses of P450 RGS can be used to predict both the dry weight concentrations of PAH, and the TOC-normalized PAH levels.

Analyses of AVS and SEM were not useful for predicting the potential toxicity of metals in sediments. Most of the sediments produced AVS to SEM ratios above 1.0, yet those with the highest ratios were seldom found to produce significant biological effects. Station F2, with a high ratio, was one of the stations producing significant effects on oyster larvae (TUc = 16). Station A2, with a moderately high ratio, produced a 40% mortality for the amphipods. However, station B3, with the highest AVS to SEM ratio, produced no strong effects on any species. Since there was significant mortality (40%) in amphipods exposed to sediments from stations F1 and F4, with rather low levels of toxicants, the low TOC of these sediments may have resulted in increased bioavailability.

TABLE 7—*ANOVA p Values*

By Offshore Stations (A - E)		By Alongshore Stations (1-5)	
Test	prob	Test	prob
Boron	0.1212	AVS (Moles)	0.0000
Magnesium	0.1877	Total PAHs (ppb)	0.0000
Aluminum	0.1919	Barium	0.0004
Cobalt	0.1953	P450-FOLD IND.	0.0006
Potassium	0.2120	Total Toxic Metals	0.0023
Copper	0.2162	Zinc	0.0027
Tin	0.2347	TOC (dry wt.)	0.0044
Iron	0.2366	Vanadium	0.0066
Sodium	0.2483	Zinc(ppm in SEM)	0.0069
Calcium	0.2686	Total Metals(ppm in SEM)	0.0071
Beryllium	0.2921	Cobalt	0.0089
Silver(ppm in SEM)	0.2949	EC50-Microtox	0.0161
Chromium(ppm in SEM)	0.3070	Nickel(ppm in SEM)	0.0172
Silver	0.3421	Copper(ppm in SEM)	0.0189
Cadmium(ppm in SEM)	0.3512	Lead(ppm in SEM)	0.0224
Manganese	0.3594	Manganese	0.0240
Nickel	0.3640	Iron	0.0279
Chromium	0.3815	Potassium	0.0290
Solids	0.4117	Magnesium	0.0426
Total Toxic Metals	0.4196	Microtox (200/EC50)	0.0442
Mercury	0.4398	Copper	0.0461
Vanadium	0.4509	Arsenic(ppm in SEM)	0.0665
Microtox (200/EC50)	0.4760	Aluminum	0.0785
P450-FOLD IND.	0.5074	Nickel	0.0860
Arsenic(ppm in SEM)	0.5199	Boron	0.0901
Cadmium	0.5394	Sodium	0.1020
Mercury(ppm in SEM)	0.5548	Lead	0.1093
Arsenic	0.5561	Silver(ppm in SEM)	0.1612
Beryllium(ppm in SEM)	0.5671	Solids	0.1613
Barium	0.6093	Chromium	0.1703
Copper(ppm in SEM)	0.6195	Arsenic	0.1837
Amphipod Mortality	0.6985	Mercury	0.2091
Total Metals(ppm in SEM)	0.7169	Chromium(ppm in SEM)	0.2332
Zinc(ppm in SEM)	0.7310	Cadmium(ppm in SEM)	0.3741
Zinc	0.7353	Tin	0.3903
Bivalves (EC50)	0.7533	Silver	0.4096
EC50-Microtox	0.7678	Bivalves (EC50)	0.4182
TOC (dry wt.)	0.7865	Cadmium	0.5394
Lead(ppm in SEM)	0.7872	Mercury(ppm in SEM)	0.5548
Lead	0.8373	Beryllium(ppm in SEM)	0.5671
Nickel(ppm in SEM)	0.9272	Beryllium	0.6010
Total PAHs (ppb)	0.9349	Amphipod Mortality	0.6591
AVS (Moles)	0.9989	Calcium	0.8321

TABLE 8 — *Correlation of P450 RGS with Chemical Parameters.*

** = 0.01   *** = 0.001

Compound	Correlation with P450	z	Significance	r Squared
Total Polycyclic Aromatic Hydrocarbons	0.779	0.00	***	0.607
C1-Chrysenes	0.772	0.00	***	0.596
C2-Chrysenes	0.772	0.00	***	0.596
Benzo(a)pyrenes	0.771	0.00	***	0.594
C1-Fluoranthenes	0.771	0.00	***	0.595
Chrysene	0.767	0.00	***	0.588
Benzo(g,h,i)perylene	0.765	0.00	***	0.586
Pyrene	0.761	0.00	***	0.579
Benzo(k)fluoranthene	0.759	0.00	***	0.577
Indeno(1,2,3-cd)pyrene	0.755	0.00	***	0.571
Dibenzothiophene	0.733	0.00	***	0.537
Benzo(b)fluoranthene	0.728	0.00	***	0.530
Total Organic Carbon	0.707	0.00	***	0.500
Total Simultaneously Extracted Metals	0.705	0.00	***	0.497
Total Metals	0.696	0.00	***	0.484
SEM Zinc	0.691	0.00	***	0.478
Zinc	0.691	0.00	***	0.478
Benzo(a)anthracene	0.684	0.00	***	0.468
C3-Chrysenes	0.673	0.00	***	0.453
Copper	0.673	0.00	***	0.453
SEM Copper	0.673	0.00	***	0.453
Nickel	0.630	0.00	***	0.398
Lead	0.605	0.00	***	0.366
SEM Lead	0.605	0.00	***	0.366
Chromium	0.575	0.00	***	0.331
SEM Chromium	0.575	0.00	***	0.331
Fluoranthene	0.551	0.00	**	0.304
C4-Chrysenes	0.549	0.00	**	0.301
Arsenic	0.533	0.00	**	0.284
SEM Arsenic	0.519	0.00	**	0.270
Acid Volatile Sulfides	0.490	0.01	**	0.240
Silver	0.486	0.01	**	0.237
Total Solids	-0.654	0.00	***	0.428

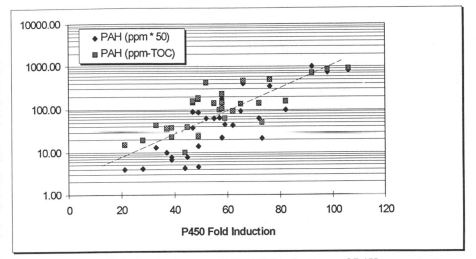

FIG. 13 — *Relationship between P450 RGS induction and PAH concentrations.*

Significance of Chemical Contamination

The SCCWRP investigation of 1987 (Anderson et al. 1988) demonstrated biological effects at both Chollas Creek and Paleta Creek. This study found very low amphipod mortality at these stations (A1 and C1). SCCWRP found 7.6 ppm of total PAH at Chollas Creek and 12.1 ppm at Paleta Creek. In this investigation we found 8.09 ppm and 14.55 ppm, respectively, for the same stations. This indicates that the chemical contamination has not changed much in approximately 6 years, but does not help explain the higher survival of the amphipods at these stations.

Long and Morgan (1990) compiled a massive amount of data on toxicity and chemistry of sediments to first develop estimated Effects Range Low (ERL) and Effects Range Median (ERM) for specific sediment contaminants. Since that time the data base has increased considerably, and Long et al. (1994) has revised these estimated concentrations of contaminants in sediment that have been associated with effects on marine species. Table 9 presents the ERM values from this recent manuscript, indicating concentrations above which one would expect to see an impact on the biota. Also shown in Table 9 are the data from stations sampled in this investigation, where the measured concentrations are at or above the latest ERM values. Station B1, which produced significant effects on each of the biological tests used in this study, contained concentrations of copper, mercury, silver, zinc, benzo(a)pyrene, and total high molecular weight PAHs above the ERM. Station D1 contained levels of copper, mercury, silver, benzo(a)pyrene, dibenzo(a,h)anthracene, and total high molecular weight PAHs above the ERM. A few other stations showed levels of some metals somewhat above the ERM, but not organics. The U.S. EPA has only distributed three sediment criteria documents (dated 1991 draft) on PAHs (Table 10). The state of Washington has utilized the apparent effects threshold (AET) values produced from studies in Puget Sound to establish sediment quality criteria. Most of the TOC normalized values derived from the analyses of NRaD samples were observed to be substantially below

TABLE 9— Concentrations (ppm) of Metals and Organics at Stations Above ERM Values.

	ERM	Station						
	(ppm)	B1	D1	C1	D2	E1	E2	B3
Arsenic	70							
Cadmium	9.6							
Chromium	370							
Copper	270	486	358				400	
Lead	218							
Mercury	0.71	1.5	1.5		1.2	1.0		2.0
Nickel	51.6							
Silver	3.7	5	4					6
Zinc	410	440		516				
Benzo(a)pyrene	1.600	2.900	2.000					
Dibenzo(a,h)anthracene	0.260		0.370					
Total High Molecular wt. PAHs	9.600	18.407	15.578					
Total PAHs	44.792							

TABLE 10 — Comparison of Available Sediment Quality Criteria (mg PAH/kg organic carbon) to NRaD Data

Component	EPA 1991 Criteria (Range)	Washington State Criteria	NRaD Station B1	NRaD Station D1
acenaphthene	240 (110-520)	16	0	0
phenanthrene	160 (74-340)	100	10.7	9.0
fluoranthene	1340 (620-2880)	160	24.8	33.2
Total benzofluoranthenes		230	168.9	247.1
benz(a)anthracene		110	32.8	43.8
chrysene		110	48.3	101.1
benzo(a)pyrene		99	100.0	112.4
dibenz(a,h)anthracene		12	5.9	20.8
Total HPAH		960	612.5	841.2

the criteria listed in Table 10. Even the most highly contaminated stations (B1 and D1) contain levels of individual PAHs well below the EPA values listed in Table 10. There were four instances where the NRaD values are above the Washington State Sediment Quality Criteria. It should be noted that Washington state has derived higher values for sediment cleanup criteria (Ginn and Pastorok 1992).

Recommendations

Since this study has demonstrated that stations B1 and D1 are suspected of containing concentrations of contaminants that may be producing biological effects, some additional studies are recommended. One of the more sensitive biological measures described in the recent literature is an interstital water test with echinoderm embryo development (Carr and Chapman 1992). By using interstitial water to test for P450 RGS, and effects on oyster larvae and echinoderm embryos, it may be possible to obtain closer agreement between toxicity measurements at the most contaminated stations. It may also be possible to determine a sediment EC_{50} value for the most toxic sediments, which will be more useful in estimating the ecological risk associated with these stations. Station B1 and D1 sediments may be appropriate for use in a sediment Toxicity Identification Evaluation (TIE). Solvent extracts of these sediments could be applied to high pressure liquid chromatography with selected solvents and columns, producing a number of fractions containing specific PAHs, as well as other low-level organic contaminants. These fractions could then be screened, using the P450 RGS approach, to determine the most toxic fraction. It may then be possible to identify by GC/MS the few specific components associated with the toxic effects.

References

Allen, H.E., G. Fu and B. Deng, 1993, "Analysis of Acid-Volatile Sulfide (AVS) and Simultaneously Extracted Metals (SEM) for the Estimation of Potential Toxicity in Aquatic Sediments," *Environmental Toxicology Chemistry,* Vol. 12, pp. 1441-1453.

American Society for Testing Materials, 1993, "Standard Guide for Conducting Static Acute Toxicity Tests Starting with Embryos of Four Species of Saltwater Bivalve Molluscs," E 724 - 89, *Annual Book of ASTM Standards,* Vol. 11.04, pp. 430-447.

American Society for Testing Materials, 1993, "Standard Guide for Conducting 10-Day Static Sediment Toxicity Tests with Marine and Estuarine Amphipods," E 1367 - 92, *Annual Book of ASTM Standards,* Vol. 11.04, pp. 1138-1163.

Anderson, J.W., S.S. Rossi, R.H. Tukey, T. Vu and L.C. Quattrochi, 1995, "A Biomarker, P450 RGS, for Assessing the Potential Toxicity of Organic Compounds in Environmental Samples, " *Environmental Toxicology Chemistry, Vol.* 14, pp. 1159-1169.

Anderson, J. W., 1995, "The Induction of P450 RGS by Sediment Extracts from Samples Collected in San Diego Bay, Charleston Harbor, and the Southern California Bays," Final Report to NOAA, Bioeffects Branch, Seattle, WA, 23 pp.

Anderson, J.W., S.M. Bay, and B.E. Thompson, 1988, "Characteristics and Effects of Contaminated Sediments from Southern California," Final Report to the California state Water Resources Control Board, Southern California Coastal Water Research Project, Contribution No. C-297, Westminster, CA.

Anderson, J.W., S.M. Bay, and B.E. Thompson, 1989, "Characteristics and Effects of Contaminated Sediments from Southern California," In: Proceedings Oceans 1989, Vol 2, september 18-21, Seattle, WA, pp. 449-451.

Battelle Northwest/Marine Sciences Laboratory, 1991, "Standard Methods Manual for Environmental Sampling and Analysis in San Francisco Bay, Volume 3: Toxicological Testing Methods: Marine and Estuarine," Prepared for the U.S. Army Corps of Engineers, Contract DE-AC06-76RLO 1830.

Carr, R.S. and D.C. Chapman, 1992, "Comparison of Solid-Phase and Pore-Water Approaches for Assessing the Quality of Marine and Estuarine Sediments," Chemical Ecology, Vol. 7, pp. 19-30.

EPA/COE, 1991, "Evaluation of Dredged Material Proposed for Ocean Disposal: Testing Manual," U.S. EPA and Army Corps of Engineers Publication, EPA - 503/8-91/001, February, 1991, Washington, D.C., 186 pp.

Finney, D.J., 1978, "Statistical Methods in Biological Assay," 3rd Ed, Charles Griffin & Co. Ltd, London, 508 pp.

Ginn, T.C. and R.A. Pastorok, 1992, "Assessment and Management of Contaminated Sediments in Puget Sound," In: Sediment Toxicity Assessment, G.A. Burton, Jr., Ed., Lewis Publishers, Boca Raton, Florida.

Hewlett, P.S. and R.L. Plackett, 1979, "Interpretation of Quantal Responses in Biology," University Park Press, Baltimore, 82 pp.

Long, E.R., D.D. MacDonald, S.L. Smith and F.D. Calder, 1995, "Incidence of adverse biological effects within ranges of chemical concentrations in marine and estuarine sediments," Environmental Management, Vol. 19, pp. 81-97.

Long, E.R. and L.G. Morgan, 1990, "The Potential for Biological Effects of Sediment-Sorbed Contaminants Tested in the National Status and Trends Program," NOAA Technical Memorandum NOS OMA 52, Seattle, WA.

Plumb, R.H., Jr., 1981, "Procedure for Handling and Chemical Analysis of Sediment and Water Samples," Technical Report EPA/CE-81-1, from the Great Lakes Laboratory, State University College at Buffalo, NY, for the U.S. EPA/Corps of Engineers Technical Committee on Criteria for Dredged and Fill Material. Published by the the U.S. Army Corps of Engineers Waterways Experiment Station, Vicksburg, MS.

SAS, 1982, "SAS User's Guide: Statistics," SAS Institute, Inc., New York, 920 pp.

Science Applications International Corporation (SAIC), 1994, "Sediment Characterization Study, Pier and Berthing Areas, U.S. Naval Station, San Diego," Vol I., Draft Report Submitted To: Department of the Navy, Southwest Division, San Diego, CA. Contract No. N68711-93-C-1527.

Sokal, R. R. and F.J. Rolf, 1969, "Biometry," W. H. Freeman, San Francisco, 76 pp.

Steel, D.J.H. and J.H. Torrie, 1980, "Principles and Procedures of Statistics," 2nd ed. McGraw-Hill Book Co., NY., 327 pp.

Brian P. Bradley,[1] Drew C. Brown,[2] Tina N. Iamonte,[3] Susan M. Boyd[3] and Michael C. O'Neill[4]

PROTEIN PATTERNS AND TOXICITY IDENTIFICATION USING ARTIFICIAL NEURAL NETWORK MODELS

REFERENCE: Bradley, B. P., Brown, D. C., Iamonte, T. N., Boyd, S. M., and O'Neill, M. C., **"Protein Patterns and Toxicity Identification,"** *Environmental Toxicology and Risk Assessment: Biomarkers and Risk Assessment—Fifth Volume, ASTM STP 1306*, David A. Bengtson and Diane S. Henshel, Eds., American Society for Testing and Materials, 1996.

ABSTRACT: Proteins extracted, separated, and visualized can provide detailed information about an organism and its environment. We have used an artificial neural network model to identify significant exposures of a cladoceran (*Daphnia magna*) to alcohol and pesticides, of a copepod (*Eurytemora affinis*) to heat and salinity, of an earthworm (*Lumbricus terrestris*) to sulfur mustard and of a small fish (*Oryzias latipes*) to groundwater concentrations. The method depends on systematic differences or tendencies in numbers and amounts of proteins present in different treatments or environments. We illustrate how neural computing might be useful in retrieving the information contained in the hundreds or thousands of proteins expressed in test organisms. Such information could apply to prediction of toxicity, identification of toxicity and to characterizing environments in general.

KEYWORDS: protein patterns, toxicity, neural networks

[1]Professor, Biological Sciences Department, University of Maryland Baltimore County, Baltimore, MD 21228

[2]Research Associate, Biological Sciences Department, University of Maryland Baltimore County, Baltimore, MD 21228

[3]Graduate Student, Biological Sciences Department, University of Maryland Baltimore County, Baltimore, MD 21228

[4]Associate Professor, Biological Sciences Department, University of Maryland Baltimore County, Baltimore, MD 21228

INTRODUCTION

There is great interest in the use of biological indicators to predict and in some cases diagnose physical, chemical, and physiological stress. The range of responses encompassing what are sometimes referred to as biomarkers is continually increasing (Dhingra et al. 1993; Ernst and Peterson 1994; Grandjean et al. 1994; Omland et al. 1994; Peakall and Walker 1994; Smith and Suk 1994). Biomarkers based on classes of proteins or on the enzymatic activities of proteins are well known (Stegmann et al. 1992).

Among the variety of protein indicators are the heat shock proteins, which have many attractive properties as environmental indicators and have been the subject of many reviews (Lindquist and Craig 1988; Schlesinger 1990; Nover 1991; Stegmann et al. 1992; Welch 1993). They are now often referred to as stress proteins (Sanders, 1993) together with related proteins inducible by other stressors (Cai et al. 1993; Ryan and Hightower 1994). We have studied HSP_{70} in this laboratory in a range of species (Bradley and Ward 1989; Hakimzadeh and Bradley 1989; Bradley 1990, 1992; Brown et al. 1995). The heat shock proteins are induced by a wide variety of agents (Welch 1993) and so are general and not specific indicators of stress.

We propose here that proteins in addition to the heat shock proteins (or stress proteins, however they may be defined) may be available as candidates for a fingerprint or profile to indicate specific conditions. The presence of thousands of proteins and the means to process the information from the patterns makes a total protein analysis attractive in principle.

The keys to success are the detection of enough protein information and the ability to draw inferences from it. If the protein patterns are specific to the stressors of interest and they can be objectively recognized, then relevant environmental conditions can be diagnosed. We have accumulated some evidence for specificity of protein expression in daphnids (Bradley et al.1994), in copepods (Hakimzadeh and Bradley 1989; Bradley et al.1992; Gonzalez and Bradley 1995) and in earthworms and medaka, as described in this paper. Other evidence of specificity comes from bacteria (Van Bogelen et al. 1987; Adamowicz et al. 1991; Blom et al. 1992) and human leucocytes (Jellum et al. 1983). Some of the specificity reported is at the individual protein level, for example zona radiata proteins (Oppen-Berntsen et al. 1994)) and onco-fetal proteins (Carsberg et al.1995). The medical literature has other such examples, including the acute-phase proteins (Lockwood et al. 1994).

The methods of extracting and visualizing proteins from test and reference organisms are well established in our laboratory and elsewhere. The methods of analysis are based on pattern recognition in either one or two dimensional separations of proteins. Many of the papers just cited depended on two dimensional separation and we have used that method also (Bradley et al. 1994). As an alternative method to visual or automated examination of 2D patterns we have investigated protein pattern recognition using artificial neural network models (A.N.N.). The procedures are powerful, iterative and allow large numbers of inputs (proteins) to be reduced to a significant few. Among these significant inputs, those proteins contributing most to the diagnosis (either by their presence or by their absence) can be identified. Thus A.N.N. analyses could lead to multiple immunoassays based on the key proteins.

In this paper we review methods of extracting and visualizing the proteins. We explain how neural networks may be useful as a method of interpreting the protein patterns. The methods are illustrated with results summarized from several systems.

METHODS

There are three main methods for detecting proteins expressed in test or control organisms: 1) To visualize all separated proteins we use **silver staining** (Bradley *et al.* 1992); 2) Specific proteins can be identified in **immunoassays** using specific antibodies (Brown *et al.* 1995); 3) Proteins currently being synthesized by the organism can be identified by **metabolic labelling** with isotope-labelled amino acids (Gonzalez and Bradley 1995).

In this paper we discuss results using the first and third methods. In the first two experiments (described later) organisms were exposed to treatments for 5 to 48 hours and labelled with 50 μCi ^{35}S-methionine (NEN Life Sciences Products, Boston, MA; specific activity 1175 Ci/mmol) added to 150 μL water for the final 4 hours of exposure. Whole individuals were frozen in liquid nitrogen, and samples were stored at -80°C. Soluble proteins were extracted by mechanical homogenization in a stabilizing buffer with protease inhibitor [phosphate-buffered saline (PBS), pH 7.4, with 10 mM phenylmethylsulfonyl fluoride (Sigma, St. Louis, MO), a protease inhibitor and 0.1 mM dithiothreitol (Sigma), a sulfhydryl protectant]. The soluble protein concentration was measured on a Spectronic 601 spectrophotometer (Milton Roy) using the method of Bradford (1976). The radioactively labelled proteins were measured by trichloroacetic acid precipitation and liquid scintillation counting (LKB Wallac 1217 Rackbeta) of an aliquot. Gels for autoradiography were loaded with equal counts of radioactivity (approximately 50,000 c.p.m. for each sample).

In the other three experiments, also described later, exposures to treatments ranged from 5 hours to 9 months. Tissue (from earthworms) or whole organisms (daphnids and medaka) were frozen in liquid nitrogen and stored at - 80°C. Protein extraction and concentration measurement was as described above. Gels in this case were loaded with equal amounts of protein.

Proteins were separated by size (one dimensional, 1D) on SDS-PAGE (sodium dodecyl sulfate-polyacrylamide gel electrophoresis) gels using a Biorad miniProtean II apparatus (BioRad Labs, Richmond, CA). Samples were heated 5 minutes in denaturing sample buffer [Tris (ICN Biomedicals Inc., Irvine, CA), β-mercaptoethanol (Sigma, St. Louis, MO), and SDS (Laemmli 1970)] before electrophoresis. Acrylamide and bis concentrations in the gels were 12% and 0.3%, respectively. A cocktail of molecular weight standards (BRL Life Technologies, Gaithersburg, MD) was run on each gel. At the end of electrophoresis, gels were silver stained for total protein by fixing in acidic ethanol, washing in ethanol and water and soaking in a silver nitrate solution (0.1%). Bands were visualized by oxidizing the silver bound to the proteins with formaldehyde. A typical silver stained gel is shown in Figure 1. Gels of proteins labelled with ^{35}S-methionine and visualized by autoradiography would appear similar.

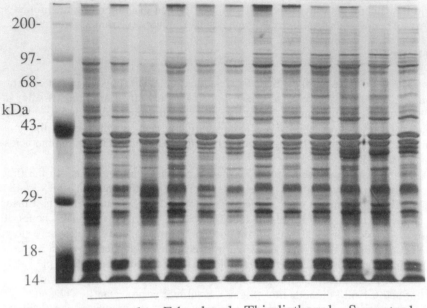

Std   Controls   Eth. glycol   Thiodiethanol   S-mustard

Figure 1   One dimensional SDS-PAGE gel of proteins extracted from earthworms
                exposed to ethylene glycol, thiodiethenol and sulfur mustard.

        To extend the separation in a second direction, 2D gels were run also using the
Biorad miniProtean II cell. The added dimension was achieved by first separating the
proteins based on isoelectric point (pI), according to O'Farrell (1975). The first
dimension gel solution (in tubes) contained 4% acrylamide and a 2% mixture of
ampholytes of 5-7 and 3-10 pI (BioRad). After separation in the O'Farrell tube gels,
the proteins were separated again by standard SDS-PAGE as described earlier. Other
important details are given in O'Farrell (1975). Our modifications are described in
Hakimzadeh and Bradley (1989). A typical 2D gel is shown in Figure 2.

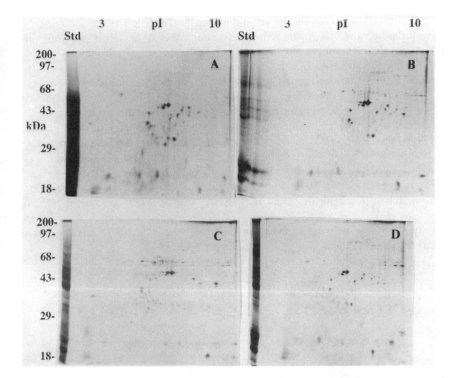

Figure 2   Two dimensional 5DS-PAGE gel using pooled extracts from control worms (A), exposed to ethylene glycol (B), to thiodiethenol (C) and to sulfur mustard (D). Data were from experiment III (see methods).

In the first two experiments (I and II), grids were superimposed on the gels and the data digitized visually based on the presence or absence of protein bands. The binary data were then presented to a neural network model.

In the latter three experiments (III, IV, V), gels were scanned with a Molecular Dynamics Personal Laser Densitometer®. With ImageQuant® (Molecular Dynamics, Sunnyvale, CA) software a grid was superimposed on the figure (# lanes X 50 channels), and a table of channel pixel volume-percents converted to binary scale was used in the neural net model.

An artificial neural network (A.N.N.) is a simulation of the type of parallel processing done in the animal brain. A major application of ANNs is in solving classification problems, where categories are recognized by the set of input data (cf. discriminant functions). The key step is training the neural network by presenting it with input samples and their expected output classification, in order to adjust the weights of connections between the inputs and outputs. The criterion for success is not how well the network learns the training data but rather how well it performs on new (test) data. If the training set is large enough and general enough then the designed network should be applicable to other data.

Neural networks are being used extensively in engineering and their use is beginning to be explored in medicine (Jorgensen *et al.* 1996). This reference contains an excellent general description of neural networks. The authors illustrate how multivariate statistics (principal components analysis) can be used to eliminate redundant variables and show how the performance of ANN in a medical diagnosis problem is superior to linear discriminant analysis and equal to that of quadratic discriminant analysis. The particular network used in this study was a back propagation network (Werbos 1974; Rumelhart and McClelland 1986). We used the version from Neural Works Professional II Software, (NeuralWare, Inc., Pittsburgh, PA).

A simple trained network is shown in Figure 3, where treatment 2 is defined (diagnosed) by inputs 2 and 4.

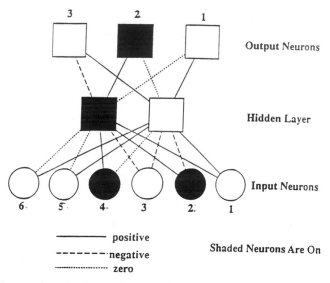

Figure 3   A trained neural network

Binary inputs, 0 or 1, enter the network at the input (buffer) layer. Each node in this layer has a weighted connection to each neuron in the hidden layer. The weights are initially random and are corrected by a gradient descent algorithm to reduce error. Each hidden layer neurons sums its weighted active (input value = 1) inputs; the neuron's output is determined by passing the sum through a sigmoidal transfer function with an output range of 0 to 1. Each output neuron has a weighted connection to each hidden neuron. Each output neuron sums and renormalizes the product of the weight and the output value of each hidden neuron to which it is connected in order to produce its output value.

In the present application, protein patterns on gels are digitized and converted to base 2 to become the binary **input** for the neural network. However any variables, even qualitative, may be used when converted to binary form. **Output** neurons may correspond to any classification. In these experiments the outputs represent chemical treatments or concentrations and physical stressors. One outcome of neural net analysis is the identification of chemicals and their concentrations. The diagnostic tool is the trained network.

A second outcome of neural net analysis is identification of the proteins (or other input variables) which are important, either by their presence or their absence, in differentiating among the stressors in the experiment. For this the weightings of the inputs associated with a particular treatment are used to identify these key inputs (proteins). This step makes feasible the development of multiple immunoassays to a set of proteins specific for a stressor of interest. Description of the methods and the preliminary results are beyond the scope of this paper but we wished to point out this added feature of neural networks.

The results of A.N.N. analyses of five experiments are summarized in this paper:

I. *Daphnia magna*: In this simple experiment, daphnids were exposed to no treatment at 20°C (controls), 34°C (heat), or 1.5% ethanol (EtOH) at 20°C for 5 hours and were labelled with ^{35}S-methionine (50μci) for the last 4 hours. Animals were frozen in sets of 5 to result in 6 replicates within each treatment. The 1 D autoradiographs were then visually digitized.

II. *Eurytemora affinis*: Estuarine copepods were exposed to 8 combinations of salinity and temperature stresses (2-20ppt and 15°C or 30°C). The newly proteins were labelled with ^{35}S-methionine (50μci) during 4 hours of the stress, and 1D autoradiographs were visually digitized.

III. *Lumbricus terrestris*: Earthworms were injected behind the clitellum with ethylene glycol (solvent control), thiodiethanol (Aldrich Chemical Co.) (a sulfur mustard breakdown product) at 2 mg/g in ethylene glycol (Sigma, St. Louis, MO), sulfur mustard also at 2 mg/g in ethylene glycol or not injected at all (control). There were 6 individuals in each of the 4 treatments; exposure was for 5 hours; tissue from the lining of the coelomic cavity was taken from each worm and soluble proteins were separated on one and two dimensional gels (see Figure 2). The silver stained 1D gels were digitized using Imagequant® as described earlier.

IV. *Daphnia magna*: In a second daphnid experiment, six replicate samples (3-5 animals per sample) were taken from populations exposed to 3.5 mg/L 2,4 dinitrophenol (Sigma, St. Louis, MO.), 0.5 mg/L pentachlorophenate (Sigma), and culture water (controls) at each of two exposure times, 8 and 48 hr. Earlier 4 hr. exposures showed no effects on protein patterns. Soluble proteins were separated on one and two dimensional gels, silver stained. The 1 D gels were digitized as described earlier.

V. *Oryzias latipes*: The Japanese medaka fish were exposed for 9 months to 4 concentrations of continuously flowing groundwater on site at a U.S. Army facility. The concentrations were 0, 1, 5 and 25%, diluted in reference creek water. 30 fish were exposed to each treatment. Proteins were separated in 1D gels, silver stained and digitized as described earlier.

The main question asked of all the data was whether assignment by A.N.N. to treatment group was significantly non-random, biased towards correct assignment. The test used was a dichotomous, directional chi-square goodness-of-fit test. All correctly assigned individuals were in one class, all incorrect in the other. No attempt was made to determine goodness-of-fit treatment by treatment.

RESULTS

One dimensional gels (Fig. 1) were run in all experiments and were the main source of data. 2D gels (Fig. 2) were run to display differences among treatments in experiments III and IV.

Table 1 shows output from the A.N.N. analysis of the first daphnid experiment, based on digitized data from 1D gels.

TABLE 1 -- <u>Analysis of heat and ethanol effect on Daphnia magna;</u>
<u>sample output of learning and test sets</u>

Learning Set			
Output Classes →	3	2.	1
Input Classes 1	0.0353	0.0376	0.9462
	0.0353	0.0376	0.9462
2.	0.0458	0.9364	0.0472
	0.0458	0.9364	0.0472
3	0.9299	0.0640	0.0432
	0.9299	0.0640	0.0432

Test Set			
Classes			
Found Actual			
1 1	0.0353	0.0376	0.9462
1 1	0.0353	0.0376	0.9462
1 1	0.0353	0.0376	0.9462
1 1	0.0672	0.0197	0.9450
2. 2	0.0458	0.9364	0.0472
2. 2.	0.0491	0.9317	0.0475
2 2	0.0458	0.9364	0.0472
2 2	0.0499	0.9255	0.0509
3 3	0.9299	0.0640	0.0432
3 3ˉ	0.9299	0.0640	0.0432
3 3ˉ	0.9299	0.0650	0.0432
3 3ˉ	0.9299	0.0640	0.0426

Key to Classes

1   Control
2. Heat (34°C)
3   Ethanol (1.5%)

The numbers shown are the output values, based on connection weights from the second layer summed and transformed, for each output neuron. Because there are 3 treatments, there are 3 classes. Samples from class 1 have a high output value for class 1, and so on. Because some patterns (input vectors) were identical after digitizing the data by hand, the output values are identical also. According to these data, the neural net program learned the patterns (high output values for each class of input vectors) and the trained network successfully assigned all the test samples to the correct class.

Similar analyses were run in the other four experiments. The success rates of the neural net analyses all summarized in Table 2. For comparison the expected numbers of correct assignment, if assignment is random, are shown in the right-most column. For example, in the earthworm experiment a completely random assignment would be a 4 x 4 table with one individual in each cell, resulting in 4 of 16 "correct" assignments.

TABLE 2 --Summary of neural network analyses

Species	Treatments (no. including control)	Correct recognition of treatment	Random expectation
Daphnid	Heat, ethanol (3)	24/24	8/24
Copepods	Heat, salinity (8)	12/14	2/14
Earthworms	Ethylene glycol, TDE, S-mustard (4)	10/16	4/16
Daphnids	PCP; 2,4D; Control (3)	26/36	12/36
Medaka	4 levels groundwater (4)	63/118	30/118

Note: The numbers in the table do not always reflect the size of the experiment. In the last two cases two different nets were run and the results were pooled. In no case did test sets overlap with training sets.

The diagnosis of treatment was significantly (P<.01) biased away from random towards correct, in every experiment.

Patterns in the copepod data from Gonzalez and Bradley (1995), with 8 salinity-temperature classes, were correctly classified in 12 of 14 cases, based on the classes with the highest output values (as reported for daphnids in Table 1). The earthworm experiments (III) resulted in 10 of 16 correct diagnoses. When the controls were combined vs the toxics combined, the assignment was correct in all 16 test animals. This result is corroborated by the set of 2D gels shown earlier in Figure 2.

A second experiment with daphnids was run using two chemicals which had no observable effects at 4hr, whether using neural nets or 2D gels. The results from 8 and 48 hr. exposures showed 26 of 36 test samples properly assigned to classes. The assignment by chemical, but not by exposure time, was correct in 3 cases and in 5 cases an 8 hr. chemical exposure was diagnosed as a control. Only two of 36 results were false positives.

al. 1993; Grover and Resnick 1993). Two dimensional gels provide useful visual displays and sophisticated image analyses are available (Giometti *et al.* 1992; Myrick *et al.* 1993a, 1993b) with over 3000 proteins documented in human keratinocytes alone (Celis *et al.* 1993). We have used 2D gels to demonstrate some interactions in the complex effluent from a paper mill (Bradley *et al.* 1994). A second promising technique for data transfer allowing automated separation of proteins in a large number of samples, is one form or another of capillary electrophoresis (CE). The resolution of CE compares favorably with high resolution agarose gel electrophoresis and the need for a densitometer is eliminated (Jenkins and Guerin 1995).

The second reason is that there is abundant evidence for specific protein differences from bacteria (Adamowicz *et al.* 1991; Blom *et al.* 1992), from urine (Barregard 1993), from human leucocytes (Jellum *et al.* 1983) from fibroblasts (He *et al.* 1994) and from cerebrospinal fluid (Johnson *et al.* 1992). Even exhaled air contains protein information (Sheideler *et al.* 1993).

The third reason is that neural networks are well established in other fields and are being continuously studied. Among the questions under review are the size of the training set required to construct a generally useful model, the structure of the model itself (number of hidden neurons), the approach to local rather than global optima and the rationale for particular cutoff choices of output values (Table 1). Although there is no algorithm for constructing the perfect model, we do have a clear criterion for success, namely whether the trained network works under the conditions for which it is intended.

Conservation of protein signal, and therefore the generalization of the learning by the neural network, is a concern. It is possible that the critical proteins in the signal are not present in all environments. If however, there is a definitive signal, we believe the neural network can be trained to detect it. We need to provide very general learning sets so that all irrelevant inputs can be discarded. For broad applications, the total protein profile may be reduced to a few key proteins, so the method becomes similar to the widespread biomarker approach.

Another concern is the functional relevance of the protein profiles. The range of applications of this and other biomarkers will be wider when they have been validated against better accepted endpoints. To be of practical use some linkages must be made to ecologically relevant responses (Lagadic *et al.* 1994) and to conventional endpoints of bioassays (Hulka *et al.* 1994; Shore and Douben 1994; Taioli *et al.* 1994). Even without such validation, biological indicators, including protein profiles, may have value in providing data on bioavailability of, and on exposure to, toxins.

Assuming the response is robust and relevant, additional applications of the protein profile analyses are possible. These include health and environmental monitoring, specific toxicity identification (Webster *et al.* 1994; Ernst and Peterson 1994), early warning of contaminant or disease impacts (Austoker 1994; Kimbrough 1994; Miller *et al.* 1994) and development of *in situ* diagnostic kits based on immunoassays of key proteins identified by the neural networks.. The latter proteins may well include some well established biomarkers such as the cytochromes P 450, metallothioneins or even some stress proteins.

It should be pointed out in conclusion that the analytical methods suggested here must be developed for each application. A library of protein profiles would not

The results from the Medaka experiment (V) are shown in detail in Table 3. This experiment was useful as a demonstration of the ability of the protein signal to differentiate, at least partially, among concentrations of chemicals in groundwater. The major contaminant was assumed to be zinc. The table shows the results of assigning fish to treatment classes according to their protein profiles.

TABLE 3 -- Assignments of test fish (Medaka) to treatments using a neural network, trained on the protein profiles of the learning set of fish

Actual Treatments	Assigned Treatments			
	Control	1%	5%	25%
Control	12	6	2	9
1% Groundwater	10	12	2	2
5%	4	3	21	4
25%	3	2	8	18

Assignment to classes is significantly ($P<.01$) non-random, as reported earlier, especially at higher groundwater concentrations. The fit improves when the two low and the two high concentrations are combined, forming two classes. The control (creek) water itself contained a low (unmeasured) level of zinc. (Tom Shedd, pers. comm.)

DISCUSSION

The results of the neural net analyses indicate a significant bias towards correct assignment to treatment. Treatments could be identified by modal frequencies so the neural networks seemed to be learning something useful. The results may have been better in the first two experiments because digitizing was subjective (although done without regard to class) but even here there must have been useful specific information. When digitizing was automated, in the latter experiments, the results, while promising, were hardly definitive. Nevertheless we believe the method described here should be further investigated, for several reasons.

The first reason is that we may expect greater precision with greater numbers of test organisms in the training sets (more generalized learning) and, more importantly, with better transfer of data from the proteins to the neural nets. One technique to vastly increase the number of proteins visualized is two-dimensional electrophoresis (Giometti et al. 1992; Tracy et al. 1992; Caudill et al. 1993; Celis et

be available, at least not immediately. For each application, the feasibility of the assays must be established, perhaps by 2D gels displaying protein variation among treatments of interest. Next, if large scale automated analyses were needed, artificial neural networks would be trained with the appropriate background conditions present. Finally, if field assays were desired, key proteins would be identified, using the network decompiling methods alluded to, and multiple immunoassays prepared. This third step has yet to be demonstrated.

References

Adamowicz, M., P.M. Kelley and W. Nickerson. 1991. Detergent (sodium dodecyl sulfate) shock proteins in *Escherichia coli.*, *Journal of Bacteriology*, **173**:229-0233.

Austoker, J. 1994. Current trends and some prospects for the future - 1. *British Medical Journal*, **309(6952)**: 449-452.

Barregard, L. 1993. Biological monitoring of exposure to mercury vapor. *Scandinavian Journal of Work Environment & Health*, **19 (SUPPL. 1)**: 45-49.

Blom, A., W. Harder and A. Matin. 1992. Unique and overlapping stress proteins of *E. coli. Applied Environmental Microbiology*, **58**:331-334.

Bradford, M. 1976. A quantitative method for measuring soluble protein levels. *Analytical Biochemistry*, **72**:248-254.

Bradley, B.P. 1990. Stress Proteins: Their detection and uses in biomonitoring ASTM 13th *Symposium on Aquatic Toxicology*. ASTM STP 1096 (W.G. Landis and W.H. van der Schalie, Eds.) American Society for Testing and Materials, Philadelphia.

Bradley, B.P. 1992. Are the stress proteins specific indicators of exposure or effect? *Marine Environmental Research*, **35**:85-88.

Bradley, B.P., J.-A. Bond, C.M. Gonzalez and B.E. Tepper. 1994. Complex mixture analysis using protein expression as a qualitative and quantitative tool. *Environmental Toxicology and Chemistry*, **13**:1043-1050.

Bradley, B.P., C.M. Gonzalez, and M.A. Lane. 1992. A molecular mechanism of adaptation in an estuarine copepod. *Netherlands Journal of Sea Research*, **30**:1-6.

Bradley, B.P. and J.B. Ward. 1989. Detection of a major stress protein using a peptide antibody. *Marine Environmental Research*, **28**:471-475.

Brown, D.C., B.P. Bradley and M. Tedengren. 1995. Genetic and environmental regulation of HSP₇₆ expression. *Marine Environmental Research*, **39**:181-184.

Cai, J.W., B.W. Henderson, J. W. Shen and J.R.Subjeck. 1993. Induction of glucose regulated proteins during growth of a murine (tumor). *Journal of Cell Physiology*, **154**: 229-237.

Carsberg, C.J., K A. Myers, G. S. Evans, T. D. Allen and P.L. Stern. 1995. Metastasis-associated 5T4 oncofetal antigen is concentrated at microvillus projections of the plasma-membrane. *Journal of Cell Science*, **108**: 2905-2916.

Caudill, S. P., J. E. Myrick and M. K. Robinson. 1993. Exploratory data analysis in two-dimensional electrophoresis. *Applied and Theoretical Electrophoresis*, **3(3-4)**: 133-136.

Celis, J. E., H. W. Rasmussen, E. Olsen, P. Madsen, H. Leffers, B. Honore, K. Dejgaard, P. Gromov, H. J. Hoffmann, and M. Nielsen. 1993. The human keratinocyte two-dimensional gel protein database: update. *Electrophoresis*, **14(11)**: 1091-198.

Dhingra, K., V. Vogel, N. Sneige, A. Sahin, M. Aldaz, G. N. Hortobagyi and W. Hittelman. 1993. Strategies for the application of biomarkers for risk assessment and efficacy in breast cancer chemoprevention trials. *Journal of Cellular Biochemistry Supplement*, **17G**: 37-43.

Ernst, W. H. D. and P. J. Peterson. 1994. The role of biomarkers in environmental assessment: 4. Terrestrial plants. *Ecotoxicology*, **3(3)**: 180-192.

Giometti, C.S., J. Taylor and S.L. Tollaksen. 1992. Mouse liver protein database: A catalog of proteins detected by two-dimensional gel electrophoresis. *Electrophoresis,* **13**:970-991.

Gonzalez, C.R.M. and B.P. Bradley. 1995. Are there salinity stress proteins? *Marine Environmental Research*, **39**:205-208.

Grandjean, P., P. Weihe and J. B. Nielsen. 1994. Methylmercury: Significance of intrauterine and postnatal exposures. *Clinical Chemistry*, **40(7 PART 2)**: 1395-1400.

Grover, P. K. and M. I. Resnick. 1993. Two-dimensional analysis of proteins in unprocessed human urine using double stain. *Journal of Urology*, **150(3)**: 1069-1072.

Hakimzadeh, R. & B.P. Bradley. 1989. The heat shock response in the copepod *Eurytemora affinis* (Poppe). *Journal of Thermal Biology* , **15**:67-77.

He, C., B. A. Merrick, L. L. Witcher, R. M. Patterson, D. R. Daluge and J. K.

Selkirk. 1994. Phenotypic change and altered protein expression in x-ray and thylcholanthrens-transformed C3H10T1 2 fibroblasts. *Electrophoresis*, **15**: 726-34.

Hulka, B. S., E. T. Liu and R. A. Lininger. 1994. Steroid hormones and risk of breast cancer. *Cancer* (Philadelphia), **74(3 SUPPL.):** 1111-1124.

Jellum, E., A.K. Thorsrud and F.W. Karasek. 1983. Two-dimensional electophoresis for determining toxicity of environmental substances. *Analytical Chemistry*, **55**:2340-2344.

Jenkins, M.A. and M.D. Guerin. 1995. Quantification of serum proteins using capillary electrophoresis. *Annals of Clinical Biochemistry*, **32**: 493-497.

Johnson, G., D. Brane, W. Block, D. P. Van Kammen, J. Gurklis, J. L. Peters, R. J. Wyatt, D. G. Kirch, H. A. Ghanbari and C. R. Merril. 1992. Cerebrospinal fluid progtein variations in common to Alzheimer's disease schizophrenia. *Applied and Theoretical Electrophoresis*, **3(2)**: 47-53.

Jorgensen, J.S., J.B. Pedersen and S. M. Pedersen. 1996. Use of neural networks to diagnose acute myocardial infarction. 1. Methodology. *Clinical Chemistry*, **42**: 604-612.

Kimbrough, R. D. 1994. Determining acceptable risks: Experimental and epidemiological issues. *Clinical Chemistry*, **40 (7 PART 2)**: 1448-1453.

Laemmli, U. K. 1970. Cleavage of structural proteins during the assembly of the head of Bacteriophage T. *Nature*, **227**:680-685.

Lagadic, L., T. Caquet and F. Ramade. 1994. The role of biomarkers in environmental assessment. 5. Invertebrate populations and communities. *Ecotoxicology*, **3(3)**: 193-208.

Lindquist, S. and Craig, E.A. 1988. The Heat-shock proteins. *Annual Reviews of Genetics* **22**:631-77.

Lockwood, J. F., M. S. Rutherford, M. J. Myers and L. B. Schook. 1994. Induction of hepatic acute-phase protein transcripts: differential effects of acute and subchronic dimethylnitrosamine exposure in vivo. *Toxicology and Applied Pharmacology* , **125**: 288-95.

Miller, M. J., D. C. Parmelee, T. Benjamin, S. Sechi, K. L. Dooley and F. F. Kadlubar. 1994. Plasma proteins as early biomarkers of exposure to carcinogenic aromatic amines. *Chemical and Biological Interactions*, **93(3)**: 221-34.

Myrick, J. E., S. P. Caudill, M. K. Robinson and I. L. Hubert. 1993. Quantitative two-dimensional electrophoretic detection of possible protein biomarkers of occupational exposure to cadmium. *Applied and Theoretical Electrophoresis*, 3(3-4): 137-146.

Myrick, J. E., P. F. Lemkin, M.K. Robinson and K. M. Upton. 1993. Comparison of the Bio Image Visage 2000 and the GELLAB II two-dimensional electrophoresis image analysis systems. *Applied and Theoretical Electrophoresis*, 3(6): 335-46.

Nover, L. 1991. Heat shock response. CRC Press, Boca Raton, Florida.

O'Farrell, P. 1975. High resolution two-dimensional electrophoresis of proteins. *Journal of Biological Chemistry*, 250: 4007-4021.

Omland, O., D. Sherson, A. M. Hansen, T. Sigsgaard, H. Autrup, E. Overgaard. 1994. Exposure of iron foundry workers to polycyclic aromatic hydrocarbons: Benzo(a)pyrene-albumin adducts and 1-hydroxypyrene as biomarkers for exposure. *Occupational and Environmental Medicine*, 51: 513-518.

Oppen-Berntsen, D. O., S. O. Olsen, C. J. Rong, G. L. Taranger, P. Swanson and B. T. Walter. 1994. Plasma levels of eggshell Zr-proteins, estradiol-17-beta, and gonadotropins during an annual reproductive cycle of Atlantic salmon (*Salmo salar*). *Journal of Experimental Zoology*, 268: 59-70.

Peakall, D. B. and C. H. Walker. 1994. The role of biomarkers in environmental assessment: 3. Vertebrates. *Ecotoxicology*, 3: 173-179.

Rumelhart, D.E. and J.L. McClelland. 1986. Parallel distributed processing. Vol. 1, Foundations. MIT Press, Cambridge, MA.

Ryan, J. A. and L. E. Hightower. 1994. Evaluation of heavy-metal ion toxicity in fish cells using a combined stress protein and cytotoxicity assay. *Environmental Toxicology and Chemistry*, 13(8): 1231-1240.

Sanders, B.M. 1993. Stress proteins in aquatic organisms: An environmental perspective. *Critical Reviews in Toxicology*, 23:49-75.

Schlesinger, M.J. 1990. Heat-Shock Proteins: A Mini review. *Journal of Biological Chemistry*, 265 (21):12111-12114.

Sheideler, L., H.G. Manke, U. Schwulera, O. Inacker, and H. Hammule. 1993. Detection of nonvolatile macromoleules in breath: a possible diagnostic tool? *American Review of Respiratory Disease*, 148:778-784.

Shore, R. F. and P. E. Douben. 1994. Predicting ecotoxicological impacts of environmental contaminants on terrestrial small mammals. *Reviews in Environmental Contamination and Toxicology*, **134**: 49-89.

Smith, M. T. and W. A. Suk. 1994. Application of molecular biomarkers in epidemiology. *Environmental Health Perspectives*, **102 Suppl 1**: 229-35.

Stegmann, J.J., M. Brouwer, R.T. DiGuilio, L. Forlin, B.A. Fowler, B.M. Sanders and P.A. Van Veld. 1992. Molecular responses to environmental contamination: enzyme and protein systems as indicators of chemical exposures and effects. In R.J. Huggett, R.A. Kimerle, P.H. Merle, Jr. and H.L. Bergman, eds., *Biomarkers: Biochemical, Physiological and Histological Markers of Anthropogenic Stress*, Lewis, Boca Raton, FL, pp. 235-310.

Taioli, E., P. Kinney, A. Zhitkovich, H. Fulton, V. Voitkun, G. Cosma, K. Frenkel, P. Toniolo, S. Garte and M. Costa. 1994. Application of reliability models to studies of biomarker validation. *Environmental Health Perspectives*, **102(3)**: 306-9.

Tracy, R. P., D. S. Young, H. D. Hill, G. W. Cutsforth and D. M. Wilson. 1992. Two-dimensional electrophoresis of urine specimens from patients with disease. *Applied and Theoretical Electrophoresis*, **3(2)**: 55-65.

Van Bogelen, R.A., P.M. Kelley and F.C. Neidhardt. 1987. Differential induction of heat shock, SOS and oxidation stress regulons and accumulation of nucleotides in *E. Coli. Journal of Bacteriology.* **169**:26-32.

Webster, P. W., A. D. Vethaak and W. B. van Muiswinkel. 1994. Fish as biomarkers in immunotoxicology. *Toxicology*, **86(3)**: 213-32.

Welch, W.J. 1993. How cells respond to stress. *Scientific American*, **268(5)**:56-64.

Werbos, P.J. 1974. Beyond regression: New tools for prediction and analysis in the behavior science. Ph.D Thesis, Harvard University, Cambridge, MA.

Mark J. Melancon,[1]

DEVELOPMENT OF CYTOCHROMES P450 IN AVIAN SPECIES AS A BIOMARKER FOR
ENVIRONMENTAL CONTAMINANT EXPOSURE AND EFFECT: PROCEDURES AND BASELINE
VALUES

REFERENCE: Melancon, M. J., **"Development of Cytochromes P450 in Avian Species
as a Biomarker for Environmental Contaminant Exposure and Effect: Procedures and
Baseline Values,"** *Environmental Toxicology and Risk Assessment: Biomarkers and Risk
Assessment—Fifth Volume, ASTM STP 1306,* David A. Bengtson and Diane S. Henshel, Eds.,
American Society for Testing and Materials, 1996.

ABSTRACT: As in mammals and fish, birds respond to many environmental
contaminants with induction of hepatic cytochromes P450. In order to
monitor cytchromes P450 in specific avian species, for assessing the
status of that species or the habitat it utilizes, it is necessary to
have background information on the appropriate assay conditions and the
responsiveness of cytochrome P450 induction in that species. Assay of
four monooxygenases which give resorufin as product, using a
fluorescence microwell plate scanner, has proven to be an effective
approach. Information is provided on the incubation conditions and
baseline activity for twenty avian species at ages ranging from pipping
embryo to adult. Induction responsiveness is presented for sixteen of
them. This information can serve as a guide for those who wish to
utilize cytochrome P450 as a biomarker for contaminant exposure and
effect to aid in selection of appropriate species, age, and
monooxygenase assay(s).

KEYWORDS: cytochrome P450, birds, monooxygenase, liver, biomarker

Cytochromes P450 (P450s) are a class of hemoproteins that were
found in the 1960s to be induced in mammalian species by a number of
pharmacologic agents and environmental contaminants (Conney 1971). Soon
afterward it was demonstrated that hepatic P450s were induced in fish by
widespread contaminants such as PCBs and polycyclic aromatic
hydrocarbons (Kleinow et al 1987, Melancon et al 1988). Because
persistent lipophilic chemicals such as PCBs reached the aquatic
environment and bioaccumulated in fish, there has been widespread
application of using P450 induction measurements in fish as a biomarker
for exposure to certain contaminants(Payne et al. 1987, Stegeman et al.
1992). Use of P450 induction as a biomarker for contaminant exposure in
wildlife, including birds, has developed more recently (Rattner et al.
1989, Ronis and Walker 1989). The early biomonitoring related studies
of cytochrome P450 in avian species generally dealt with piscivorous
species that were known to be exposed to high levels of contaminants
from consuming contaminated fish.

[1]Research Chemist and Group Leader, Environmental Contaminants
Research Branch, Patuxent Environmental Science Center, National
Biological Service, U.S. Department of the Interior, 12011 Beech Forest
Road, Laurel, MD 20708.

MONITORING GOALS AND SAMPLING STRATEGY

Because the Department of the Interior has management responsibilities for both extensive land holdings and trust species such as migratory birds and anadramous fish, monitoring protocols are required not just for the species of interest but for additional species to cover a variety of habitats. Studies with birds therefore may be designed to provide information about a location, or about a species, or about both.

The time of year at which sampling is done and the life stage(s) sampled are both very important regardless of the goal (evaluating habitat or species or both) of the sampling. Because the baseline P450s and the response to inducers of P450 can vary with age and life stage of the birds, it is necessary to characterize P450 and responsiveness of birds comparable to the ages to be utilized in field biomonitoring applications. The life stages usually examined are pipping embryo, 10-30 day old young, subadult and nonbreeding adult. The time of year of sampling is determined by the species, the life stage and the location to be evaluated. These choices reflect attempts to maximize collection of comparable samples with interpretable P450 differences. Sampling pipping embryos provides greater age uniformity to sampling because the evidence of pipping is more accurate than trying to time incubation of multiple nests in the field, and avoids repeated nest disturbance. Collection of an egg also has a smaller negative impact on the population of birds under study than collecting an adult bird. The egg burden of contaminants is known to have come from the hen, but the source of these contaminants for the hen must be determined. The use of young birds requires accurate information of the hatching date so that they can be collected before fledging and at the same age. Young birds grow very rapidly and a two-week-old bird may weigh ten times as much as the pipping embryo. Because of this, the contaminant burden from the embryo stage has, at the very least, been significantly diluted by growth of the bird, and may also have been decreased by metabolism and excretion. Unless the original body burden of contaminants was high, P450 induction observed in the nestling is probably due to its diet. Here again, the effect of collecting a prefledging bird should have a smaller negative impact on the population of birds under study than collecting an adult bird. The diet of the subadult may well differ from that of the nestling and would therefore evaluate different aspects of the habitat without concerns about the hormonal complications in breeding adults. Sampling of adults must take into account major hormonal changes such as breeding.

The life stage utilized also affects the sample size of liver available and the size of carcass available for contaminant analysis. Because many of the contaminants that induce P450 may impact reproduction, sampling that can be related to reproductive success is an important consideration.

To monitor habitat, one can use resident wild birds or release birds for recapture. In order to effectively utilize a species for monitoring, information must be available about the P450 response in that species and how best to measure it. In cases where the species itself is the target of the monitoring, it is important to know how responsive different life stages of the species are to the contaminants of concern and select samples that will maximize one's ability to assess exposure and effects. When the habitat is the target of the monitoring there is more flexibility and it is possible to select a species that is responsive to the impacts of concern and the life stage that is most effective.

EXPERIMENTAL INDUCTION OF CYTOCHROMES P450

Regardless of the species to be studied it is desirable to obtain uncontaminated organisms for the purpose of studying responsiveness of P450 to prototype inducing agents and the appropriate assay conditions. The difficulty of obtaining uncontaminated individuals differs from species to species, and for different life stages. Collecting eggs from areas known to be low in contaminants with subsequent mechanical incubation and dosing at appropriate times before pipping is a convenient way to approach the study of pipping embryos. The complicating factors are the location of the uncontaminated eggs, timing of the egg collection and transportation, and successful mechanical incubation. The availablility of captive populations of the subject species are a convenience but not a necessity for embryo studies.

Nestlings can be studied by injecting inducing agents into individual birds in the nest in the field in uncontaminated locations. In this case the availablility of captive populations of the subject species are a convenience but not a necessity for such studies. The raising of mechanically incubated individuals to eventually provide uncontaminated subadults or adults is a reasonable approach for precocial hatchlings, but not for altricial hatchlings which require parental feeding. Thus far responses to inducing agents have been examined in subadults and adults of precoccial species mainly in birds raised from mechanically incubated eggs and from captive flocks. The common and scientific names of the twenty species reported on here are presented in Table 1, along with the life stages utilized and their sources. In addition to expanding the types of waterfowl and waterbirds, other types of birds such as passerines and raptors were studied. Florida sandhill cranes were studied as surrogates for the endangered Mississippi sandhill cranes (*Grus canadensis pulla*).

The representative P450 inducers utilized are phenobarbital (PB), 3,4,5,3',4'-pentachlorobiphenyl (PCB 126) (as classified by Balschmiter and Zell 1980), and 3-methylcholanthrene (MC) in eggs and PB, β-naphthoflavone (BNF), MC, and PCB 126 in young birds, subadults and adults. The doses of inducers used were high enough to increase the likelihood that a response would be observed. This is typical for studies in new species and the doses are similar to those used for early studies in mammals and fish (in most cases dose responses would be worked out in field validation studies). PB was generally administered at 20-100 mg/kg body weight on days 3, 2 and 1 before sacrifice of young birds, subadults and adults and at 0.2 to 5 mg/egg on days 3, 2 and 1 before the estimated time of pipping. BNF was generally administered at 20-100 mg/kg body weight on days 4 or 3 before sacrifice of nestlings, subadults and adults. MC was administered to eggs at 20 to 500 µg/egg 2-3 days before estimated time of pipping and at 20 mg/kg to adults on day 3 before sacrifice. The wider range of values for eggs represents dose-response studies which were not done in the older individuals. Exact amounts of these materials administered are presented with the response data.

SAMPLE COLLECTION AND STORAGE

When developing methods for field application, most samples are handled in the same manner that field samples will be handled. Livers are removed as quickly as possible after sacrifice, the whole liver if 0.25g or less or a 0.25-0.5g sample if larger is placed in a tube with a few drops of glycerol and snap frozen in liquid nitrogen. Whenever possible two or three liver samples from each bird are frozen spearately. For large birds, such as adult ducks, multiple liver samples are taken. When only a small portion of the liver is utilized it is best to sample the same part of the liver from each bird (i.e. tip of left lobe). The samples are then stored in liquid nitrogen until

TABLE 1--Avian species and ages studied and their sources

Species	Scientific name	Age	Source
Mallard	*Anas platyrhynchos*	adult	commercial breeder
Black duck	*Anas rubripes*	adult	PESC[1]
Wood duck	*Aix sponsa*	pipping embryo	field-North Carolina
Lesser scaup	*Aythya affinis*	6 month	commercial-from field eggs
Double-crested cormorant	*Phalacrocorax auritis*	14 day, pipping embryo	field-Minnesota
Black-crowned night heron	*Nycticorax nycticorax*	13 day, pipping embryo	field-Virginia
Great blue heron	*Ardea herodias*	pipping embryo	field-Wisconsin
Florida sandhill crane	*Grus canadensis*	30 day	PESC
Black necked stilt	*Himantopus mexicanus*	30 day	field-California
American avocet	*Recurvirostra americana*	30 day	field-California
Red-winged blackbird	*Agelaius phoenicius*	adult	field-PESC
European starling	*Sturnus vulgaris*	12 day	field-Ilinois
Tree swallow	*Tachycineta bicolor*	pipping embryo	field-midwest
Barn swallow	*Hirundo rustica*	12 day, pipping embryo	field-midwest
Bobwhite quail	*Colinus virginianus*	adult,1 day	PESC
American kestrel	*Falco sparverius*	adult, 10 day, pipping embryo	PESC
Screech owl	*Otus asio*	adult	PESC
Forster's tern	*Sterna forsteri*	adult	field-California
Caspian tern	*Sterna caspia*	adult	field-California
Western sandpiper	*Calidris mauri*	adult	field-Texas

[1]From captive flock or captured at the Patuxent Environmental Science Center

~~Microsome preparation and assay.~~ After samples in the field are snap frozen in liquid nitrogen they are transported or shipped to Patuxent Environmental Science Center (PESC) in liquid nitrogen or on dry ice where they are then stored in liquid nitrogen. Previous to the summer of 1994 samples were stored at PESC in an ultracold mechanical freezer at -80°C.

APPROACHES FOR CYTOCHROME P450 ASSESSMENT

There are a variety of ways to assess the P450 status of organisms including birds. In vitro methods generally utilize subcellular liver fractions such as microsomes or 9,000 to 11,000 g supernatants. Monooxygenase activities may be assayed in either the supernatant or microsomes whereas determination of total cytochromes P450, gel electrophoresis and western blot utilize microsomes. Messenger RNA for cytochromes P450 is determined in liver homogenates. Although animals are generally sacrificed to obtain the liver samples, it is possible to obtain adequate liver samples by biopsy (Melancon et al. 1994). In vivo assessment of cytochrome P450 status by phenobarbital (PB) sleep time (Halbrook and Kirkpatrick 1990) or by metabolism of an administered chemical such as caffeine is also possible, but have been little used, and the latter would require considerable development in each species. The latter three methods are much more time consuming and expensive, but in the case of endangered birds may be necessary.

Many assays for P450-associated monooxygenase activities with different specificities for various inducers are available. Arylhydrocarbon hydroxylase activity is an effective indicator of P450 induction, but it requires the routine use of benzo(a)pyrene, and in its most sensitive form, the use of radioactive benzo(a)pyrene (Van Cantfort et al. 1977). Although an effective method, its usefulness is reduced by the expense of disposing of radioactive waste and the health hazard associated with routine use of benzo(a)pyrene. Benzphetamine-N-demethylase is a specific assay for PB-type induction (Anders and Mannering 1966), but it is relatively insensitive, inconvenient, and time-consuming, and because of the requirement for large quantities of microsomes, is not readily applicable to small samples. There are a number of assays that generate fluorescent products such as resorufin or umbelliferone by dealkylase reactions. These have varying specificities for the different cytochromes P450 and have typically been performed on spectrofluorometers in 1 cm² cuvettes at appropriate temperatures. Generally these instruments hold a small number of cuvettes and the assays cannot readily be automated. Ethoxyresorufin-O-dealkylase (EROD), pentoxyresorufin-O-dealkylase (PROD) and benzyloxyresorufin-O-dealklyase (BROD) assays were performed with slight variations from the original published methods (Burke and Mayer 1974, 1983, Burke et al. 1977, 1985). The recent availability of fluorescence microwell plate scanners has provided the opportunity to automate monooxygenase assays that generate a fluorescent product.

MICROSOME PREPARATION

Liver samples are defrosted on crushed ice and homogenized in four mls ice-cold buffer (1.15% potassium chloride in 0.01 M sodium/potassium phosphate, pH 7.4) per g of tissue using a Polytron (at setting 5 for 20 sec) while maintaining the tube in a beaker of crushed ice. In order to maintain an adequate volume for the Polytron to function effectively and without excessive frothing, the minimum volume of buffer used is 1.0 ml even when the sample is less than 0.25 g. The supernatant from a 20 min, 11,000g centrifugation of the homogenate is centrifuged at 100,000g for 60 min to obtain the microsomal pellet. Because the field samples processed are generally 0.5 g or less they are generally resuspended in 2.0 ml per g of tissue weight of ice-cold buffer (0.05 M sodium/

potassium phosphate, 0.001 M disodium ethylenediamine tetraacetate, pH
7.6) using a motor-driven stainless steel and teflon pestle in a glass
homogenizing vessel. Smaller samples are resuspended in 4.0 ml or 10.0
ml buffer per g of tissue to ensure that there is adequate volume for
effective resuspension and to reduce loss to vessel walls, etc.

MONOOXYGENASE ASSAY PROCEDURES

Because of the small volume (an effective working volume of
approximately 0.26 ml) of the wells in a 96 microwell plate, the amount
of microsomes needed for assay is also small. Use of such a
fluorescence microwell plate scanner began at PESC in 1990 and became
the only approach used for the resorufin-based monooxygenase assays in
1991. Other laboratories are also using this type of instrument for
environmental studies (Eggens and Galgani 1992, Kennedy et al. 1992).
Currently, four resorufin generating dealkylases are assayed on this
instrument. They are benzyloxyresorufin-O-dealkylase (BROD),
ethoxyresorufin-O-dealkylase (EROD), methoxyresorufin-O-dealkylase
(MROD), and pentoxyresorufin-O-dealkylase (PROD). Data are
automatically placed into computer files which are transferred to a
spreadsheet for necessary calculations.
    Because the microsomes are assayed on the same day they are
prepared, the assays are run before protein concentrations are
determined. The quantity of microsomes assayed is therefore based on
the amount of liver used in their preparation and varies by assay,
species and life stage. The quantity of microsomes selected for each
assay is that which gives a linear response over the time of the assay,
that is proportional to the amount of microsomes added and that falls
within the range of the standard curve. Exact values are given later
with the incubation conditions. In the case of highly induced samples
it may be necessary to repeat the assay with fewer microsomes to have
fluoresecence readings that are linear for enzyme activity and fall
within the standard curve. Substrate concentrations were selected that
gave maximum velocity and were constant over the duration of the assay.
Because of the high cost of NADPH, the concentration of NADPH selected
was that which gave a reading of at least 10 fluorescence units for
uninduced samples or that for which doubling the NADPH concentration
gave less than a 20% increase in monooxygenase activity.
    As the assays are currently performed, the 96 microwell plate
contains 24 samples in triplicate, a duplicate resorufin standard curve
with 0 to 0.2 nmol per well and four wells with noninduced mallard
reference microsomes. Each well receives 200 ul of pH 7.4, 0.066M Tris
buffer (TB) containing substrate and 50 ul of TB containing microsomes.
This is preincubated in the dark at assay temperature (37°C) for 10
minutes followed by addition of NADPH in 10 µl of TB and the plate is
placed in the fluorescence microwell plate scanner. An initial reading
is taken followed by seven additional readings at 90 sec intervals
(Approximately 75 sec are required to read the plate.) After checking
fluorescence readings for proper instrument functioning and linearity
with time, the fluorescence units are translated to nmoles of product by
utilizing the resorufin standard curve. Protein concentrations are
determined by a reduced volume (by 50%) Lowry assay (Lowry et al. 1951)
and monooxygenase activity calculated as nmol or pmol product per min
per mg microsomal protein. (Because of the presence of Tris buffer in
the monooxygenase assays, it is not possible to use fluorescamine to
assay protein in the assay well.)
    The incubation conditions for these species and life stages are
given in Table 2. Most assays utilized the amount of microsomes derived
from 0.65 to 5.2 mg of liver per well, with 1.25 to 5.0 µM substrate and
0.125 or 0.25 mM NADPH.

TABLE 2--Incubation conditions for O-dealkylase assays of avian hepatic microsomes using a fluorescence microwell plate scanner

Species	Age	EROD liver[1] mg	EROD sub[2] µM	EROD NADPH mM	BROD liver mg	BROD sub µM	BROD NADPH mM	MROD liver mg	MROD sub µM	MROD NADPH mM	PROD liver mg	PROD sub µM	PROD NADPH mM
Mallard	adult	5.2	1.25	.25	2.5	1.25	.25	1.3	0.62	.125	2.6	5.0	.25
Black duck	adult	2.0	1.25	.125	2.0	1.25	.125	2.0	0.92	.125	1.3	1.5	.25
Wood duck[3]	pemb[4]	1.3	0.75	.125	1.3	1.0	.125	2.6	1.25	.125	1.3	2.5	.125
Lesser scaup	6 month	1.3	2.5	.125	2.5	1.25	.125	1.3	2.5	.125	1.3	2.5	.125
Double-crested cormorant	14 day	0.65	2.5	.125	0.55	2.5	.125						
	pemb	0.65	2.5	.125				0.65	2.5	.125	0.55	2.5	.125
Blk-crowned night heron[5]	13 day	0.65	2.5	.25	1.5	5.0	.25	1.3	2.5	.25	1.3	5.0	.25
	pemb	2.6	5.0	.25	3.5	2.5	.25	5.2	2.5	.25	5.2	10.0	.50
Grt blue heron	pemb	2.6	2.5	.25	2.6	1.25	.125	1.3	2.5	.125	1.3	5.0	.125
Fla sand-hill crane[6]	30 day	0.33	2.5	.25	1.5	2.5	.25	1.3	1.88	.125	0.52	7.5	.125
Blk necked stilt	30 day	1.3	2.5	.25	2.6	2.5	.25	2.0	2.5	.25	5.2	10.0	.25
American avocet	30 day	2.6	5.0	.25	2.6	2.5	.25	2.6	2.5	.25	5.2	5.0	.50
Red-wgd blkbird	adult	2.6	5.0	.25	2.5	1.25	.25	2.6	2.5	.125	1.3	5.0	.125
European starling[7]	12 day	1.3	2.5	.25	2.5	1.25	.25	5.2	2.5	.50			
Barn swallow	12 day	0.5	2.5	.125	0.5	1.25	.125	1.3	5.0	.125			
	pemb	5.0	1.25	.125									

Tree swallow[8]	12 day	5.0	1.25	.125	0.5	2.5	.125						
	pemb	5.0	1.25	.125									
Northern bobwhite	adult	2.6	1.25	.125	1.3	1.25	.125	5.2	2.5	.125	2.6	5.0	.25
	1 day	2.0	1.25	.125	2.6	2.5	.125	2.6	2.5	.125	2.0	2.5	.125
American kestrel[9]	adult	1.3	1.88	.125	1.3	2.5	.125	1.3	2.5	.125	1.3	10.0	.125
	10 day	0.65	1.25	.125	0.65	1.25	.125	0.65	5.0	.25	0.65	10.0	.25
	pemb	0.65	1.25	.125	0.65	1.25	.125	0.65	5.0	.25			
Screech owl	adult	0.65	2.5	.125	1.3	3.0	.25	1.3	5.0	.25	0.65	5.0	.25
Western sandpiper[10]	adult	0.25	2.5	.25	0.25	2.5	.25				0.25	2.5	.25
Forster's tern	pemb	1.3	1.25	.125	1.3	1.25	.125						
Caspian tern	pemb	1.3	1.25	.125	1.3	1.25	.125						

[1]microsomes obtained from this amount of liver; [2]substrate concentration; [3]Beeman et al. 1993; [4]pipping embryo; [5]Melancon et al. 1992; [6]Melancon et al. 1994b; [7]Melancon et al. 1994a; [8]Not determined, used values from barn swallow; [9]Melancon et al. 1993; [10]Rattner et al. 1995.

RESULTS

Baseline values are presented in Table 3. The yield of microsomal protein for these twenty avian species averaged approximately 9 to 36 mg/g liver. The wide range of microsomal protein yields shown in this table may be due in part to water loss from some samples during storage which could lead to artificially high values for microsome yield per gram of tissue for such samples. In general, baseline EROD activity was highest and PROD activity the lowest of the four O-dealkylases assayed. For many species, when assay conditions were being determined the PROD activity was so low that it was not assayed for individual birds, and PROD activity is generally not assayed in liver samples from field studies. The data for Forsters' tern, Caspian tern and Western sandpiper (all adults) were obtained solely from field-collected, field-sacrificed adult birds that were not maintained on clean diets, so they may not be true baseline values.

Results of treatment with MC-type inducers are presented in Table 4. All species and ages studied showed significant induction of at least one of the monooxygenases assayed. Scaup showed the largest induction ratio and Northern bobwhite, particularly the pipping embryos, the lowest, for the species studied. Generally EROD was most responsive, but this varied among species. For some species, such as screech owl, the induction was significant for all four assays despite being only a doubling for MROD and PROD, while others such as Black-necked stilt and American avocet, although giving ratios from four to six and one half were not significant because of small numbers of birds used and highly variable responses.

The effect of PB (Table 5) on these four monooxygenases in the nine species studied was very slight. Scaup again was most responsive, and only three of the nine species showed a significant increase. One cannot conclude that the other six species are nonresponsive to PB, because these results may be due to a lack of responsiveness for these particular P450-associated enzyme activities, but not a complete lack of induction response to PB. In an earlier study with adult Mallard ducks (using 1 cm^2 cuvettes), PB at a slightly higher dose increased EROD 3.6-fold, but increased arylhydrocarbon hydroxylase 19.8-fold and benzphetamine-N-demethylase 7.8-fold (Melancon et al. 1990).

CONCLUSIONS

Hepatic microsomal monooxygenase activity was measured in the twenty avian species studied using a fluorescence microwell plate scanner to quantify the resorufin produced. Generally PROD activity was lowest, but EROD and MROD or BROD were found at readily measureable levels. The same assays were generally most responsive to MC-type inducers. The results provide information on twenty species that would make it possible to monitor a variety of habitats. When utilizing P450 as a biomarker for contaminant exposure it is important to use positive controls to ensure that the assay selected is responsive to the contaminant of interest in the species under study. For the studies summarized here, detailed information will be presented in future publications. Some of these species are presently the objects of field studies.

TABLE 3--Hepatic microsomal protein and O-dealkylase activities
(determined using a fluorescence microwell plate scanner) for
untreated (uninduced) birds

Species	Age	Micro prot. mg/g liver	EROD	BROD	MROD	PROD
			pmol product/min/mg microsomal protein			
Mallard	adult	12.6, 1.9[1]	41.7, 16.8[1]	11.4, 4.9	58.9, 33.2	7.4, 4.1
Black duck	adult	34.7, 3.8	13.1, 4.5	10.3, 2.9	13.3, 4.3	
Lesser scaup	6 mo	19.3, 2.0	16.6, 16.6	8.0, 8.0	22.7, 25.9	1.8, 1.8
Double-crested cormorant	14 day	21.3, 4.0	44.7, 25.6		40.7, 17.0	
	pemb[2]	14.1, 2.1	21.6, 7.3	13.3, 4.0	5.2, 4.7	
Black-crowned night heron[3]	13 day	9.5, 1.7	51.6, 22.0	23.0, 14.2	41.1, 15.3	52.2, 30.0
	pemb		36.2, 26.0	16.8, 6.2		25.5, 9.4
Grt blue heron	pemb	20.1, 2.4	5.6, 3.3	5.5, 1.1	5.1, 1.7	5.0, 1.6
Fla sandhill crane[4]	30 day	8.1, 2.2	50.8, 22.4	0.1, 0.1	22.8, 12.5	1.4, 0.6
Black necked stilt	30 day	17.7, 25.4	51.7, 67.0	26.6, 33.5	15.3, 20.9	4.3, 6.4
American avocet	30 day	18.1, 2.6	38.8, 10.0	16.8, 7.0	17.8, 3.9	6.1, 1.1
Red-winged blackbird	adult	31.0, 2.4	7.4, 2.5	1.9, 0.7	23.3, 7.4	
European starling[5]	12 day	18.5, 5.0	48.3, 28.7	3.6, 0.8	22.1, 9.7	
Tree swallow	pemb	25.1, 4.5	24.3, 21.0	18.4, 17.4		
Barn swallow	12 day	35.5, 3.7	42.1, 15.8	24.1, 13.2	14.4, 5.5	
Northern bobwhite	adult	36.4, 15.0	3.1, 1.4	6.8, 2.2	2.9, 1.1	2.2, 1.3
	1 day	16.7, 3.0	32.6, 10.3		46.9, 15.2	
American kestrel[6]	adult	24.3, 7.8	44.0, 14.4	19.6, 4.8	53.9, 23.6	
	10 day	10.5, 2.1	43.4, 12.3	39.0, 15.3	21.1, 11.4	11.8, 6.0
Screech owl	adult	14.9, 2.8	116, 15.9	16.3, 3.7	105, 28.9	91.5, 11.5

Forster's tern	adult	24.8, 6.9	4.0, 1.5	
Caspian tern	adult	24.9, 7.0	6.1, 2.5	4.3, 2.0
Western sandpiper[7]	adult	9.1, 1.6	866, 597	113, 129	55.6, 31.0

[1]mean value followed by standard deviation, except individual values for black necked stilt for which n = 2, for other species n = 4-20; [2]pipping embryo; [3]Melancon et al. 1992; [4]Melancon et al. 1994b; [5]Melancon et al. 1994a; [6]Melancon et al. 1993; [7]Rattner et al. 1995.

TABLE 4--Effects of 3-methylcholanthrene (MC), polychlorinated biphenyl (PCB 126) and β-naphthoflavone (BNF) on O-dealkylase activities expressed as ratio of treated activity over control activity

Species	Age	Induction Regimen	EROD	BROD	MROD	PROD
			(treated/control)[1]			
Mallard	adult	BNF; 100 mg/kg	3.9[2]	13.9[3]	2.2[2]	4.7[3]
Black duck	adult	BNF; 50 mg/kg	4.7[2]	8.8[4]	5.8[3]	
Lesser scaup	6 month	BNF; 100 mg/kg	55.7[3]	16.7[3]	35.5[3]	24.0[3]
Double-crested cormorant	14 day	BNF; 100 mg/kg	6.7[4]		5.2[4]	
	pemb[5]	MC; 5 mg/kg	19.7[4]	12.1[4]	89.1[4]	
Great blue heron	pemb	MC; 400 µg/egg	13.1[4]	5.9[4]	6.5[4]	3.0
Fla sandhill crane[6]	30 day	BNF; 100 mg/kg	7.9[4]	>15[4]	5.1[4]	8.4[4]
Black necked stilt	30 day	BNF; 50 mg/kg	4.1	4.2	3.0[2]	5.8[3]
American avocet	30 day	BNF; 50 mg/kg	6.5	5.5	3.3	9.1[2]
Red-winged blackbird	adult	BNF; 100 mg/kg	5.5[3]	10.3[4]	0.6[2]	
European starling[7]	12 day	BNF; 50 mg/kg	3.2[4]	4.4[4]	0.7[3]	
Barn swallow	12 day	BNF; 100 mg/kg	6.4[3]	7.6[3]	1.3	
Northern bobwhite	adult	BNF; 100 mg/kg	4.8[3]	1.1	4.9[3]	2.0
	1 day	PCB126; 70 ug/kg	2.1[2]		1.5	
American kestrel	adult	BNF; 100 mg/kg	2.2[2]	4.6[4]	1.2	
	10 day	PCB126; 50 µg/kg	10.7[4]	11.3[4]	4.9[4]	1.9[3]
Screech owl	adult	BNF; 100 mg/kg	4.0[3]	5.6[3]	2.2[3]	2.1[3]

[1]ratio based on activity calculated as pmol product/min/mg microsomal protein; [2]$p < 0.05$; [3]$p < 0.01$; [4]$p < 0.001$; n = 3-19; [5]pipping embryo; [6]Melancon et al. 1994b; [7]Melancon et al. 1994a

TABLE 5--Effects of phenobarbital on O-dalkylase activities
expressed as ratio of treated activity over control activity

Species	Age	Induction Regimen	EROD	BROD	MROD	PROD
			(treated/control)[1]			
Mallard	adult	3 X 70 mg/kg	1.5	0.9	1.5	0.8
Black duck	adult	3 X 70 mg/kg	2.6[2]	1.1	1.0	
Lesser scaup	6 month	3 X 70 mg/kg	10.4[3]	1.3	4.6[4]	2.8
Double-crested cormorant	pipping embryo	50 mg/kg	1.1	1.1	1.1	
Great blue heron	pipping embryo	80 mg/kg	1.2	1.7	1.0	0.9
Red-winged blackbird	adult	3 X 75 mg/kg	0.9	0.8	0.9	
European starling[5]	12 day	3 X 50 mg/kg	4.4[2]	1.3	2.7[2]	
Amer. kestrel	adult	3 X 70 mg/kg	1.1	1.0	1.2	
Screech owl	adult	3 X 70 mg/kg	0.9	0.8	0.9	0.8

[1]ratio based on activity calcuated as pmol product/min/mg microsomal
protein; [2]$p<0.001$; [3]$p<0.01$; [4]$p<0.05$, n = 8-13; [5]Melancon et al. 1994a

ACKNOWLEDGEMENTS

The author wishes to acknowledge the many individuals who have
participated in various aspects of the studies summarized in this
manuscript. These include coworkers within NBS and USFWS, Barnett
Rattner, Dave Hoffman, Tom Custer, Leonard LeCaptain, Randy Hines, John
Eisemann, Mary Maxey, Carolyn Marn, Roger Hothem, Larry Blus, Chuck
Henny, Dan Sparks, Diane Beeman, and Jim Fleming, graduate student, Amy
Yorks, and volunteers, Kathy Guger, Dan Hockett, Sarah Ford, Matthew
Mann, Heather Wheat, Julie Isackson, Dawn Myren, Cynthia Peters, Doug
Bruggeman, Jim Riggs, Kristin Koppenhaver, Krishna Niles, and Lauren
Schultheiss. The author also thanks Barnett Rattner, David Hoffman,
Gary Heinz, and John Eisemann for reviewing the manuscript.

REFERENCES

Anders, M. W. and Mannering, G. J., Kinetics of the inhibition of the N-
demethylation of ethylmorphine by 2-diethylamino-2,2-diphenylvalerate
HCl (SKF-525A) and related compounds. Molecular Pharmacology 2, 1966,
pp 319-327.

Balschmiter, K. and Zell, M., Analysis of polychlorinated biphenyls by
capillary gas chromatography. Fresenius Zeitschrift fOur analytische
Chemie 30, 1980, pp 20-31.

Beeman, D. K., Melancon, M. J. and Fleming, W. J. The cytochrome P450
monooxygenase system of the wood duck as a potential biomarker for
dioxin exposure. Proceedings of the Fourteenth Annual Meeting of the
Society of Environmental Toxicology and Chemistry, 1993, pp 270.

Burke, M. D. and Mayer, R. T., Ethoxyresorufin: direct fluorimetric
assay of a microsomal O-dealkylation which is preferentially inducible

by 3-methylcholanthrene. Drug Metabolism and Disposition 2, 1974, pp 583-588.

Burke, M. D. and Mayer, R. T., Differential effects of phenobarbitone and 3-methylcholanthrene induction on the hepatic microsomal metabolism and cytochrome P-450-binding of phenoxazone and a homologous series of its n-alkyl ethers (alkoxyresorufins). Chemical-Biological Interactions 45, 1983, pp 243-258.

Burke, M. D., Prough, R. A. and Mayer, R. T., Characteristics of a microsomal cytochrome P-448-mediated reaction. Drug Metabolism and Disposition 5, 1977, pp 1-8.

Burke, M. D., Thompson, S., Elcombe, C. R., Halpert, J., Haaparanta, T. and Mayer, R. T., Ethoxy-, pentoxy- and benzyloxyphenoxazones and homologues: a series of substrates to distinguish between different induced cytochromes P-450. Biochemical Pharmacology 34, 1985, pp 3337-3345.

Conney, A. H., Environmental factors influencing drug metabolism, in Fundamentals of Drug Metabolism and Drug Disposition, LaDu, B. N., Mandel, H. G. and Way, E. L. Eds., Williams and Wilkins, Baltimore, 1971, pp 253-278.

Eggens, M. L. and Galgani, F., Ethoxyresorufin-O-deethylase (EROD) activity in flatfish: fast determination with a fluorescence plate-reader. Marine Environmental Research 33, 1992, 213-221.

Halbrook, R. S. and Kirkpatrick, R. L., Use of barbiturate-induced sleeping time as an indicator of exposure to environmental contaminants in the wild, in Biomarkers of Environmental Contamination, McCarthy, J.F. and Shugart, L.R. Eds., Lewis Publishers, Boca Raton, FL, 1990, pp 151-164.

Kennedy, S. W., Lorenzen, A., James, C. A. and Norstrom, R. J., Ethoxyresorufin-o-deethylase (EROD) and porphyria induction in chicken embryo hepatocyte cultures - a new bioassay of PCB, PCDD and related chemical contamination in wildlife. Chemosphere 25, 1992, pp 193-196.

Kleinow, K. M., Melancon, M. J. and Lech, J. J., Biotransformation and induction: Implications for toxicity, bioaccumulation and monitoring of environmental xenobiotics in fish. Environmental Health Perspectives 71, 1987, pp 105-119.

Lowry, O. H., Rosebrough, N. J. Farr, A. L.and Randall, R. J.,   Protein measurement with the Folin phenol reagent. Journal of Biological Chemistry 193, 1951, pp 265-275.

Melancon, M. J., Binder, R. L. and Lech, J. J., Environmental induction of monooxygenase activity in fish, in Toxic Contaminants and Ecosystem Health; A Great Lakes Focus, Evans, M.S. Ed., John Wiley & Sons, New York, 1988, pp 215-236.

Melancon, M. J., Eisemann, J. D. Maxey, M. E. and McKee, M. J., Monooxygenase activity in dosed and field-collected nestling starlings (Sternus vulgaris). Proceedings of the Fourteenth Annual Meeting of the Society of Environmental Toxicology and Chemistry, 1994, pp 82.

Melancon, M. J., Gee, G. F., Olsen, G. H., Eisemann, J. D. and Maxey, M. E., Induction of cytochromes P450 in sandhill crane (Grus Canadensis) chicks. Proceedings of the Fourteenth Annual Meeting of the Society of Environmental Toxicology and Chemistry, 1994, pp 179.

Melancon, M. J., Hoffman, D. Hines, R. and Eisemann, J., Induction of cytochromes P450 in nestling kestrels by 3,3',4,4',5-pentachlorobiphenyl (PCB 126). Proceedings of the Fourteenth Annual Meeting of the Society of Environmental Toxicology and Chemistry, 1993, pp 281.

Melancon, M. J., Rattner, B. A. and LeCaptain, L. J.: Comparative induction of cytochromes P450 by 3-methylcholanthrene (MC) and phenobarbital (PB) in mallard duck (MD) and in Fisher-344 rat (FR). Proceedings of the Eleventh Annual Meeting of the Society of Environmental Toxicology and Chemistry, 1990, p. 155.

Melancon, M. J., Rattner, B. A, Rice, C. P., Hines and Eiseman, J., Hepatic microsomal monooxygenase activity in Black-Crowned Night Herons (BCNHS) from the Chesapeake Basin. Proceedings of the Thirteenth Annual Meeting of the Society of Environmental Toxicology and Chemistry, 1992, p. 77.

Payne, J. F., Fancey, L. L., Rahimtula, A. D. and Porter, E.L., Review and perspective on the use of mixed-function oxygenase enzymes in biological monitoring. Comparative Biochemistry and Physiology 86C, 1987, pp 233-245.

Rattner, B. A., Capizzi, J. L., King, K. A., LeCaptain, L. and Melancon, M. J., Exposure and effects of oilfield brine discharges on western sandpipers (Calidris mauri) in Nueces Bay, Texas. Bulletin of Environmental Contamination and Toxicology 54, 1995, pp 683-689.

Rattner, B. A., Hoffman, D. J. and Marn, C. M., Use of mixed-function oxygenases to monitor contaminant exposure in wildlife. Environmental Toxicology and Chemistry 8, 1989, 1093-1102.

Ronis, M. J. J. and Walker, C. H., The Microsomal Monooxygenases of Birds, in Reviews in Biochemical Toxicology, V. 10, Hodgson, E., J.R. Bend and R.M. Philpot, eds., Elsevier Science Publishing Co., Inc., 1989, pp 301-384.

Stegeman, J. J., Brouwer, M., Di Giulio, R. T., Forlin, L., Fowler, B. A., Sanders, B. M. and Van Veld, P. A., Enzyme and protein synthesis as indicators of contaminant exposure, in Biomarkers: Biochemical, Physiological, and Histological Markers of Anthropogenic Stress, Huggett, R.J., Kimerle, R.A., Mehrle, P.M., Jr. and Bergman, H.L. Eds., Lewis Publishers, Chelsea, MI, 1992, pp 235-335.

Van Cantfort, J., De Graeve, J. and Gielen, J. E., Radioactive assay for aryl hydrocarbon hydroxylase. Improved method and biological importance. Biochemical and Biophysical Research Communications 79, 1977, pp 505-512.

Joe N. Lucas[1] and Tore Straume[1]

Chromosome Translocations Measured by Fluorescence In-Situ Hybridization: A Promising Biomarker

REFERENCE: Lucas, J. N. and Straume, T., **"Chromosome Translocations Measured by Fluorescence In-Situ Hybridization: A Promising Biomarker,"** *Environmental Toxicology and Risk Assessment: Biomarkers and Risk Assessment—Fifth Volume, ASTM STP 1306,* David A. Bengtson and Diane S. Henshel, Eds., American Society for Testing and Materials, 1996.

ABSTRACT: A biomarker for exposure and risk assessment would be most useful if it employs an endpoint that is highly quantitative, is stable with time, and is relevant to human risk. Recent advances in chromosome staining using fluorescence *in situ* hybridization (FISH) facilitate fast and reliable measurement of reciprocal translocations, a kind of DNA damage linked to both prior clastogenic exposure and to risk. In contrast to other biomarkers available, the frequency of reciprocal translocations in individuals exposed to whole-body radiation is stable with time post exposure, has a rather small inter-individual variability, and can be measured accurately at the low levels. Here, we discuss results from our studies demonstrating that chromosome painting can be used to reconstruct radiation dose for workers exposed within the dose limits, for individuals exposed a long time ago, and even for those who have been diagnosed with leukemia but not yet undergone radiotherapy or chemotherapy.

KEY WORDS: chromosome; translocation; FISH; persistence; radiation

There is a need for reliable methods to assess past clastogenic exposures and to assess risk. This is particularly the case for a large number of individuals exposed to various levels of ionizing radiation as a result of nuclear accidents such as Chernobyl, atmospheric nuclear testing prior to the early 1960's, past human experimentation by US Government agencies, the atom bombs dropped on Hiroshima and Nagasaki, various medical radiological procedures, occupational exposures, and a variety of other radiation-related exposures for which dosimetry information may be poor or absent.

[1]Professor & Senior Scientist, Lawrence Livermore National Laboratory, University of California, P.O. Box 808, Livermore, CA 94550.

The efforts in our laboratory have centered principally on the development and validation of a technology referred to as "chromosome painting" for use in human exposure and risk assessment. This technology employs fluorescence in situ hybridization (FISH) with whole chromosome probes to rapidly and accurately detect chromosome abnormalities such as stable translocations [1] in human cells. For a description of FISH see Lucas et al. 1992a. The development of this technology began at the Lawrence Livermore National Laboratory during the early 1980's (Pinkel et al. 1986) and has now developed into the method of choice world-wide for the detection of chromosome translocations in humans (e.g., see Lucas et al. 1992a; Nakano et al. 1993; Bauchinger et al. 1993; Straume et al. 1995; National Research Council 1995).

METHODOLOGY

The method employs lymphocytes obtained from a small blood sample taken from the individual to be evaluated. The lymphocytes are cultured and metaphase spreads made on glass slides using standard cytogenetic methods (Evans et al. 1979). A cocktail of composite chromosome-specific DNA probes are used in combination with pan-centromeric probes to discriminate between translocations and dicentrics (e.g., see Lucas et al. 1992a; Straume and Lucas 1993). Chromosome painting is generally performed using DNA probes specific for only a sub-set of the genome, e.g., painting chromosomes 1, 2, and 4 results in the detection of 35% of all translocations (Lucas et al 1992a). Here, genome refers to the full compliment of chromosomes in a cell. Comparisons with results from conventional cytogenetic methods requires scaling-up the chromosome painting results to full genome equivalents. As described below, we have shown that such scaling can be performed accurately by assuming that radiation results in a random distribution of chromosome breaks.

To visualize interchromosomal exchanges, the metaphase chromosomes are stained yellow with probes for the selected target chromosomes and red for the non-target chromosomes (e.g., see Fig. 1 in Lucas et al. 1992a). With the additional application of blue pan-centromeric probes, the discrimination between translocations and dicentrics is made possible. Thus, exchange aberrations are recognized as bi-color (part red and part yellow) chromosomes, and are scored as reciprocal translocations if the two derivative chromosomes each have one blue-stained centromere and as dicentrics if the derivative chromosomes have two centromeres and a bi-color acentric fragment.

As indicated above, full genomic translocation frequencies are accurately obtained after selectively painting only a small fraction of the genome. This important finding was determined by comparing in the same individuals reciprocal translocation frequencies measured using FISH and G-banding (Lucas et al. 1992a). The frequencies measured using

---

[1]Here, translocations are defined as complete exchanges between two chromosomes resulting in two monocentric derivative chromosomes. Dicentrics are defined as complete exchanges between two chromosomes resulting in one dicentric derivative chromosome and an acentric fragment.

FISH for chromosomes 1, 2 and 4 (i.e., 22% of the genome) were converted to full genome equivalents and then plotted against translocation frequencies measured by G-banding for all chromosomes for the same individuals. The results demonstrated that FISH provided reciprocal translocation frequencies that did not differ significantly from those measured by the standard G-banding method.

G-banding, which is universally accepted as an accurate method of detecting chromosome translocations, is much too labor intensive for exposure and risk assessment applications. The demonstration that the much faster FISH method provided identical results when scaled to full genome, provided a new practical biomarker for applications that require the scoring of large numbers of cells and individuals.

Much of our recent work has centered on the validation of the FISH technology for radiation dose reconstruction and the development of the data required to translate a measured frequency into a dose. Most of these efforts have been summarized in Straume and Lucas 1995 and are further expanded here.

HUMAN STUDIES

To date, we have evaluated four individuals previously exposed to penetrating whole-body radiation, either accidentally or during normal work situations. Each of these four cases were exposed to different kinds of radiation, patterns of exposure, and dose rates. All, however, had in common exceptionally good independent dosimetry against which our biodosimetry results could be compared.

The first case, a radiation worker exposed occupationally during the 1950's, 1960's, and early 1970s was also evaluated biodosimetrically using four different assays, including translocations measured by chromosome painting (Straume et al. 1992). This worker's whole-body, fully penetrating exposure was always within occupational dose limits. In 1989, the best-estimate dose obtained from the measured translocation frequency was 0.49±0.21 Sv, in good agreement with the total integrated dose recorded in his official dosimetry record from badge readings of 0.56±0.20 Sv (Straume and Lucas 1995). These results suggested that stable biomarkers could be detected in workers, even those exposed within the dose limits.

The second case, a tritium worker accidentally inhaled tritium oxide in 1985 that resulted in a whole-body dose of 0.44 Sv based on urinalysis and 0.42 Sv based on dicentric aberrations measured within one month of the acute inhalation exposure (Lloyd et al. 1986). Our biodosimetry performed for this same individual in 1992 (six years after exposure) using chromosome painting to measure stable reciprocal translocations (Lucas et al. 1992b) resulted in 0.44 Sv, essentially identical to the dosimetry results obtained immediately after the accident from urinalysis and dicentrics (Straume and Lucas 1995).

The third case was a worker exposed to photons and particle radiation from high-energy accelerator operations during 30-years of work in that environment. This individual was a dosimetry expert and kept meticulous records of his exposure history. His integrated dose-equivalent from personnel dosimeters was 0.33±0.04 Sv which compares very well with our biodosimetry results (0.3±0.1 Sv) from the frequency of translocation in his blood lymphocytes measured during the past year.

The fourth case was a radiation worker exposed during the past decade to external gamma radiation from ^{137}Cs and some internal contamination by radiocesium. The external and internal exposure resulted in essentially uniform whole-body radiation dose. Two independent dosimetry methods were employed on this worker: (1) electron paramagnetic resonance (EPR) dosimetry was performed on the individual's tooth enamel by scientists in the Ukraine, and (2) chromosome painting was performed on the individual's blood lymphocytes. Dosimetry results from the two independent methods show good agreement, i.e., 0.3±0.1 Sv for EPR and 0.33±0.12 Sv for translocations measured using FISH.

Taken together, these case studies suggest that the frequency of translocations in human lymphocytes provide an accurate measure of prior low-level exposure to ionizing radiation in whole-body exposed individuals, regardless of the temporal pattern of the exposure or the kind of radiation involved. Additional individuals with independent, good dosimetry are being sought to continue these very important validation studies.

Chromosome translocation studies have also been performed on large numbers of individuals such as atom-bomb survivors and radiation accident victims. However, in those cases, the independent dosimetry is uncertain and cytogenetic analyses were not made soon after the radiation exposure. It is nevertheless informative that cytogenetic follow-up for those populations (which unfortunately began many years after the exposure occurred) has shown that the translocation frequencies measured in blood lymphocytes of exposed individuals do not change with time when the same individuals are re-sampled many years later (Straume and Lucas 1995; Salassidis et al. 1995; Littlefield et al. 1984). Individuals and groups from which temporal stability information has been obtained are shown in Fig. 1. It is seen that prior to our efforts, there was a multi-year gap in the translocation stability data between exposure and the first measurement.

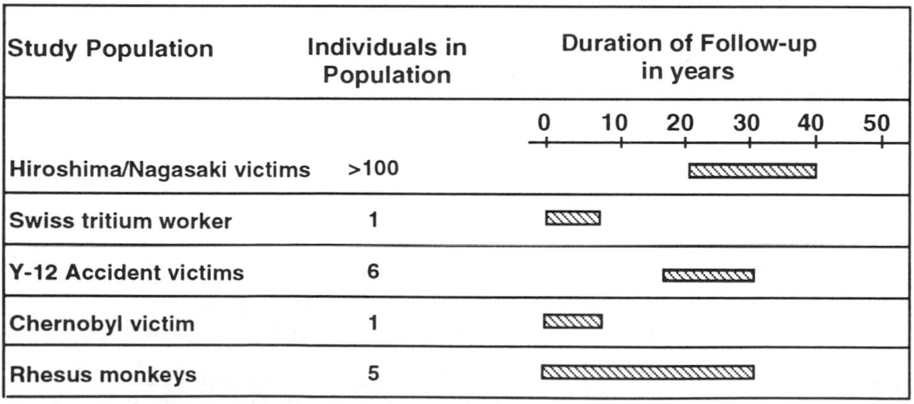

Study Population	Individuals in Population	Duration of Follow-up in years					
		0	10	20	30	40	50
Hiroshima/Nagasaki victims	>100				▨▨▨▨▨		
Swiss tritium worker	1	▨▨					
Y-12 Accident victims	6			▨▨▨▨			
Chernobyl victim	1	▨▨					
Rhesus monkeys	5	▨▨▨▨▨▨▨▨					

FIG 1. Duration of follow-up in various groups evaluated for chromosome translocations. Plotted from data in Straume and Lucas 1995.

NON-HUMAN PRIMATE STUDIES

Rhesus monkeys were exposed in 1965 to whole-body (fully penetrating) radiation in connection with NASA studies (Hardy 1991). Some 28 years later, in 1993, near the end of their lifespan, we performed biodosimetry on blood lymphocytes from six of the primates and compared our results with the actual doses delivered to the animals in 1965 (in one individual, biodosimetry was also performed on skin fibroblasts). Results are listed in Table 1 and show very good agreement between the actual treatment dose given in 1965 and the dose estimated biodosimetrically from the translocation frequency in 1993. From the Table, it is observed that the biological dose estimates are within 25% of the actual doses for all six animals, and for four of the six animals our biodosimetry differs by less than 10% from the given doses. Given the fact that almost 30 years had elapsed since exposure, these results are promising indeed.

TABLE 1--<u>Dose reconstruction for rhesus monkeys irradiated 28 years</u> <u>previously.</u>*

Treatment dose(Sv)	Biodosimetry dose (Sv)	Biodosimetry dose/ treatment dose	Percent difference
0.56	0.59	1.05	5
1.13	0.99	0.88	12
1.13	1.05	0.93	7
2.25	1.70	0.76	24
2.25	2.13	0.95	5
2.00	1.90	0.95	5
2.25	1.84	0.82	18

*Lucas et al. 1996.

IN VITRO **STUDIES**

The use of a biomarker for quantitative evaluation of exposure and dose assessment requires good calibration curves. Such curves provide a relationship between biomarker frequency and dose, and must therefore be obtained for relevant exposure conditions. For radiation-induced chromosome aberrations, calibration curves are generally obtained using lymphocytes exposed *in vitro* (blood obtained from a healthy donor and irradiated in a culture vial), which have been shown to be identical to those exposed *in vivo* (e.g., Brewen and Gengozian 1971).

Studies currently underway in our program will provide many of the *in vitro* calibration curves necessary for radiation biological dosimetry using the chromosome painting technology. For example, we have recently obtained a full-range calibration curve for ^{60}Co gamma-ray-induced translocations measured by FISH in human lymphocytes (Lucas et al. 1995), and we are currently working on a curve for ^{137}Cs gamma rays, which will provide a means for dose reconstruction at Chernobyl where radiocesium contamination is producing most of the population dose. We are also working on human calibration curves for tritium beta rays and orthovoltage x rays. This effort is particularly timely now, as the FISH technology is becoming more generally employed in dose reconstruction.

BIODOSIMETRY FOR LEUKEMIA PATIENTS

A substantial amount of genetic damage appears in the blood cells of leukemia patients due to the well known phenomenon of genetic instability of cancer cells. This is of particular significance for biological dosimetry because such genetic instability in the malignant lymphocytes can mask the genetic damage that may have been caused by radiation or other clastogens prior to the disease. We have developed a new approach that may be used to measure pre-cancer-induced chromosomal aberrations in patients with B-cell leukemia by totally separating the unaffected T lymphocytes from the malignant B lymphocytes (Lucas et al. 1994). Results suggest that pre-leukemia exposure to radiation may be biodosimetrically quantified from translation frequencies in a certain subset of blood lymphocytes of leukemia patients as long as the blood sample is obtained prior to radiotherapy or chemotherapy (Lucas et al., 1994). This method fills an important need in the determination of prior exposures that may have contributed to the induction of leukemia or lymphoma.

OTHER CONSIDERATIONS

Variables such as spontaneous translocation frequencies in unexposed individuals and non-uniform body dose in exposed individuals are also being addressed. We have measured about two dozen unexposed controls of varying ages, from ~20 to more than 60 years of age. The translocation frequencies range from ~2 to 10 per 1000 cells (Bender et al. 1988; Straume and Lucas 1995). Further work is needed to fully quantify the effect of variables such as age and natural background radiation.

When the dose distribution is highly non-uniform within the body, biodosimetry results can be difficult to evaluate. For example, inhalation or ingestion of radioiodine results in dose primarily to the thyroid. In that case, biodosimetry using blood lymphocytes would not be appropriate. Also, radiation exposures to body extremities such as fingers or hands would result in very few damaged blood lymphocytes. We are working on the development of biodosimetry assays for specific organs that would be particularly useful in assessing partial body exposures.

CONCLUSION

When the human case studies are considered together with the results for non-human primates, the overall biodosimetry data are now beginning to provide a strong basis for the use of chromosome translocations detected by FISH in retrospective dosimetry and risk assessment. This is true no matter how long ago the exposure occurred or whether the exposure was received acutely or chronically.

ACKNOWLEDGMENT

This work was performed under the auspices of the U. S. Department of Energy by the Lawrence Livermore National Laboratory under contract number W-7405-Eng-48. We are especially grateful for the support of DOE/EH.

REFERENCES

Bauchinger, M., Schmid, E., Zitzelsberger, H., Braselmann, H., and Nahrstedt, U., 1993, "Radiation-induced chromosome aberrations analysed by two-color fluorescence in situ hybridization with composite whole chromosome-specific DNA probes and a pancentromeric DNA probe", International Journal of Radiation Biology, 64, pp. 179-184

Bender, M. A., Awa, A .A., Brooks, A. L., Evans, H. J., Groer, P. G., Littlefield, L. G., Pereira, C., Preston, R. J., and Wackholtz, B. W., 1988, "Current status of cytogenetic procedures to detect and quantify previous exposures to radiation", Mutation Research, 196, pp. 103-159

Brewen, J. G., and Gengozian, N., 1971, "Radiation-induced human chromosome aberrations. II. Human in vitro irradiation compared to in vitro and in vivo irradiation of marmoset leukocytes", Mutation Research, 13, pp. 383-391

Evans, H. C., Buckton, K. E., Hamilton, G. E., Carothers, A., 1979, "Radiation-induced chromosome aberrations in nuclear-dockyard workers", Nature, 277, pp. 531-534

Hardy, K. A., 1991, "Dosimetry methods used in the studies of the effects of protons on primates: a review", Radiation Research, 126, pp. 120-126

Littlefield, L.G., Sayer, A. M., Colyer, S., Joiner, E.E., Outlaw, J., and Dry, L., 1984, "Persistent radiation-induced chromosome lesions in lymphocytes of the Y-12 accident survivors: Evaluation 25 years post-exposure", Mamilian Chromosome Newsletter, 25, p. 18

Lucas, J. N., Awa, A., Straume, T., Poggensee, M., Kodama, Y., Nakano, M., Ohtaki, K., Weier, U., Pinkel, D., Gray, J., and Littlefield, G., 1992a, "Rapid translocation frequency analysis in humans decades after exposure to ionizing radiation ", International Journal of Radiation Biology, 62, pp. 53-63

Lucas, J. N., Hill, F., Burk, C., Fester, T., Straume, T., 1995, "Dose-response curve for chromosome translocations measured in human lymphocytes exposed to ^{60}Co gamma rays", Health Physics, 68, pp. 761-765

Lucas, J. N., Poggensee, M., Straume, T., 1992b, "The persistence of chromosome translocations in a radiation worker accidentally exposed to tritium", Cytogenetics and Cell Genetics, 60, pp. 255-256

Lucas, J. N., Swansbury, G., Clutterbuck, R., Hill, F., Burk, C., and Straume, T., 1994, "Discrimination between leukemia- and non-lekemia-induced chromosomal abnormalities in the patient's lymphocytes", International Journal of Radiation Biology, 66, pp. 185-189

Lucas, J. N., Hill, F. S., Burk, C. E., Cox, A. B., Straume, T., 1996, "Stability of translocation frequency following whole-body irradiation measured in rhesus monkeys", International Journal of Radiation Biology, (in press)

Nakano, M., Nakashima, E., Pawel, D.J., Kodama, Y., and Awa, A., 1993, "Frequency of reciprocal translocations and dicentrics induced in human blood lymphocytes by X-irradiation and determined by fluorescence in situ hybridization", International Journal of Radiation Biology, 64, pp. 565-569

National Research Council, 1995, Radiation Dose Reconstruction for Epidemiologic Uses. US National Academy of Sciences Press, Washington, DC., pp. 52-54

Pinkel, D., Straume, T., and Gray, J. W., 1986, "Cytogenetic analysis using quantitative, high sensitivity, fluorescence hybridization", Proceedings of the National Academy of Sciences (USA), 83, pp. 2934-2938

Salassidis, K., Georgiadou-Schumacher, G., Braselmann, H., Muller, P., Peter, R.U., Bauchinger, M., 1995, "Chromosome painting in highly irradiated Chernobyl victims: a follow-up study to evaluate the stability of symmetrical translocations and the influence of clonal aberrations for retrospective dose estimation", International Journal of Radiation Biology, 68, pp. 257-262

Straume, T. and Lucas, J. N., 1993, "A comparison of the yields of translocations and dicentrics measured using fluorescence in situ hybridization", International Journal of Radiation Biology, 64, pp.185-187

Straume, T. and Lucas, J. N., 1995, "Validation studies for monitoring of workers using molecular cytogenetics", Biomarkers in Occupational Health: Progress and Perspectives (M. L. Mendelsohn, J.P. Peeters, and M.J. Normandt, Eds.), Joseph Henry Press, Washington DC, pp. 174-193

Straume, T., Lucas, J. N., Tucker, J. D., Bigbee, W. L., and Langlois, R. G., 1992, "Biodosimetry for a radiation worker using multiple assays", Health Physics, 62, pp. 122-130

J. McHugh Law[1], Debra J. McMillin[2], David H. Swenson[2], and Jay C. Means[2]

QUANTIFICATION OF DNA ADDUCTS IN SMALL FISH EXPOSED TO ALKYLATING AGENTS

REFERENCE: Law, J. M., McMillin, D. J., Swenson, D. H., and Means, J. C., "Quantification of DNA Adducts in Small Fish Exposed to Alkylating Agents," *Environmental Toxicology and Risk Assessment: Biomarkers and Risk Assessment—Fifth Volume, ASTM STP 1306*, David A. Bengtson and Diane S. Henshel, Eds., American Society for Testing and Materials, 1996.

ABSTRACT: It is widely believed that most chemical carcinogens act by binding to cellular genetic material and causing somatic mutations. Chemical modification of DNA (e.g., the formation of DNA adducts) is the first in a series of stages that lead to mutation, cell transformation, and tumor development.

Sensitive methods for detection of DNA adducts are essential for mechanistic studies of mutagenesis and carcinogenesis and for biomonitoring of populations at risk for environmentally caused cancer. DNA adducts may be detected with such methods as ^{32}P-postlabeling, immunoassays, HPLC with fluorescence detection, and gas chromatography/mass spectrometry, with varying degrees of sensitivity and structural specificity. Alkylation at the N-7 position of guanine is a preferential site of attack for most alkylating agents, but may be of little biological consequence, while adduct formation at the O^6 position of guanine (less common) is most highly correlated with carcinogenesis.

We have examined the suitability of western mosquitofish (*Gambusia affinis*) as a native sentinel species for monitoring environmental exposures to mutagens and carcinogens. Mosquitofish are a native species to the U.S. and are also widely distributed in warm waters throughout the world. These fish are ideal for monitoring local exposures because they are non-migratory and are found in a wide variety of habitats. In the laboratory, they are easily cultured using techniques developed for other small fish species and appear resistant to infectious diseases. Thus, methods may be directly assessed under controlled conditions before being applied to field situations.

In these studies, mosquitofish were exposed to a model alkylating agent, methylazoxymethanol acetate, at 10 ppm in the ambient water for 2 h. Fish were then transferred to clean water and held for up to 72 h. Livers were excised, pooled for 5 fish, and DNA was extracted and prepared for analysis. Liver DNA extracts were assessed for levels of N-7 and O^6-methylguanine by isotope dilution GC/mass spectrometry, using deuterated analogs of methylguanine adducts as standards. Detection limits for the assay

[1] Assistant Professor, North Carolina State University, College of Veterinary Medicine, Department of Microbiology, Pathology, and Parasitology, 4700 Hillsborough Street, Raleigh, NC 27606.

[2] Research Associate, Associate Professor, and Professor, respectively, Louisiana State University, School of Veterinary Medicine, Department of Veterinary Physiology, Pharmacology, and Toxicology, Baton Rouge, LA 70803.

were approximately 1.6 femtomoles of adduct per mg DNA (about 1 adduct per 2 million bases). Approximately 55-185 pg (330-1100 femtomoles) O^6-methylguanine per mg DNA were measured in exposed fish in the first 72 h after exposure. These lesions were correlated with a 33% liver tumor incidence after 25 weeks in parallel experiments.

KEYWORDS: DNA adducts, 7-methylguanine, O^6-methylguanine, GC/mass spectrometry, methylazoxymethanol acetate, liver, carcinogenesis, mosquitofish, *Gambusia affinis*

Chemical carcinogenesis is a complex, multistage process thought to involve genetic and epigenetic damage to susceptible cells that subsequently gain a selective growth advantage over neighboring cells as the result of activation of protooncogenes and/or inactivation of tumor suppressor genes (Harris 1991). An approach to assessing genotoxic damage that integrates all of the various factors involved in chemical exposure, uptake, biotransformation, etc., is to compare levels of specific covalent adducts of DNA in the target tissue. It is generally accepted that most chemical carcinogens act by interacting with the genetic material of the cell, in particular the DNA template (Lawley 1984). Chemical modification of DNA is the first in a series of steps that lead to mutation, cell transformation, and tumor development (Wogan 1988). In fact, it has been suggested that any chemical that forms DNA adducts, even at low levels, has the potential to be mutagenic and carcinogenic (de Serres 1988). DNA adduct determinations can therefore provide crucial information on metabolic pathways as well as chemical effects on DNA structure, transcription, synthesis, and repair. Adduct analyses, along with appropriate measures of mutation rates, can also provide direct information relevant to the somatic mutation theory and DNA adducts can be considered dosimeters of exposure to chemicals in cancer risk assessments (Beland and Poirier 1989).

Alkylating agents are archetypal carcinogens, in that most other carcinogens are active only after being metabolized to alkylating or aralkylating agents (Lawley 1984). Substitution at the N-7 position of guanine is a preferential site of attack for most alkylating agents, while attack at the O^6 position of guanine (less common) is most highly correlated with carcinogenesis (Beranek et al. 1980; Lawley 1984; Loveless 1969; Swenson and Lawley 1978). Agents that cause alkyl-DNA or aryl-DNA adducts can be divided into two major classes: (1) those compounds or their metabolites that form bulky chemical adducts of the purine and pyrimidine bases, represented by such classical chemical carcinogens as benzo(a)pyrene, aflatoxin, 7,12-dimethylbenz(a)anthracene, and 2-acetylaminofluorene; and (2) agents that form simple base modifications, differing from bulky adducts in that they do not distort the DNA helix (Dresler 1989). This second group includes such classical alkylating mutagens as N-methyl-N-nitrosourea (MNU), methyl methanesulfonate (MMS), N-methyl-N'-nitro-N-nitrosoguanidine (MNNG), N-ethyl-N-nitrosourea (ENU), ethyl methanesulfonate (EMS), and diethylnitrosamine (DEN) or their metabolites. Although simple base modifications can block DNA replication, more often they directly produce promutagenic adducts in DNA (Dresler 1989; Miller 1983; Singer and Kusmierek 1982).

Methylazoxymethanol acetate (MAM-Ac), a model alkylating carcinogen, forms methyl DNA adducts following esterase-mediated release of a highly reactive methyl carbonium ion (Feinberg and Zedeck 1980). Metabolism leads to the final formation of methanol, acetic and formic acids and nitrogen gas. MAM-Ac has been shown to be carcinogenic in several mammalian animal models and to cause liver neoplasia in several fish species (Hawkins et al. 1985; Stanton 1966). For example, a 2 h pulse exposure to 10 mg/L MAM-Ac in the ambient water resulted in a 33% incidence of liver tumors in western mosquitofish by 25 weeks after exposure, and more than a 50% incidence after 40 weeks (Law et al. 1994).

There is increasing interest in the use of small fish models for carcinogenicity testing, for investigations of basic carcinogenic mechanisms, and as sentinel species for monitoring health risks associated with aquatic environments (Hawkins et al. 1988a; Hawkins et al. 1988b; Hoover 1984). Unlike many rodent models, fish have an extremely low background incidence of tumors and are relatively inexpensive to breed and maintain (Couch and Harshbarger, 1985). However, because most published studies to date have been performed with exotic or non-native species or with larger cold water fish species difficult to rear in the laboratory, there is a need for a freshwater, temperate-zone small fish species that could serve as an environmental sentinel and also be amenable to laboratory culture for validation of biological markers (Couch and Harshbarger, 1985).

The western mosquitofish is a small, native, freshwater fish that is distributed from New Jersey to Florida and from Florida to the Texas/Mexico coasts and has been introduced world-wide as a mosquito control agent (Dees 1961). Mosquitofish are easily cultured using techniques developed for other small fish species such as the guppy (*Poecilia reticulata*). They breed prolifically and appear resistant to many infectious diseases. They have been shown in previous studies to express measurable changes in a variety of biomarkers following contaminant exposure and, thus, may prove useful for both controlled laboratory investigations as well as field studies, enabling substances to be tested under validated conditions in the field (Law 1995).

Direct measurement of DNA adducts may be employed as a biomarker of both exposure and effects in organisms exposed to genotoxic agents (Shugart et al. 1992). Biomarkers such as DNA adducts may afford a temporally and spatially integrated measure of bioavailable pollutants not provided by chemical analyses of water, soils, or tissues, thus giving information that is more relevant to evaluating ecological or health risks (McCarthy and Shugart 1990). The application of DNA adduct analysis in fish has been reviewed recently by Maccubbin (1994). Formation and persistence of O^6-ethylguanine in rainbow trout exposed to DEN were reported by Fong and co-workers using HPLC with fluorescence detection (Fong et al. 1988). Few studies, however, have attempted to measure specific adduct levels in small fish species exposed to small (i.e., non-bulky) alkylating carcinogens. This could be due to the fact that many existing methods are not sensitive enough to utilize the small amounts of tissue available from these species. Accurate, sensitive, and structurally selective measurements of DNA adduct levels have been obtained using stable isotope-labeled analogs of analytes as internal standards with analysis by selected ion monitoring GC/MS (Dizdaroglu 1993).

The present study was designed to use these techniques to measure DNA adduct formation and persistence in the liver of western mosquitofish (*Gambusia affinis*) exposed to MAM-Ac in order to further validate the use of this species both in laboratory and as a sentinel species in field studies.

METHODS

Experimental Design

Experiments were performed to investigate the extent and kinetics of DNA alkylation and subsequent DNA repair following a single, short, pulse exposure to MAM-Ac. The exposure designs and sample preparation sequence are shown schematically in Fig. 1. All specimens used in this study were the progeny of laboratory-maintained western mosquitofish caught originally in Ocean Springs, Mississippi, USA. Adult fish ranging from 9 to 14 months old were randomized and selected for use. The fish were

Experimental Protocol:

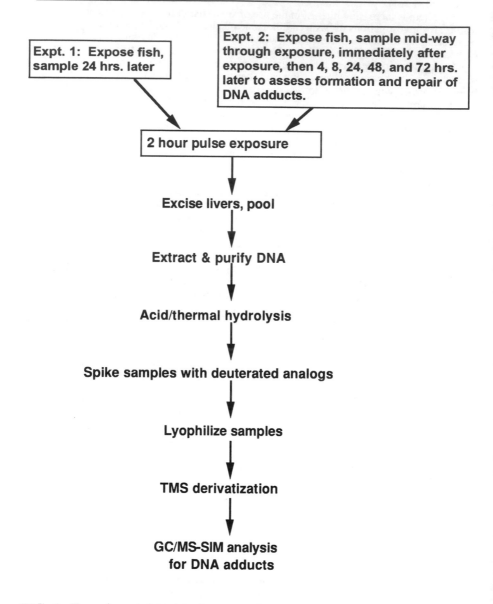

FIG. 1--Experimental protocol.

acclimated for a minimum of two weeks in 40-L aquaria containing dechlorinated, organic-free water maintained at 27±1°C by a recirculating water bath. The aquarium room was maintained on a 12 h light/12 h dark cycle with incandescent lighting. The fish were fed commercial flake food (Prime Tropical Flakes-Yellow, Zeigler Brothers, Inc., Gardners, PA, USA) two times daily. Water quality was monitored and tank maintenance performed once weekly.

Exposure

Two basic protocols, differing only in post-exposure sampling times (Fig. 1) and numbers of specimens used, were followed in these experiments. Randomly selected adult fish ranging from 30 to 35 mm in length were used. Specimens were randomly distributed into 4 L Pyrex beakers containing dechlorinated, organic-free water (pH 8.7, dissolved oxygen 9.0 mg/L) maintained at 27±1°C in a heated recirculating waterbath contained within a ventilated laboratory hood.

In experiment 1, a total of 15 test fish (in one beaker) and 10 unexposed controls (in a second beaker) were used (Table 2). In experiment 2, a total of 70 test fish (divided evenly into two beakers) and 10 unexposed controls (in a third beaker) were used (Table 3). The test fish were exposed for 2 h to methylazoxymethanol acetate (MAM-Ac; Sigma Chemical Company, St. Louis, Missouri, USA, water miscible liquid, density =1.27 g/ml) at 10 mg/L, then rinsed and transferred to carcinogen-free water in separate 40-liter aquaria maintained at 27±1°C. This exposure protocol was designed to parallel the conditions used in an earlier study (Law et al. 1994) in which we diagnosed liver tumors in mosquitofish 25 weeks after exposure to MAM-Ac. At each designated sampling time, fish were randomly selected and euthanized by stunning in ice water followed by decapitation. In experiment 1, the 15 test specimens (pooled for analysis into 3 groups of 5 fish each: *Exposed 1, 2, and 3* in Table 2) and 10 control animals (2 groups of 5 fish each: *Control 1 and 2*) were sampled 24 h after the exposure. In experiment 2, 5 test fish from each of the 2 test beakers were sampled halfway through the 2 h exposure (*-1a, -1b* in Table 3). At the end of the 2 h exposure, duplicate groups of 5 control fish each (*Control a and Control b*) and 5 exposed fish from each of the 2 test beakers (*0a and 0b*) were sampled. Duplicate groups of 5 test fish each were then sampled at 4, 8, 24, 48, or 72 h post-exposure (*4a and 4b, 8a and 8b*, etc.). Feeding of the fish resumed following the exposure period.

DNA Extraction and Purification

Livers were immediately excised, pooled for duplicate 5 fish groups into 2 mL polypropylene microtubes, weighed, and flash-frozen in liquid nitrogen. DNA was extracted and purified according to standard methods (Strauss 1987), with some modifications. Briefly, the frozen liver tissue was pulverized within each microtube, then suspended in approximately 1 mL of a digestion buffer consisting of 100 mM NaCl, 10 mM TrisCl (pH 8), 25 mM EDTA (pH 8), 0.5% sodium dodecyl sulfate, and 0.1 mg/mL proteinase-K. Samples were then incubated with shaking at 50°C for 14-16 h. A reagent blank which contained all reagents and materials except liver tissue was also prepared. Organic extraction was performed twice using 1 mL of biotechnology grade phenol:chloroform:isoamyl alcohol (25:24:1, pH 8.0, Amresco, Solon, Ohio, USA). The extracted DNA was then precipitated by addition of isopropanol and 7.5 M ammonium acetate, followed by centrifugation at 13,000 x g. The DNA pellet was then rinsed in 70% ethanol and briefly air-dried.

Hydrolysis and Derivatization

Isolated DNA samples were hydrolyzed in 0.5 mL of 60% formic acid (Mallinckrodt, Paris, Kentucky, USA) in evacuated, PFTE-sealed, conical bottom, glass vials at 75°C for 30 min. After cooling, all samples were spiked with a mixture of four deuterium-labeled adduct standards (see below). Standard blanks were also prepared at this time by adding both the deuterated and a non-deuterated guanine adduct standard mixture to clean vials. Nanopure grade water (2 mL) was added to each tube except the standard blanks. Samples and blanks were lyophilized and trimethylsilyl derivatives were produced using a mixture of 80 µL of bis(trimethylsilyl)-trifluoroacetamide (BSTFA)/1% trimethylsilylchlorosilane (Alltech, Deerfield, Illinois, USA) and 20 µL of acetonitrile under nitrogen at 75°C for 30 min. After cooling, derivatized mixtures were injected directly onto the gas chromatograph (GC). Lyophilized mixtures of standard methylated and ethylated guanine bases and their deuterium-labeled analogs were silylated in the same fashion and used to create standard response curves.

Stable Isotope-Labeled Standards

7-methylguanine (7-MG) was purchased from Sigma. 7-ethylguanine (7-EG), O^6-methylguanine (O-MG), and O^6-ethylguanine (O-EG) were prepared using published procedures (Beranek et al. 1980; Farmer et al. 1973). Procedures specific for the synthesis of methyl derivatives were modified to yield ethyl derivatives by selecting the corresponding ethyl donating agent. Deuterium-labeled analogs of the four analytes were prepared from the corresponding fully-deuterated methyl or ethyl donating agents. For the synthesis of deuterium-labeled 7-alkylguanines, 2'-deoxyguanosine 5'-monophosphate (Aldrich Chemical Company, Milwaukee, Wisconsin, USA) was dissolved in DMSO and stirred overnight with iodomethane-d_3 (Sigma) or iodoethane-d_5 (Aldrich). The resulting product was precipitated in ethyl acetate and purified by recrystalization. For the synthesis of the deuterated O^6-alkylguanines, either methyl-d_3 alcohol-d (Aldrich) or ethyl-d_5 alcohol-d (Aldrich) was first reacted with sodium metal to form $Na^+O^-CD_3$ or $Na^+O^-C_2D_5$. These products were heated with 2-amino-6-chloropurine (Aldrich) at 70°C overnight in sealed vials. The reactant solutions were neutralized with 3.5 mM glacial acetic acid, solvents removed by evaporation, and the resulting products purified by recrystalization.

The identity and purity of the methylated and ethylated guanine bases and their stable-labeled analogs were confirmed by GC/MS (see below), HPLC with fluorescence detection (Beranek et al. 1980), and UV spectrophotometry (Balsiger and Montgomery 1960). The identity of the derivatized methyl adducts was verified by comparison with reference mass spectra (NIST/EPA/NIH Spectral Library, U.S. Department of Commerce) for 7-methyl-N-(trimethylsilyl)-6-[(trimethylsilyl)oxy]-7H-purin-2-amine.

Quantitative Analysis

The derivatized adduct standards and corresponding alkylated bases isolated from control and exposed biological samples were analyzed using a Hewlett-Packard GC/MS system. A HP 5890 Gas Chromatograph equipped with a 30 m by 0.25 mm ID DB-5 column (J&W Scientific) with a liquid film of 0.25 µm was directly interfaced with a HP 5970 Mass Selective Detector. The column was initially held at 100°C for 3 min and then temperature programmed to 300°C at a rate of 7°C/min, following the method of Dizdaroglu (Dizdaroglu 1993). The transfer line was held at 300°C. Initial spectral identifications and confirmations were carried out using the scanning mode (50-550 amu, at 1.3 scan/s). Three ions were selected for each of the 8 analytes based upon relative abundance and the lack of mass spectral interferences such as column bleed. A selected ion monitoring (SIM) method was then developed based on retention times and characteristic ions of each component. Samples and standards were introduced to the GC using a HP 7673 liquid autosampler set to deliver 2 µL aliquots into a split/splitless injection liner packed with deactivated glass wool and held at 250°C. The electron multiplier was operated at 400 volts above the tune value. Peak areas were determined from the primary (most abundant) ion using a signal-to-noise ratio of at least 2:1 for peak identification.

RESULTS

Table 1 shows the chromatographic and mass spectral parameters for each analyte. Trimethylsilyl-guanine adducts and their deuterated analogs were initially analyzed separately by GC/MS. Examples of extracted ion chromatograms within selected retention time windows for the non-deuterated adduct standards are given in Fig. 2. Their corresponding spectra are shown in Fig. 3. Gas chromatographic retention times of the derivatized adduct standards were very similar to (± <0.05 min) their respective deuterated analogs.

Standard curves were prepared by plotting amount ratios (non-deuterated versus deuterated) over a range representing an average of 30 femtomoles (5 pg) to 6.1 nanomoles (10 ng) of alkylguanines on column. Duplicate dilutions at nine levels of the non-deuterated compound containing a constant amount of its deuterated analog were prepared by lyophilization and derivatization. The primary ion for quantitation was detected at all levels. Regression statistics were generated by plotting amount ratios against response ratios. The standard curves resulted in linear responses (R^2 = 0.998 or greater) across all data points and indicated detection limits as low as femtomoles (10^{-15} moles) on column of DNA adduct. An average sample detection limit of 0.025 ng/mg (150 femtomoles/mg) tissue for both methyl adducts was calculated based upon 10 times the minimum detected level (0.0051 ng), for a 100 mg tissue sample size, a final 100 µl derivatized volume, and a 2 µl injection volume.

Results of DNA adduct analyses from experiment 1, in which levels of 7-MG and O-MG were quantified in fish after a 2 h exposure to MAM-Ac, are shown in Table 2 and Fig. 4. Based on an average of 2 µg of DNA isolated per mg of liver tissue (Strauss 1987), approximately 10 pg (61 femtomoles) O-MG and approximately 50 pg (303 femtomoles) 7-MG per µg DNA were obtained at 24 h post-exposure. Levels of 7-MG were significantly higher in the exposed fish than the controls. No O-MG was detected in the control fish in this experiment.

Results from experiment 2, which were designed to investigate the kinetics of DNA adduct formation and repair over time, are shown in Table 3 and Fig. 5. Recoveries of internal standards were lower than expected. Further investigation has established that the low recoveries were due not to poor or inconsistent extraction of DNA but rather to low yields of derivatized bases associated with effects of residual moisture in the samples and some small losses due to non-specific binding on the chromatographic column. The former problem has now been overcome with better techniques for removal and exclusion of water in the samples prior to and during derivatization and the latter problem has been overcome by use of a column dedicated to DNA adduct analysis. Since recoveries of the deuterated internal standards were lower than expected, statistical inferences could not be made between the groups at each time point. However, variances calculated for both experiments demonstrate that the levels of 7-MG increase rapidly soon after exposure to MAM-Ac, then begin to decline by 48 and 72 h post-exposure. In experiment 2 (Table 3), the levels of 7-MG rose five-fold relative to unexposed controls after one hour and to levels ten-fold higher in the case of 7-MG by 4 h post-exposure. In contrast, although O-MG was detected at levels ten-fold above unexposed controls within the first hour of exposure, levels of O-MG did not appear to substantially increase or decrease by 72 h post-exposure.

TABLE 1--Retention times and characteristic mass fragments of guanine adducts.

Adduct	Retention Time	m/z	Relative Abundance[†]
d_3 O^6-methylguanine	21.83	297	100%
		312	33%
		298	24%
O^6-methylguanine	21.86	294	100%
		309	35%
		295	24%
d_3 7-methylguanine	22.54	297	100%
		312	21%
		298	25%
7-methylguanine	22.56	294	100%
		309	22%
		295	21%
d_5 O^6-ethylguanine	22.31	313	*93%
		328	93%
		329	25%
O^6-ethylguanine	22.38	308	*67%
		323	79%
		324	20%
d_5 7-ethylguanine	22.84	313	100%
		328	22%
		329	13%
7-ethylguanine	22.87	308	100%
		323	20%
		324	52%

*The most abundant masses for the deuterated and non-deuterated O^6 ethylguanines were 280 and 281, respectively, masses seen in liquid phase background bleed of the GC column. Therefore, these masses were not used for SIM analyses.

[†]Spectra obtained under standard tune conditions.

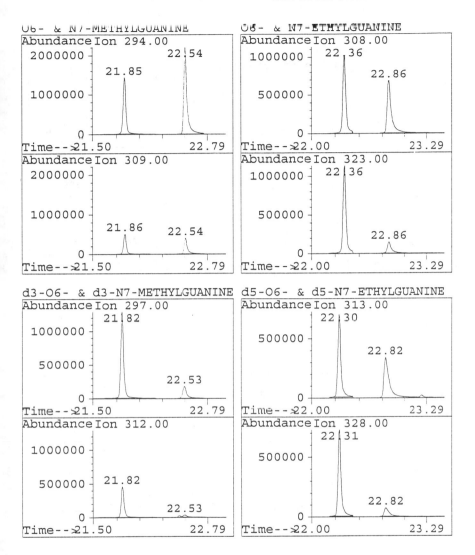

FIG. 2--Extracted ion chromatograms of the four DNA adduct standards and their deuterated analogs.

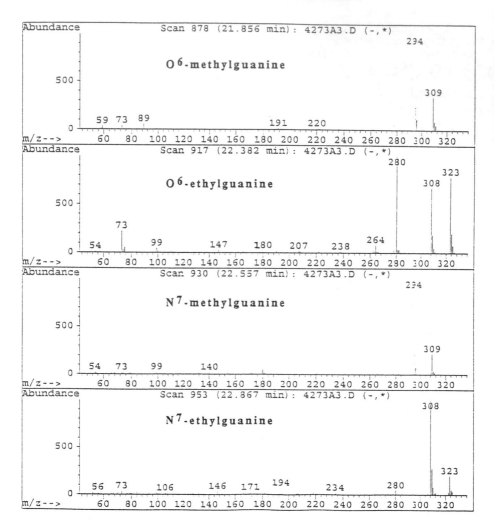

FIG. 3--Mass spectra of the four DNA adduct standards.

TABLE 2--Alkylguanine adduct concentrations in liver DNA of western mosquitofish 24 hr after exposure to 10 ppm MAM-Ac. Results are given for samples of 5 pooled fish from control or exposed groups. Percent recovery of deuterium-labeled standards is also given.

SAMPLE	TISS WT.	Liver tissue concentrations, corr. for recovery				Recovery of deuterated internal standards			
		O-MG	7-MG	O-EG	7-EG	dO-MG	d7-MG	dO-EG	d7-EG
	mg	ng/mg	ng/mg	ng/mg	ng/mg	%	%	%	%
Reag. Blank	...	nd	nd	nd	nd	85%	28%	79%	46%
Control 1	133	nd	0.27	nd	nd	27%	25%	22%	32%
Control 2	167	nd	0.29	nd	nd	30%	27%	24%	32%
Exposed 1	176	0.17	0.36	nd	nd	22%	33%	17%	35%
Exposed 2	152	0.089	0.58	nd	nd	44%	61%	33%	67%
Exposed 3	120	0.11	0.83	nd	nd	52%	77%	40%	83%
MEAN EXPOSED		0.12	0.82						
STD DEV-EXPOSED		0.044	0.14						

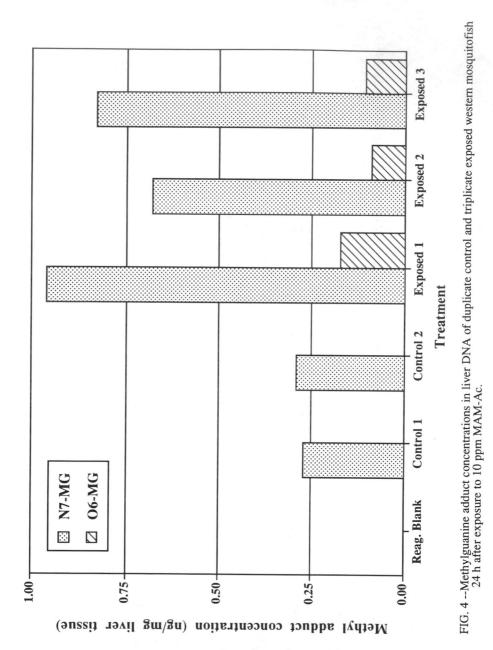

FIG. 4 --Methylguanine adduct concentrations in liver DNA of duplicate control and triplicate exposed western mosquitofish 24 h after exposure to 10 ppm MAM-Ac.

TABLE 3--Alkylguanine adduct concentrations in duplicate (a and b) samples of liver DNA of western mosquitofish before, mid-way through (-1), and after 2 hr pulse exposure to 10 ppm MAM-Ac. The "0, 4, 8, 24, 48, and 72" time points denote time (hrs) of sampling following removal of fish specimens to carcinogen-free water. Percent recovery of deuterium-labeled standards is also given.

TIME POST-EXPOSURE (hrs)	TISS. WT. mg	Liver tissue concentrations, corr. for recovery				Recovery of deuterated internal standards			
		O-MG ng/mg	7-MG ng/mg	O-EG ng/mg	7-EG ng/mg	dO-MG %	d7-MG %	dO-EG %	d7-EG %
Reagent Blank A	66*	0.030	nd	0.010	nd	90%	6%	81%	20%
Reagent Blank B	79*	0.051	0.23	0.050	0.17	40%	3%	31%	7%
Control a	87	0.033	0.28	nd	nd	21%	4%	31%	nd
Control b	87	nd	0.40	nd	0.017	17%	27%	17%	43%
-1a	59	0.37	nd	0.021	nd	16%	nd	23%	4%
-1b	83	0.15	1.2	0.032	0.090	20%	31%	17%	60%
0a	60	0.12	0.91	0.028	nd	16%	5%	31%	nd
0b	74	0.25	1.5	nd	0.050	17%	23%	14%	38%
4a	65	0.11	3.8	0.043	nd	35%	3%	48%	8%
4b	95	0.16	2.7	nd	0.025	16%	14%	17%	14%
8a	76	0.13	2.7	0.033	nd	16%	16%	27%	21%
8b	70	0.30	3.5	nd	0.051	21%	45%	17%	65%
24a	62	nd	2.1	nd	0.16	2%	3%	4%	5%
24b	65	0.36	4.1	nd	0.048	15%	36%	15%	46%
48a	52	0.13	1.7	nd	nd	18%	2%	26%	0%
48b	60	0.30	2.7	0.25	0.46	40%	36%	29%	61%
72a	65	0.11	1.2	nd	nd	19%	2%	29%	nd
72b	99	0.28	1.6	nd	0.038	9%	16%	9%	28%

*average of liver sample weights from each specimen group used for calculation of reagent blank adduct concentrations.

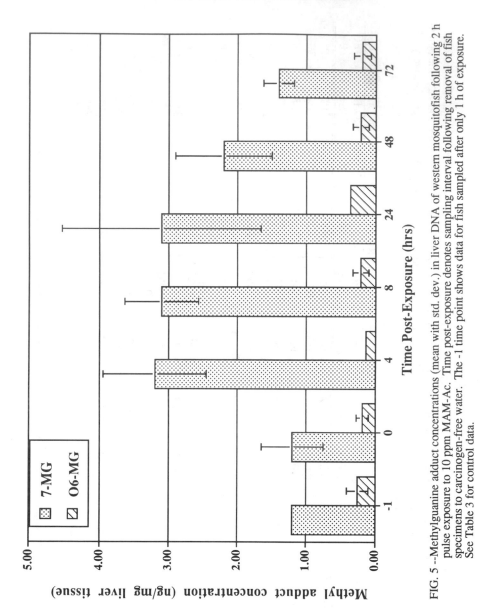

FIG. 5 --Methylguanine adduct concentrations (mean with std. dev.) in liver DNA of western mosquitofish following 2 h pulse exposure to 10 ppm MAM-Ac. Time post-exposure denotes sampling interval following removal of fish specimens to carcinogen-free water. The -1 time point shows data for fish sampled after only 1 h of exposure. See Table 3 for control data.

DISCUSSION

The present study was designed to measure DNA adduct formation and persistence in the liver of western mosquitofish (*Gambusia affinis*) exposed to MAM-Ac. Such baseline information will help to further validate the use of this sentinel species in both laboratory and field studies. Continued development and application of this GC/MS-SIM method for use in other alternative test animals, including other small fish species, and using other alkylating agents, could provide useful mechanistic information on alkylating carcinogenesis in these animals.

MAM-Ac has been shown in histopathology studies to be carcinogenic for several small fish species, including mosquitofish, medaka, guppy, sheepshead minnow, Gulf killifish, inland silverside, Rivulus, and fathead minnow (Aoki and Mastsudaira 1977; Couch and Harshbarger 1985; Fournie et al. 1987; Harada and Hatanaka 1988; Hawkins et al. 1985; Law et al. 1994). However, there are no previous reports concerning *in vivo* alkylation of fish liver DNA by this compound.

Most early studies on carcinogen-DNA adduct formation in aquatic species relied upon the use of radiolabeled carcinogens (Maccubbin 1994). However, studies designed to measure DNA adducts in multiple tissues in whole animals, especially involving previous and/or possibly unknown exposures to environmental mutagens or carcinogens, require alternative methods that do not involve pre-administration of radiolabeled compounds. While ^{32}P-post-labeling may be used to sensitively detect the presence of adducts, the attribution of labeled material to specific pre-cursor compounds in a mixture of unknown agents is not possible. Since stable-isotope-labeled compounds were used in the isotope dilution GC/MS method applied in these studies, this method could be used in both field and laboratory studies, allowing for direct measurements of environmental exposures. GC/MS with selected ion monitoring is a highly versatile method which can identify and quantify specific adducts at extremely low detection limits (femtomole levels) (Maccubbin 1994). A similar method was used by Malins *et al* to detect hydroxyl radical-induced DNA adducts in liver neoplasms of feral English sole from Puget Sound (Malins 1993; Malins et al. 1990).

Other methods that have been used to measure adducts in aquatic species include ^{32}P-postlabeling, immunoassays, and HPLC with fluorescence detection (Cadet and Weinfeld 1993; Maccubbin 1994). ^{32}P-postlabeling, while extremely sensitive, cannot identify the exact chemical structures for specific adducts detected. Immunochemical methods can be sensitive and very specific; however, they are by nature limited to the detection of adducts against which specific monoclonal antibodies have been developed. In addition, these two methods are not useful for detection of unknown adducts. A newer immunochemical method in which specific DNA adducts are isolated by the use of monoclonal antibodies and selective nitrocellulose membranes, then quantitated by polymerase chain reaction, shows some promise (Hochleitner et al. 1991).

MAM-Ac, the aglycone of cycasin, was chosen for this study because its carcinogenic effects in non-human primates, rodents, and small fish species are relatively well-characterized. It is a potent alkylating agent that can kill crucial, dividing cells in developing embryos or neonates as well as cause neoplasia (Johnston et al. 1979). Further, the compound, like many environmental carcinogens, requires metabolic activation for maximum carcinogenic effectiveness. Several target organs are involved in MAM-Ac carcinogenesis. Old World monkeys developed hepatocellular carcinomas, intrahepatic bile duct adenocarcinomas, renal carcinomas and adenomas, squamous cell carcinomas of the esophagus, adenocarcinomas of the small intestine, and adenomatous polyps of the colon in response to chronic MAM-Ac administration (Sieber et al. 1980). Rodents developed liver, kidney, and intestinal tract neoplasia (Laquer and Spatz 1968; Zedeck and Sternberg 1977), along with central nervous system disorders and teratogenic effects such as microencephaly (Spatz 1969). Metabolic activation of MAM-Ac in mammalian species is thought to occur primarily through the action of NAD^+-dependent esterases (Grab and Zedeck 1977).

Fish respond to aqueous MAM-Ac exposure with cytotoxic and neoplastic lesions, the majority of which have been reported in the liver (Hawkins et al. 1985; Law et al. 1994). However, exocrine pancreatic neoplasms (Fournie et al. 1987) and eye neoplasms, thought to be related to retinoblastoma of humans (Hawkins et al. 1986), have been reported. Liver lesions include cytotoxicity, megalocytosis, spindle cell proliferation, foci of cellular alteration, hepatocellular carcinomas, and cholangiocellular carcinomas (Law 1995). Because of this background information, we chose to limit our adduct analyses to the liver.

Table 3 and Fig. 5 show general trends of carcinogen-DNA adduct formation and repair with time following an aqueous pulse exposure to MAM-Ac. However, recoveries of the internal standards will need to be improved with this methodology to lessen sample variability, as well as larger sample numbers used, before definitive conclusions can be drawn concerning DNA repair rates in mosquitofish. Maximal concentrations of 7-MG were detected in liver samples at 4 h post-exposure (PE) and declined through the last sampling period, suggesting in general that repair of this lesion is initiated within 72 h after cessation of exposure. As shown in previous studies with mammalian species (Lawley 1984; Swenson 1983), 7-MG is probably not a critical mutagenic lesion in fish. Nevertheless, its detection could be useful in biomonitoring studies since this adduct is formed early after exposure and at higher levels than other methyl-DNA adducts (Lawley 1984).

Concentrations of O-MG in DNA averaged 12% of the corresponding 7-MG concentrations in DNA at each of the 7 sampling times (Table 3, Fig. 5), which is similar to O-MG:7-MG ratios reported *in vitro* for another methylating agent (N-methyl-N-nitrosourea, 9 to 11%) by Lawley (1984). Alkylation at the O^6 position is thought to have considerably greater biological consequences. This lesion fixes guanine in an unfavorable tautomeric configuration that tends to base-pair with thymine rather than cytosine, leading to transition mutations (Swenson 1983). Once formed, O-MG adducts did not appear to undergo significant repair by 72 h PE. Other workers have concluded that fish have relatively slow rates of repair of alkylguanine adducts at the O^6 position (Maccubbin 1994). Fong *et al* (1988) found in rainbow trout exposed to 250 ppm diethylnitrosamine that, although O^6-alkylguanine-DNA alkyltransferase activity was present, the rate and extent of removal of O-EG was low. They suggested that the enzyme was depleted rapidly and was probably not induced in the liver. The same study demonstrated that 7-ethylguanine and O^6-ethylguanine were removed from liver DNA in a biphasic manner. That is, concentrations of these adducts decreased rapidly from 0 to 12 h PE, but increased slightly between 24 and 48 h PE; no significant decreases in adduct concentrations were found from 12 to 96 h after DEN exposure (Fong et al. 1988). Compounds that must be metabolically activated *in vivo* can show complicated kinetics with regard to DNA adduct formation and repair (Becker and Shank 1985). Depending upon the exposure method, target organ enzyme levels, and depuration from tissue depots such as fat or blood, the opposing processes of adduct formation and repair may occur simultaneously. The results suggest that a more detailed investigation of DNA-repair enzymes, their repair capacities and their reaction kinetics be conducted in this species.

A complicating factor in MAM-Ac-induced carcinogenesis following a single pulse of the chemical is its dual proliferative and anti-proliferative effects. Tumor initiation requires at least one round of cell proliferation for "fixation" of an initiating event such as a mutation arising from DNA adduct formation (Farber and Sarma 1987; Maronpot 1991). MAM-Ac caused nucleolar structural abnormalities as early as 15 min following intravenous administration in rats (Zedeck et al. 1972; Zedeck et al. 1974), suggesting that the compound may interfere with cell replication. Opposing this are the cytotoxic effects of

MAM-Ac which stimulate cell proliferation in the liver through regenerative hyperplasia. In mammalian systems, cell proliferation is no longer effective in tumor initiation after 96 h and most lesions are repaired by that time (Ishikawa et al. 1980; Ying et al. 1982). In mosquitofish, therefore, the formation of critical potentially mutagenic liver cell lesions such as alkylguanine adducts, followed by a round of cell proliferation, would likely occur before 96 h for fixation of tumor initiation to occur. Alternatively, DNA repair mechanisms may be comparatively slower in this species. This awaits further investigation.

Considerable differences in concentrations of methylguanine adducts at 24 h PE were found in identically treated groups of fish in the first set of experiments (Fig. 4). These differences may be attributed to method/instrumental error from both sample preparation/extraction, sample matrix effects, and instrument variability, as well as to biological variability (i.e., individual fish will have different rates of carcinogen metabolism).

Not determined in these experiments was the contribution of RNA to the total number of guanine adducts in each sample. However, the DNA isolation procedure used (Strauss 1987), was selected to specifically minimize the amount of RNA in the extracts.

Carcinogen-DNA adducts formed by aqueous exposure to the alkylating agent, MAM-Ac, were detected at femtomole levels in a small fish model using an isotope dilution GC/mass spectrometry method. Levels of O-MG ranging from approximately 55-185 pg (330-1100 femtomoles) per μg DNA, measured in the first 72 h after exposure, were correlated with a 33% liver tumor incidence after 25 weeks in parallel experiments (Law et al. 1994). Although further studies are needed with this and other carcinogens representing different mechanistic classes and with other small fish species, the method appears to be useful for studies of carcinogens and mutagens in aquatic environments. These findings, along with additional mechanistic studies such as investigations of oncogene activation, tumor suppressor gene inactivation and cellular messages which trigger apoptosis which are currently underway in our laboratory, should also serve to further demonstrate the utility of the western mosquitofish as both an environmental sentinel organism and as a model for carcinogenicity testing in the laboratory.

REFERENCES

Aoki, K. and Mastsudaira, H., "Induction of hepatic tumors in a teleost (*Oryzias latipes*) after treatment with methylazoxymethanol acetate: brief communication," Journal of the National Cancer Institute, 59, 1977, 1747-1749.

Balsiger, R. W. and Montgomery, J. A., "Synthesis of potential anticancer agents. XXV. Preparation of 6-alkoxy-2-aminopurines," Journal of the American Chemical Society, 25, 1960, 1573-1575.

Becker, R. A. and Shank, R. C. "Kinetics of formation and persistence of ethylguanines in DNA of rats and hamsters treated with diethylnitrosamine," Cancer Research, 45, 1985, 2076-2084.

Beland, F. A. and Poirier, M. C., "DNA adducts and carcinogenesis," The Pathobiology of Neoplasia, A. E. Sirica, Ed., Plenum Press, New York, 1989, pp. 57-80.

Beranek, D. T., Weis, C. C., and Swenson, D. H., "A comprehensive quantitative analysis of methylated and ethylated DNA using high pressure liquid chromatography," Carcinogenesis, 1, 1980, 595-606.

Cadet, J. and Weinfeld, M., "Detecting DNA damage," Analytical Chemistry, 65, 1993, 675A-682A.

Couch, J. A. and Harshbarger, J. C., "Effects of carcinogenic agents on aquatic animals: an environmental and experimental overview," Environmental Carcinogenesis Reviews, 3, 1985, 63-105.

Dees, L. T., "The mosquitofish, *Gambusia affinis*," Fishery Leaflet 525, Bureau of Commercial Fisheries, Fish and Wildlife Service, U.S. Department of the Interior, September, 1961.

de Serres, F. J., "Banbury Center DNA adducts workshop, meeting report," Mutation Research, 203, 1988, p. 55.

Dizdaroglu, M., "Quantitative determination of oxidative base damage in DNA by stable isotope-dilution mass spectrometry," FEBS Letters, 1993, 315, 1-6.

Dresler, S. L., "DNA repair mechanisms and carcinogenesis" The Pathobiology of Neoplasia, A. E. Sirica, Ed., Plenum Press, New York, NY, 1989, pp. 173-197.

Farber, E. and Sarma, D. S. R., "Hepatocarcinogenesis: a dynamic cellular perspective," Laboratory Investigation, 56, 1987, 4-22.

Farmer, P. B., Foster, A. B., Jarman, M., and Tisdale, M. J., "The alkylation of 2'-deoxyguanosine and of thymidine with diazoalkanes," Biochemical Journal, 135, 1973, 203-213.

Feinberg, A. and Zedeck, M. S., "Production of a highly reactive alkylating agent from the organospecific carcinogen methylazoxymethanol by alcohol dehydrogenase," Cancer Research, 40, 1980, 4446-4450.

Fong, A. T., Hendricks, J. D., Dashwood, R. H., Van Winkle, S., and Bailey, G. S., "Formation and persistence of ethylguanine in liver DNA of rainbow trout (*Salmo gairdneri*) treated with diethylnitrosamine by water exposure," Food and Chemical Toxicology, 26, 1988, p. 699.

Fournie, J. W., Hawkins, W. E., Overstreet, R. M., and Walker, W. W., "Neoplasms of the exocrine pancreas in guppies *(Poecilia reticulata)* after exposure to methylazoxymethanol acetate," Journal of the National Cancer Institute, 78, 1987, 715-725.

Grab, D. J. and Zedeck, M. S. "Organ-specific effects of the carcinogen methylazoxymethanol related to metabolism by nicotinamide adenine dinucleotide-dependent dehydrogenases," Cancer Research, 37, 1977, 4182-4189.

Harada, T. and Hatanaka, J., "Liver cell carcinomas in the medaka *(Oryzias latipes)* induced by methylazoxymethanol acetate," Journal of Comparative Pathology, 98, 1988, 441-452.

Harris, C. C., "Chemical and physical carcinogenesis: advances and perspectives for the 1990s," Cancer Research, 51 (Suppl.), 1991, 5023s-5044s.

Hawkins, W. E., Fournie, J. W., Overstreet, R. M., and Walker, W. W., "Intraocular neoplasms induced by methylazoxymethanol acetate in Japanese medaka (Oryzias latipes)," Journal of the National Cancer Institute, 76, 1986, 453-365.

Hawkins, W. E., Overstreet, R. M., Fournie, J. W., and Walker, W. W., "Development of aquarium fish models for environmental carcinogenesis: tumor induction in seven species," Journal of Applied Toxicology, 5, 1985, 261-264.

Hawkins, W. E., Overstreet, R. M., and Walker, W. W., "Carcinogenicity tests with small fish species," Aquatic Toxicology, 11, 1988a, 113-128.

Hawkins, W. E., Overstreet R. M., and Walker, W. W., "Small fish models for identifying carcinogens in the aqueous environment," Water Resources Bulletin, 24, 1988b, 941-949.

Hochleitner, K., Thomale, J., Yu.Nikitin, A., and Rajewsky, M. F., "Monoclonal antibody-based, selective isolation of DNA fragments containing an alkylated base to be quantified in defined gene sequences," Nucleic Acids Research, 19, 1991, 4467-4472.

Hoover, K. L., Use of Small Fish Species in Carcinogenicity Testing, National Cancer Institute Monograph 65, NIH Publication No. 84-2653, National Cancer Institute, Bethesda, Maryland, 1984.

Ishikawa, T., Takayama, S., and Kitagawa, T., "Correlation between time of partial hepatectomy after a single treatment with diethylnitrosamine and induction of adenosine triphosphatase-deficient islands in rat liver," Cancer Research, 40, 1980, 4261-4264.

Johnston, M. V., Grzanna, R., and Coyle, J. T., "Methylazoxymethanol treatment of fetal rats results in abnormally dense noradrenergic innervation of neocortex," Science, 203, 1979, 369-371.

Laquer, G. L. and Spatz, M., "Toxicology of cycasin," Cancer Research, 28, 1968, 2262-2267.

Law, J. M., Hawkins, W. E., Overstreet, R. M., and Walker, W. W., "Hepatocarcinogenesis in western mosquitofish (Gambusia affinis) exposed to methylazoxymethanol acetate," Journal of Comparative Pathology, 110, 1994, 117-127.

Law, J. M., Mechanisms of Chemically-induced Hepatocarcinogenesis in Western Mosquitofish (Gambusia affinis), Doctoral Dissertation, Louisiana State University, 1995.

Lawley, P. D., "Carcinogenesis by alkylating agents," Chemical Carcinogens, C. E. Searle, Ed., American Chemical Society Monographs, Washington, DC, 1984, pp. 325-484.

Loveless, A., "Possible relevance of O-6 alkylation of deoxyguanosine to the mutagenicity and carcinogenicity of nitrosamines and nitrosamides," Nature, 223, 1969, 206-207.

Maccubbin, A. E., "DNA adduct analysis in fish: laboratory and field studies, "Aquatic Toxicology: Molecular, Biochemical, and Cellular Perspectives, D. C. Malins and G. K. Ostrander, Eds., Lewis Publishers, Boca Raton, Florida, 1994, pp. 267-294.

Malins, D. C. "Identification of hydroxyl radical-induced lesions in DNA base structure: biomarkers with a putative link to cancer development," Journal of Toxicology and Environmental Health, 40, 1993, 247-261.

Malins, D. C., Ostrander, G. K., Haimanot, R., and Williams, P., "A novel DNA lesion in neoplastic livers of feral fish: 2,6-diamino-4-hydroxy-5-formamidopyrimidine," Carcinogenesis, 11, 1990, 1045-1047.

Maronpot, R. R., "Chemical carcinogenesis," Handbook of Toxicologic Pathology, W. M. Haschek and C. G. Rousseaux, Eds., Academic Press, Inc., San Diego, 1991, pp. 91-130.

McCarthy, J. F. and Shugart, L. R., Biomarkers of Environmental Contamination, Lewis Publishers, Boca Raton, Florida, 1990.

Miller, J. H., "Mutational specificity in bacteria," Annual Review of Genetics, 17, 1983, 215-238.

Shugart, L., Bickham, J., Jackim, G., et al., "DNA alterations," Biomarkers: Biochemical, Physiological, and Histological Markers of Anthropogenic Stress, R. J. Huggett, R. A. Kimerle, P. M. Mehrle, Jr., and H. L. Bergman, Eds., Lewis Publishers, Boca Raton, Florida, 1992, pp. 125-154.

Sieber, S. M., Correa, P., Dalgard, D. W., McIntire, K. R., and Adamson, R. H., "Carcinogenicity and hepatotoxicity of cycasin and its aglycone methylazoxymethanol acetate in nonhuman primates," Journal of the National Cancer Institute, 65, 1980, 177-183.

Singer, B. and Kusmierek J. T., "Chemical mutagenesis," Annual Review of Biochemistry, 52, 1982, 655-693.

Spatz, M., "Toxic and carcinogenic alkylating agents from cycads," Annals of the New York Academy of Science, 163, 1969, 848-859.

Stanton, M. F., "Hepatic neoplasms of aquarium fish exposed to *Cycas circinalis*," Federation Proceedings, 25, 1966, p. 661.

Strauss, W. M., "Preparation of genomic DNA from mammalian tissue," Current Protocols in Molecular Biology," Vol. 1, F. M. Ausubel, R. Brent, and R. E. Kingston, Eds., John Wiley and Sons, Inc., Media, Pennsylvania, 1987, pp. 2.2.1-2.2.3.

Swenson, D. H., "Significance of electrophilic reactivity and especially DNA alkylation in carcinogenesis and mutagenesis," Developments in the Science and Practice of Toxicology, A. W. Hayes, R. C. Schnell, and T. S. Miya, Eds., Elsevier Science Publishers B.V., London, 1983, pp. 247-254.

Swenson, D. H. and Lawley, P. D., "Alkylation of deoxyribonucleic acid by carcinogens dimethyl sulphate, ethyl methanesulphonate, N-ethyl-N-nitrosourea, and N-methyl-N-nitrosourea," Biochemical Journal, 171, 1978, 575-587.

Wogan, G. N., "Detection of DNA damage in studies on cancer etiology and prevention," Methods for Detecting DNA Damaging Agents in Humans: Applications in Cancer Epidemiology and Prevention, H. Bartsch, K. Hemminki, and I. K. O'Neill, Eds., IARC Scientific Publication No. 89, International Agency for Research on Cancer, Lyon, France, 1988, pp. 32-51.

Ying, T. S., Enomoto, K., Sarma, D. S. R., and Farber, E., "Effects of delays in the cell cycle on the induction of preneoplastic and neoplastic lesions in rat liver by 1,2-dimethylhydrazine," Cancer Research, 42, 1982, 876-880.

Zedeck, M. and Sternberg, S. S., "Tumor induction in intact and regenerating liver of adult rats by a single treatment with methylazoxymethanol acetate," Chemico-Biological Interactions, 17, 1977, 291-296.

Zedeck, M. S., Sternberg, S. S., McGowan, J., and Poynter, R. W., "Methylazoxymethanol acetate: induction of tumors and early effects on RNA synthesis," Federation Proceedings, 31, 1972, 1485-1492.

Zedeck, M. S., Sternberg, S. S., Yataganas, X., and McGowan, J., "Early changes induced in rat liver by methylazoxymethanol acetate: mitotic abnormalities and polyploidy," Journal of the National Cancer Institute, 53, 1974, 719-724.

Kirby C. Donnelly, Timothy D. Phillips, Amy M. Onufrock, Shanna L. Collie, Henry J. Huebner an Kenneth S. Washburn

GENOTOXICITY OF MODEL AND COMPLEX MIXTURES OF POLYCYCLIC AROMATIC HYDROCARBONS

REFERENCE: Donnelly, K. C., Phillips, T. D., Onufrock, A. M., Collie, S. L., Huebner, H. J., and Washburn, K. S., **"Genotoxicity of Model and Complex Mixtures of Polycyclic Aromatic Hydrocarbons,"** *Environmental Toxicology and Risk Assessment: Biomarkers and Risk Assessment—Fifth Volume, ASTM STP 1306,* David A. Bengtson and Diane S. Henshel, Eds., American Society for Testing and Materials, 1996.

ABSTRACT: Polycyclic aromatic hydrocarbons (PAHs) are one of the most ubiquitous classes o environmental carcinogens; however, limited information is available to describe their potential genotoxi interactions. This manuscript reports on the interactions of PAHs in complex mixtures as determined i microbial mutagenicity assays. Samples analyzed included separate 2-, 3-, and 4-ring PAH individual mode fractions (IMFs) constructed to simulate the composition of a model coal tar. These were tested individuall and in various combinations, including a reconstituted model fraction (RMF) composed of all three IMFs. solvent extract of coal tar and a benzo(a)pyrene-amended extract of coal tar were also tested. The maximun mutagenic response of 1,089 revertants was induced by the RMF at a dose of 90 µg/plate with metaboli activation. At the four lowest dose levels, the response observed in the RMF sample was increased whe compared to the 4-ring-IMF sample alone. However, the response observed with the RMF sample at th highest dose tested (900 µg/plate) was less than was observed in the 4-ring-IMF sample tested independently When IMF samples were combined or mixed with individual chemicals, some inhibition was observed These data indicate that mixtures of PAHs can exhibit a variety of mutagenic interactions controlled by bot the metabolism of the PAHs and by their concentration in the mixture. This research was supported b NIEHS Grant No. P42-ES04917.

KEYWORDS: PAHs, *Salmonella typhimurium*, TA100, complex mixtures, coal tar, mutagenicity

[1]Assistant professor, professor, graduate research assistants, and postdoctoral research associate respectively, Department of Veterinary Anatomy and Public Health, Texas A&M University, College Station TX 77843-4458.

INTRODUCTION

The exposure of human populations to toxic organic compounds occurs mainly in the form of complex mixtures rather than individual components (NRC 1988). Information is needed to accurately characterize the potential genotoxic interactions of complex environmental mixtures. Of the many classes of organic compounds found in the environment, the polycyclic aromatic hydrocarbons (PAHs) are of special interest because they are frequently found in a variety of products including cigarette smoke, foods, and many types of complex waste mixtures. PAHs are formed during the incomplete combustion of organic materials and are introduced into the environment via natural deposition and anthropogenic processes including wood preserving, coal tar distillation, and petroleum refining. Many of the PAHs are persistent in the environment because of their high C:H ratio, low volatility, high degree of symmetry, and resistance to microbial degradation (Bingham et al. 1980).

In terms of human health, many of the PAHs are considered to be the causitive agents of a variety of adverse effects. Acute exposure to high concentrations of environmental PAHs may produce skin and respiratory irritation, as well as headache, dizziness, and nausea (Genium Publishing Company 1991). The carcinogenic potential of chronic exposure to individual PAHs, as well as complex mixtures of PAHs, is well documented (Harvey 1991; IARC, 1983; Bingham et al. 1980; Blackburn et al. 1986; Tennant et al. 1987); however, little data is available to describe potential mutagenic interactions of PAHs in a complex mixture such as coal tar. Although interactions between individual PAHs are assumed to be strictly additive for purposes of risk assessment, some studies have shown that potential synergistic or antagonistic interactions may occur (DiGiovanni and Slaga 1981; Rao et al. 1979; Kawalek and Andrews 1981; Yoshida and Fukuhara, 1983; Shoeny et al. 1983). Thus, the prediction of risk based on the presence of specific components such as benzo(a)pyrene is simplistic and may not adequately address the possible interactions of components within the mixture and the overall impact on genotoxicity (Tennant et al. 1987). Risk assessment of complex mixtures is thus a difficult task. Current Risk Assessment Guidance for Superfund (RAGS) methodology provides a standardized procedure for estimating risk (U.S. EPA 1989). Given the broad range of exposure pathways and intake variables, the RAGS methods do provide a remarkably comprehensive system; however, improvements are needed to increase the accuracy of risk assessments. Factors that continue to limit the accuracy of a risk assessment, especially for complex mixtures such as coal tar, include interpreting chemical interactions, predicting bioavailability, and estimating toxicity values for unknown chemicals. This report describes initial studies to investigate possible interactions between the components of a complex PAH mixture.

EXPERIMENTAL METHOD

Sample Descriptions

Model PAH fractions This study investigated interactions in two distinct sets of PAH containi samples. The first set was constructed to simulate a coal tar sample obtained from the Electric Po Research Institute (EPRI), Palo Alto, CA. A gas chromatography/mass spectrometry (GC/MS) anal (Hewlet Packard 5890 GC and Hewlet Packard 5790 mass selective detector; Geochemical Environmental Research Group, Texas A & M University, College Station, Texas) of the EPRI coal revealed that the crude sample contained 193.7 µg/g total PAHs (Table 1). Using this data, three PAH fractions were constructed in-house (Dr. S.H. Safe, Department Veterinary Physiology and Pharmacolo Texas A&M University, College Station, TX). Each of these three PAH fractions was formulated represent a 2-, 3-, and 4-ring mixture. The relative composition of individual PAHs in these fractions w similar to that reported for the crude EPRI mixture, except that the benzo(a)pyrene content was increase 0.55% (Chaloupka 1994) The three composite PAH mixtures (based on the number of rings containe each constituent PAH) will be referred to here as individual model fractions (IMFs). The three IMFs w combined to produce a reconstituted model fraction (RMF) that contained approximately the same percent of individual PAHs as the model EPRI coal tar. Each fraction was analyzed by GC/MS to verify composition. Each fraction was subsequently redissolved in dimethyl sulfoxide for biological analyses stored at 4° C.

Midwest coal tar sample A solvent extract was also prepared from a coal tar sample obtained fr an abandoned coal gasification site in the midwestern United States. Prior to extraction, the sample was dr in an oven at 60° C. The sample was sequentially extracted with methylene chloride and methanol usin Tecator Automatic Soxtec procedure (U.S. EPA 1991). Following each extraction, the separate methyl chloride and methanol fractions were transferred to screw-capped tubes, dried under a stream of nitrog and weighed. A dried aliquot of each extract was resuspended in methylene chloride and analyzed by GC/ to verify its composition. All samples were redissolved in dimethyl sulfoxide for biological analyses stored at 4° C.

Mutagenicity Assay

Bacterial mutagenicity of each mixture was determined using the *Salmonella*/microsome pla incorporation assay (Ames et al. 1975; Maron and Ames 1983). *Salmonella typhimurium* strains TA98 an TA100 were provided by Dr. B. N. Ames (University of California, Berkeley, CA). The samples wei tested with and without metabolic activation. Metabolic activation was achieved by using an S9 mixtu containing 30% S9 (9,000g supernatant from Aroclor 1254-induced homogenized Sprague-Dawley r liver; Molecular Toxicology, Annapolis, MD).

Samples and a benzo(a)pyrene (BAP) standard were tested in the standard plate incorporatic assay at a minimum of five dose levels on duplicate plates in two independent experiments. Positi

Table 1. PAH composition of two coal tar samples.

Chemical (ring composition)	EPRI coal tar		Midwest coal tar	
	μg/g	%*	μg/g	%*
Indan (2)	4100	3	ND	--
Naphthalene (2)	43000	31	9600	22
2-methylnaphthalene (2)	42000	31	7000	16
1-methylnaphthalene (2)	24000	18	9000	21
Acenaphthylene (2)	14000	10	8000	18
Acenaphthene (2)	1000	1	2000	5
Dibenzofuran (2)	1200	1	ND	--
Fluorene (2)	7700	6	8300	19
2-ring total	137000	71	43900	31
Phenanthrene (3)	19000	63	30000	60
Anthracene (3)	6100	20	5000	10
Fluoranthene (3)	5300	17	15000	30
3-ring total	30400	16	50000	36
Pyrene (4)	7800	30	17000	12
Benzo(a)anthracene (4)	2600	10	7000	15
Chrysene (4)	2700	10	7000	15
Benzo(b)fluoranthene (4)	1500	6	3000	7
Benzo(k)fluoranthene (4)	700	3	3000	7
Dibenzanthracene (4)	ND	--	500	1
Benzo(a)pyrene (5)	5500	21	4000	9
Benzo(e)pyrene (5)	ND	--	2000	4
Benzo(ghi)perylene (5)	ND	--	2000	4
4-ring total	26300	13	45500	33
Total PAHs	193700		139400	

% denotes percent composition of respective ring fraction or total PAHs for each ring fraction. ND = not detected.

controls included 25 µg/plate of the direct-acting 2-nitrofluorene, and 10 µg/plate of the indirect-acting BAP. Dimethyl sulfoxide served as a negative control. The plates were incubated for 72 hours at 37° C, and revertant colonies were counted with an Artek automated colony counter (Dynatek, Chantilly, VA). The integrity of the genetic characteristics in each tester strain was monitored by performing routine strain checks including sensitivity to crystal violet, ampicillin, and ultraviolet light as well as testing for the existing nutritional markers characteristic of each strain. Baseline data was established by testing each IMF, the combined IMFs (RMF), and the methanol extract of Midwest coal tar in the plate incorporation assay. The IMFs were also tested in the following combinations: 2- and 3-ring IMFs; the 2- and 4-ring IMFs; and the 3- and 4-ring IMFs. Additionally, the RMF was tested in combination with naphthalene, phenanthrene and benzo(a)pyrene. The individual PAHs for each of these mixtures were chosen based on abundance in the GC/MS analysis of the EPRI coal tar. After each bioassay was completed, the data were analyzed using the modified two-fold rule (Chu et al. 1981). A response was considered positive if the number of induced revertants exceeded twice the concurrent negative/solvent control value at two consecutive dose levels.

RESULTS AND DISCUSSION

Chemical Analysis

The composition of the EPRI and Midwest coal tar samples are given in Table 1. The total PAH concentration of the two samples are comparable. The EPRI coal tar contained 193,700 µg PAH per gram of residue, while the Midwest sample had 139,400 µg PAH per gram of residue. Much higher levels of 2-ring components were detected in the EPRI sample, while higher levels of 4-ring components were detected in th Midwest coal tar. The total 4-ring and greater content for the EPRI coal tar was 26,300 µg/g and th Midwest coal tar contained 45,500 µg/g 4-ring and greater PAHs. Higher levels of 3-ring components wer also detected in the Midwest coal tar. These data may reflect the aging of the Midwest coal tar. Since thi material had been contained in an outdoor pit for several decades, much of the lighter PAH fraction may hav been lost due to degradation and volatilization.

Biological analysis

The potential genotoxic interactions of each simulated mixture of PAHs based on the EPRI model coal tar were evaluated using tester strains TA98 and TA100 in the *Salmonella*/microsome plate incorporation assay. Although the mutagenicity data with strain TA98 were dose-dependent (not shown), more detailed analysis focused on strain TA100 mutagenicity due to that strain's stronger and more linear dose response. The mutagenicity of the positive control (BAP) and the 2-, 3-, and 4-ring IMF and RMFs in strain TA100 are presented in Table 2. The data indicate that neither the 2-ring or 3-ring IMF induced a doubling of revertants. At the highest dose tested (900 µg/plate), the RMF appeared to produce a cytotoxic response. Both the 4-ring IMF and RMF induced a mutagenic response. The response induced by the RMF was consistently higher than the 4-ring IMF when tested at equivalent doses. The maximum response induced by the 4-ring IMF was 809 revertants at a dose of 900 µg/plate (Table 2); while the RMF

Table 2. *Salmonella* TA100 mutagenicity of model PAH mixtures.

Chemical mixture	Dose (µg/plate)	Total his[+] revertants/plate[1] + 30% S9
DMSO control	--	154 ± 17
Positive control[2]	--	884 ± 288
Benzo(a)pyrene	4.5	560 ± 18
	9	1182 ± 8
	45	1004 ± 41
	90	881 ± 8
	900	955 ± 28
2-ring IMF	4.5	167 ± 14
	9	176 ± 12
	45	184 ± 1
	90	146 ± 1
	900	101 ± 6
3-ring IMF	4.5	190 ± 21
	9	216 ± 1
	45	207 ± 14
	90	226 ± 16
	900	161 ± 8
4-ring IMF	4.5	192 ± 13
	9	427 ± 89
	45	454 ± 72
	90	628 ± 123
	900	809 ± 238
RMF	4.5	671 ± 127
	9	915 ± 161
	45	954 ± 209
	90	1089 ± 37
	900	69 ± 20

[1]Data reported as mean ± standard deviation.
[2]2-nitrofluorene was employed as direct-acting positive control (without S9) at 25 µg/plate and BAP was employed as indirect-acting positive control (with 30% S9) at 10 µg/plate.

induced 1089 revertants at a dose of 90 μg/plate. At the lowest dose tested (4.5 μg/plate), the 4-ring IMF induced 192 revertants and the combined fractions (RMF) induced 671 revertants. In the bacterial mutagenicity assay, a higher frequency of mutations was observed when the non-mutagenic 2- and 3-ring fractions were combined with the mutagenic 4-ring fraction.

Testing was also conducted by combining separate IMFs and by spiking the RMF with individual chemicals representative of 2-ring (napththalene), 3-ring (phenanthrene) and greater than 4-ring (benzo(a)pyrene) compounds. The data from testing these combined and spiked fractions are presented in Table 3. The mixture of the 2- and 3-ring fractions again failed to induce a positive mutagenic response. The mutagenic response induced by the 4-ring IMF appeared to be reduced by approximately 30% when tested as a mixture with either the 2- or 3-ring fraction. At a dose of 90 μg/plate, the 4-ring fraction induced 628 revertants, while the combined 2- and 4-ring fractions induced 414 total revertants. The mixture of phenanthrene and the 4-ring fraction also induced a reduced response, although naphthalene appeared to have no effect on the 4-ring mixture. The mixture of BAP and the RMF induced a response that was lower than either component tested individually. While the RMF induced 1089 revertants and BAP induced 881 revertants at a dose of 90 μg/plate, the mixture of the RMF and BAP induced only 525 revertants.

Chemical interactions were also studied using the methanol extract of the Midwest coal tar mixed with varying doses of benzo(a)pyrene (BAP). The initial testing of the methylene chloride and methanol extracts of the Midwest coal tar indicated that the maximum mutagenic response was obtained from the methanol extract; therefore, further studies focused only on the methanol extract of the Midwest coal tar. This extract, when spiked with BAP, induced a mutagenic response at all doses tested with metabolic activation. At the three lowest doses the response observed for the mixture was accurately predicted from the individual responses (Figure 1). At a dose of 1.8 μg per plate, BAP induced 783 total revertants and the coal tar induced 100 total revertants at a dose of 50 μg per plate; when tested as a mixture, the BAP and coal tar induced 892 total revertants. At the higher dose levels, there appeared to be a reduced response in the mixture. At a dose of 90 μg per plate, BAP induced 1123 total revertants and the coal tar extract induced 537 total revertants at a dose of 1 mg per plate. When these were tested as a mixture, the observed response was only 772 revertants, or approximately one half that which would be predicted from the individual responses.

CONCLUSIONS

The purpose of this study was to investigate potential genotoxic interactions between individual PAHs and complex mixtures. Information describing potential chemical interactions is important to risk assessment as most toxicity values have been derived from testing single chemicals. Elevated responses were observed at lower doses when the 2- , 3- and 4-ring fractions were tested in combination. When individual chemicals or non-mutagenic fractions were combined with mutagenic fractions, the response was generally lower than was observed for the mutagenic fraction alone   Similar reductions were

Table 3. *Salmonella* TA100 mutagenicity of PAH mixtures.

Chemical mixture	Dose (µg/plate)	Total his[+] revertants/plate[1]	
		- S9	+ 30% S9
DMSO control	0	153 ± 11	176 ± 18
Positive control[2]	--	1182 ±7	435 ± 28
Benzo(a)pyrene	90	NT[3]	881 ± 8
2-ring	90	47±5	146±1
3-ring	90	56±1	226±16
4-ring	90	66±1	628±123
2- and 3-ring	90	124 ± 1	176 ± 1
3- and 4-ring	90	125 ± 3	426 ± 58
2- and 4-ring	90	139 ± 6	414 ± 69
Reconstituted 2-,3-,4-ring	90	35 ± 13	1089 ± 37
Naphthalene and 2-,3-,4-ring	90	126 ± 4	629 ± 37
Phenanthrene and 2-,3-,4-ring	90	115 ± 14	472 ± 35
Benzo(a)pyrene and 2-,3-,4-ring	90	133 ± 14	525 ± 28

[1]Data reported as mean ± standard deviation.
[2] 2-nitrofluorene was employed as direct-acting positive control (without S9) at 25 µg/plate and BAP was employed as indirect-acting positive control (with 30% S9) at µg/plate.
[3]Not tested.

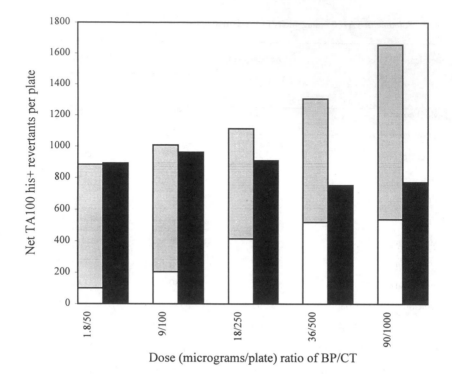

Figure 1.   Mutagenicity, as measured in strain TA100, of a BAP and coal tar (BP/CT) mixture and individual coal tar and BAP extracts. (Predicted response from individual components: BAP alone is represented by the gray column, coal tar alone by the white column; Observed response from BAP-spiked coal is represented by the black column.)

observed when BAP was combined with the RMF sample or crude extract of coal tar The data indicate that chemical interactions are highly dose-dependent and that it will be difficult to predict the genotoxic potential of a complex mixture for the purpose of risk assessment. These studies have also indicated that the genotoxicity of a complex mixture cannot be predicted from BAP content alone. In most cases the observed genotoxicity of the BAP:coal tar mixture was less than that predicted from the additive response of the BAP plus coal tar; and at the highest dose, the observed mutagenic response of the BAP:coal tar mixture was less than that of the BAP alone Additional research using *in vitro* bioassays of individual chemicals and mixtures could thus provide much-needed information to assist in risk assessment of complex mixtures

ACKNOWLEDGMENTS

The authors wish to thank Dr. L. Goldstein of the Electric Power Research Institute for supplying the model coal tar, Dr. L.-Y. He for chemical extractions and Dr. S. Safe for preparing the simulated model fractions.

REFERENCES

Ames, B. N., McCann, J., and Yamaski, E., 1975, "Methods for detecting carcinogens and mutagens with the *Salmonella*/mammalian-microsome mutagenicity test," Mutation Research, Vol. 31, pp. 347-364.

Bingham, E., Trosset, R. P. and Warshawsky, D., 1980, "Carcinogenic potential of petroleum hydrocarbons: a critical review of the literature," Journal of Environmental Pathology and Toxicology, Vol. 3, pp. 483-563.

Blackburn, G. R., Deitch, R. A., Schreiner, C. A., and Mackerer, C. R., 1986, "Predicting carcinogenicity of petroleum distillation fractions using a modified *Salmonella* mutagenicity assay," Cell Biology and Toxicology, Vol. 2, No. 1, pp. 63-84.

Chaloupka, K. J., 1994. "Complex mixtures of polynuclear aromatic hydrocarbons as Ah receptor agonists." PhD dissertation, Texas A&M University.

Chu, K. C., Patel, K. M., Lin, H. A., Tarone, R. E., Linhart, M. S., and Dunkel, V. C., 1981, "Evaluating statistical analyses and reproducibility of microbial mutagenicity assays," Mutation Research, Vol. 85, pp. 119-132.

DiGiovanni, D. J. and Slaga, T. J., 1981,"Modification of polycyclic aromatic hydrocarbon carcinogenesis," Polycyclic Hydrocarbons and Cancer, H. V. Gelboin and P. O. P. Ts'O, Eds., Academic Press, New York.

Genium Publishing Company, 1991, "Material Safety Data Sheets: Coal Tar Creosote," Sheet No. 757. Genium Publishing Company, Schenectady, NY.

Harvey, R. G., 1991, Polycyclic Aromatic Hydrocarbons: Chemistry and Carcinogenicity, Cambridge University Press, Cambridge.

Kawalek, J. C. and Andrews, A. W., 1981, "Effects of aromatic hydrocarbons on the metabolism of 2-aminoanthracene to mutagenic products in the Ames assay," Carcinogenesis, Vol. 2, No. 12, pp. 1367-1369.

Maron, D. M., and Ames, B. N., 1983, "Revised methods for the *Salmonella* mutagenicity test," Mutation Research, Vol. 113, pp. 173-215.

National Research Council (NRC), 1988. "Complex mixtures: Methods for in vivo toxicity testing," National Academy Press, Washington, DC.

Rao, T. K., Young, J. A., Weeks, C. E., Slaga, T. J., and Epler, J. L., 1979, "Effect of the co-carcinogen benzo(e)pyrene on microsome-mediated chemical mutagenesis in *Salmonella typhimurium*," Environmental Mutagenesis, Vol. 1, pp. 105-112.

Schoeny, R., Warshawsky, D., and Moore, G., 1983, "Non-additive mutagenic responses by components of coal-derived materials," Environmental Mutagenesis, Vol. 8, No. 6, p. 73.

Tennant, R. W., Margolin, B. H., Shelby, M. D., Zeiger, E., Haseman, J. K., Spalding, J., Caspary, W., Resnick, M., Stasiewics, S., Anderson, B., and Minor, R., 1987, "Prediction of chemical carcinogenicity in rodents from *in vitro* genetic toxicity assays," Science, Vol. 236, pp. 933-941.

U.S. Environmental Protection Agency (EPA), 1989, "Risk Assessment Guidance for Superfund: Human Health Evaluation Manual, Part A," OSWER DIRECTIVE 9285.4-1. Office of Emergency and Remedial Response, Washington, DC.

U.S. Environmental Protection Agency (EPA), 1991, "Development of a Soxtec Extraction Procedure for Extracting Organic Compounds from Soils and Sediments," Office of Research and Development, Environmental Monitoring Systems Laboratory: Las Vegas, NV, 1991; EPA-600/X-91-140.

Yoshida, D. and Fukuhara, Y., 1983, "Mutagenicity and co-mutagenicity of catechol on *Salmonella*," Mutation Research, Vol. 120, pp. 7-11.

W.A. Rees[1,2], S. Kwiatkowski[4], S.D. Stanley[5], D.E. Granstrom[2], J-M. Yang[6], C.G. Gairola[1,3], D. Drake[4], J. Glowczyk[4], W.E.Woods[2], and T. Tobin[1,2]

DEVELOPMENT AND CHARACTERIZATION OF AN ELISA FOR *trans*-3-HYDROXYCOTININE, A BIOMARKER FOR MAINSTREAM AND SIDESTREAM SMOKE EXPOSURE.

REFERENCE: Rees, W. A., Kwiatkowski, S., Stanley, S. D., Granstrom, D. E., Yang, J-M., Gairola, C. G., Drake, D., Glowczyk, J., Woods, W. E., and Tobin, T., **"The Development and Characterization of an ELISA for *trans*-3-hydroxycotinine, a Biomarker for Mainstream and Sidestream Smoke Exposure,"** *Environmental Toxicology and Risk Assessment: Biomarkers and Risk Assessment—Fifth Volume, ASTM STP 1306,* David A. Bengtson and Diane S. Henshel, Eds., American Society for Testing and Materials, 1996.

Abstract: *trans*-3-Hydroxycotinine is the major urinary metabolite of nicotine in man and can serve as an important biomarker of tobacco smoke exposure. A sensitive ELISA test for *trans*-3-hydroxycotinine was developed with an I-50 for this nicotine biomarker of between 1.0-3.0 ng/ml. This ELISA test has about 10 fold less affinity for cotinine and 1000-fold less affinity for nicotine and other nicotine metabolites. No matrix effects were detectable in human saliva and relatively small matrix effects (I-50 for *trans*-3-hydroxycotinine, about 25 ng/ml) in urine was observed. The assay readily detected levels of apparent *trans*-3-hydroxycotinine in urine samples from smoke-exposed mice and rats. This ELISA is therefore a sensitive test for the determination of *trans*-3-hydroxycotinine in plasma, saliva, and urine samples from humans and animals, and can be used to monitor exposure to tobacco smoke or nicotine.

Keywords: Enzyme-Linked Immunosorbant Assay, nicotine, t-3-hydroxycotinine, cotinine, metabolite

Active and passive exposure to tobacco smoke is associated with a number of health effects in exposed populations. While considerable data on health-related effects of smoking has accumulated, it has been difficult to accurately quantify tobacco smoke exposure in individuals, especially passive smokers. Various biomarkers, e.g., blood levels of nicotine and its metabolites, isocyanide, carboxyhemoglobin and urinary mutagens, etc., have been employed in attempts to assess tobacco smoke exposures. In this regard, nicotine is generally seen as a specific biomarker of tobacco smoke exposure as it is an important,

The Graduate Center for Toxicology[1], The Maxwell Gluck Equine Research Center[2], Tobacco and Health Research Institute[3], Dept. of Plastic Surgery[4], University of Kentucky, Lexington, Kentucky 40546-0099

Dept. of Chemistry University of Warsaw, Poland[4]

Truesdail Laboratories, Inc.[5], Tustin, California

Duke University Medical Center[6], Durham, N.C.

pharmacologically active constituent of tobacco and is found at significant concentrations only in tobacco plants.

On the other hand, nicotine's plasma half-life is short, and it is found only in relatively low concentrations in the blood and urine of active and passive smokers (Kyerematen et al., 1990). In experimental animals it is especially difficult to accurately assess smoke exposure not only because the nicotine concentrations are low, but also because the sample size is generally small. What is required is a highly sensitive detection method for a non-invasive biomarker of passive smoke or nicotine exposure.

trans-3-Hydroxycotinine, the major urinary metabolite of nicotine, possesses many characteristics required of a biomarker for monitoring tobacco smoke exposures. Its steady state levels in plasma are several-fold higher than those of nicotine, reaching concentrations as high as 115 to 160 ng/ml or higher in the plasma of smokers (Kyerematen et al., 1991); additionally, the steady state levels of trans-3-hydroxycotinine in human plasma are directly related to nicotine intake (Neurath et al., 1988). Another advantage is that its plasma half-life is relatively long (6 hours) (Neurath et al., 1988), which means that it can serve as an integrative biomarker of nicotine exposure. A further advantage is that trans-3-hydroxycotinine levels in human urine tend to be substantially higher than plasma levels of nicotine and persist for longer periods. These characteristics make trans-3-hydroxycotinine a potentially very useful biomarker of tobacco smoke exposure in humans (Watts et al., 1990).

As part of an effort to characterize animal models for studying the inhalation toxicity of tobacco smoke, a rapid, sensitive and inexpensive routine method to quantify the exposure of humans and animals to cigarette smoke was developed. Immunoassay, specifically Enzyme-Linked Immunosorbent Assay (ELISA), is one of the few analytical techniques that can readily detect circulating concentrations of cotinine or trans-3-hydroxycotinine (Benkirane, et al., 1991; Langone et al., 1973; Kyerematen et al., 1990). In this regard, an ELISA which detected low levels of cotinine in humans and animal fluids was previously developed.

This report details the development and characterization of a highly sensitive ELISA for trans-3-hydroxycotinine; we outline the characteristics of this ELISA, and its application to the detection of this agent in saliva specimens from man and plasma and urine specimens from laboratory animals. This trans-3-hydroxycotinine test may be used as an alternative to or in conjunction with the cotinine ELISA allowing for more accurate quantification of tobacco smoke exposure.

Published as #183 from the Maxwell H. Gluck Equine Research Center and the Department of Veterinary Science, University of Kentucky.

Published as Kentucky Agricultural Experimental Station Article #92-4-167 with approval of the Dean and Director, College of Agriculture and Kentucky Agricultural Experiment Station.

Supported by grants entitled "Detection of Nicotine and Cotinine by Enzyme-Linked Immunosorbant Assay" from the Kentucky Tobacco Research Board.

MATERIALS AND METHODS

Animals:

New Zealand White rabbits 3-4 years old were used to raise the anti-*trans*-3-hydroxycotinine antibody. Samples of plasma and urine were obtained from rats and mice following exposure to tobacco smoke as previously described (Gairola, 1986). These samples were collected as part of an ongoing study and held frozen at 4°C prior to analysis. All animal experiments were performed according to the protocols approved by the University of Kentucky Institutional Animal Care and Use Committee operated under PHS Animal Welfare Assurance A3336-01. These rabitts were fed Agway Rabbit Chow *ad lib* under 8 hours of light at 62°F.

Human Subjects:

Saliva specimens collected from the Department of Plastic Surgery, University of Kentucky were used to evaluate the assay. These samples were collected as part of a previous study concerning patient pre- and post-operative surgery health status and had been stored at 4°C for 2 years. Blind samples from 30 volunteer subjects were chosen from a total group of approximately 50 individuals for analysis. The status of the individual (smoker or non-smoker) remained unknown until the assay results were completed. A series of human urine samples from non-smokers was provided by the University of Kentucky Medical Center Clinical Toxicology Laboratories. These samples were collected for clinical evaluation and were released for analysis once the specimen had been cleared by the clinical toxicology laboratory. Four of these urine samples were pooled and the pooled sample was used for the preparation of standard curves in the matrix studies.

Hapten Synthesis and Conjugation

The *trans*-3-hydroxycotinine hapten possessing a carboxylic group in the β-position of the pyridine ring was synthesized as follows. Methyl 5-formylnicotinate was synthesized according to the procedure given by Wenkert (1970) and purified by silica-gel chromatography. This aldehyde was used in the preparation of N-methyl-5-carboxymethylpyridil nitrone and applied afterwards in the 1,3-dipolarcycloaddition to methyl acrylate. The mixture of the diastereoisomeric isoxazolidines obtained was then reduced over Nickel-Raney catalyst yielding a mixture of ($\pm$)-*cis* and ($\pm$)- *trans*-3-pyrrolidone derivatives. The separation of single diastereoisomeric racemates was reached via silica-gel chromatography. The less polar ($\pm$) -*trans*-isomer structure was assigned by comparison of its hydrogen nuclear magnetic resonance (H-NMR) spectrum with the data given in the paper of Dagne (1972) for the natural *trans*-3-hydroxycotinine. The H-NMR spectrum of the ($\pm$) *cis* isomer corresponded well with the data given in the same paper for *cis*-3-hydroxycotinine.

The resulting compound was then covalently linked to both bovine serum albumin (BSA) and horseradish peroxidase (HRP)(Zymed Labs, So. San Francisco, CA). The coupling of the carboxyl compound to the different proteins was as follows. The *trans*-3-hydroxycotinine derivative (0.3 mg) was dissolved in 0.3 ml anhydrous dimethylformamide (DMF) at 0°C with $2\mu l$ of triethylamine (Reagent 1). Reagent 2 consisted of $5\mu l$ isobutyl chloroformate per milliliter DMF (precooled to 0°C). Next, $100\mu l$ of Reagent 2 was added to Reagent 1, mixed well and allowed to stand at 0°C for 15 minutes. The protein of choice (BSA or HRP) (0.8 mg dissolved in 1.2 ml H_2O plus 0.18 ml of 50 mM Na_2CO_3) was added to the above mixture and sealed with parafilm. The reaction mixture was rotated overnight at 4°C and then dialyzed against phosphate buffered saline extensively. A portion of the purified derivative-protein mixture was taken and stored at 4°C ready for use (Wie and Hammock, 1982).

ELISA Procedures:

The *trans*-3-hydroxycotinine ELISA developed here was similar in format to those reported by Stanley and co-workers (1991). A dilute solution of Protein-A (200ul@200mg/ml)(Genzyme, Boston,MA.) was first applied to the bottom of microtiter wells (Costar Corp., Cambridge, MA), then the *trans*-3-hydroxycotinine antiserum (100ul)(used without further purification) was non-covalently coated (Voller et al., 1976) to the Protein-A coated wells. Authentic *trans*-3-hydroxycotinine and analog standards were prepared in methanol and diluted to appropriate concentrations in assay buffer (0.1M potassium phosphate buffered saline, pH 7.4 with 0.1% bovine serum albumin) or biological fluids. *trans*-3-hydroxycotinine, nicotine-N-oxide, cotinine-N-oxide, *cis*-3'-hydroxycotinine, and dimethylcotinine were kindly provided by J. Donald deBethizy (RJR-Nabisco, Winston-Salem, N.C.).

All assays were performed at room temperature. The assay was started by adding 20 μl of the standard, test, or control samples to each well, along with 180 μl of *trans*-3-hydroxycotinine-HRP conjugate solution. After an incubation period of 1 hr, the wells were washed with wash buffer (0.01M phosphate buffer, pH 7.4 with 0.05% Tween-20) and 150 μl of KY Blue ELISA substrate (ELISA Technologies, Lexington, KY.) were added to each well. The optical density (OD) of each well was read at a wavelength of 650 nm with an automated microplate reader (EL310 Microplate Autoreader, Bio-Tek Inc., Winooski, VT) approximately 30 min after addition of the substrate.

During the assay, the presence of unbound *trans*-3-hydroxycotinine in the standard or test sample competitively prevented the binding of the *trans*-3-hydroxycotinine-HRP complex to the antibody present in the antiserum. Since the reaction of KY Blue substrate with HRP was responsible for the color (blue) production in the ELISA, the apparent concentration of *trans*-3-hydroxycotinine in the sample was inversely related to the OD_{650} of the well. Apparent *trans*-3-hydroxycotinine concentrations in biological specimens were calculated based on standard curves which were run in duplicate with each individual assay.

RESULTS

Figure 1 illustrates the standard inhibition curves that were constructed to determine the sensitivity and specificity of the *trans*-3-hydroxycotinine antiserum using various metabolites of nicotine and related compounds. *trans*-3-Hydroxyotinine inhibited the ELISA with an I-50 (analyte concentration at half-maximal inhibition) of about 3.0 ng/ml, and this ELISA test also exhibited a 10 fold lower affinity for cotinine and *cis*-3-hydroxycotinine. Other tested congeners (dimethyl-cotinine, nicotine, nicotine N-oxide, nicotimamide, nicotinic acid, nikethamide, niacinamide) showed minimal cross-reactivity, and several hundred fold higher concentrations were needed to inhibit the test.

Matrix or background effects can severely limit the usefulness of ELISA tests by changing their sensitivity. Therefore the apparent shifts in I-50 values were determined when the standard curves were prepared in different biological matrices, i.e., rat plasma and urine; human saliva and urine. Standards prepared in human saliva showed virtually no matrix effects (Fig. 2) while rat plasma exhibited minimal matrix effects (Fig. 4). While the apparent I-50 for samples prepared in human urine increased about 10-fold (Fig. 2), the samples prepared in rat urine increased about 20-fold (Figure 3).

The ability of this test to detect apparent *trans*-3-hydroxycotinine was evaluated in urine samples collected from smoke-

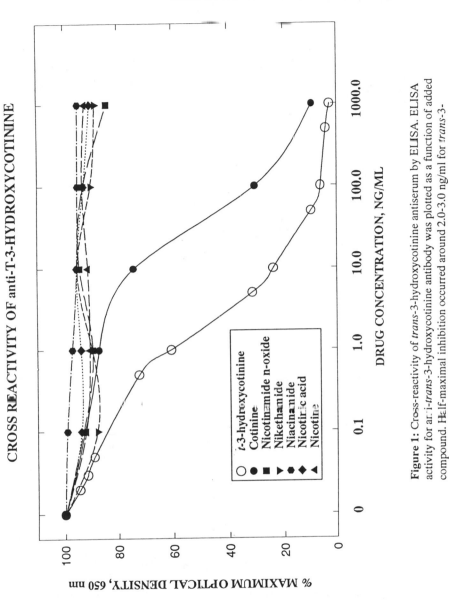

Figure 1: Cross-reactivity of *trans*-3-hydroxycotinine antiserum by ELISA. ELISA activity for an-i-*trans*-3-hydroxycotinine antibody was plotted as a function of added compound. Half-maximal inhibition occurred around 2.0-3.0 ng/ml for *trans*-3-hydroxycotinine.

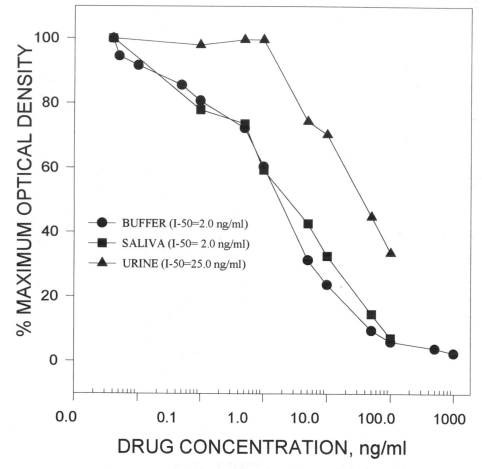

Figure 2: Sample matrix effects of *trans*-3-hydroxycotinine ELISA standard curve. The symbols show an increase of the inhibition of the ELISA by *trans*-3-hydroxycotinine in the presence of buffer, and 20ul of human saliva or urine.

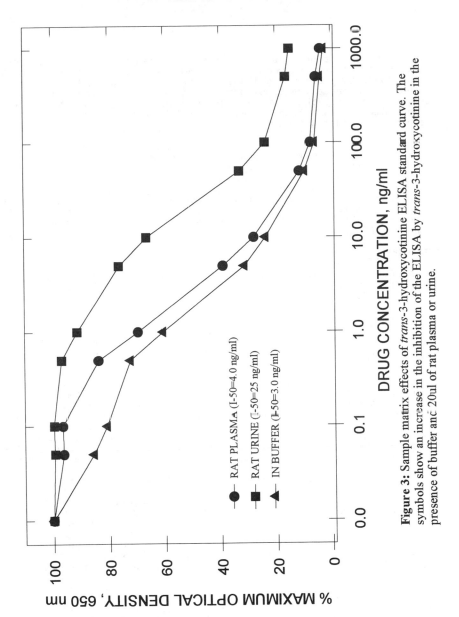

Figure 3: Sample matrix effects of *trans*-3-hydroxycotinine ELISA standard curve. The symbols show an increase in the inhibition of the ELISA by *trans*-3-hydroxycotinine in the presence of buffer and 20ul of rat plasma or urine.

exposed rats. The test clearly differentiated between the smoke exposed and unexposed groups of animals (P>.05) (Fig. 4).

This ELISA was next used to estimate the salivary concentrations of apparent *trans*-3-hydroxycotinine in human smokers and nonsmokers. The test was found to readily distinguish between these groups (P>.05). A series of 30 human saliva samples were analyzed in a blind study utilizing this test. The *trans*-3-hydroxycotinine levels of the saliva samples from smokers averaged 386.9 ng/ml, while those from the non-smokers averaged 3.6 ng/ml (Fig. 5).

Similarly, 40 urine samples from approximately 20 smoke-exposed mice (A.M. and P.M. collection) and 20 unexposed mice (A.M. and P.M. collection) were analyzed for *trans*-3-hydroxycotinine. Again, not only did this test clearly differentiate between the two groups of mice, but also between mainstream and sidestream smoke-exposed mice (P>.05). The mean concentration of apparent *trans*-3-hydroxycotinine in (P.M.) urine samples from smoke-exposed mice was 3760.4 ng/ml, with a range of 1054.2 ng/ml to 8720.8 ng/ml, while the samples from unexposed animals averaged 34.0 ng/ml (Figure 6).

DISCUSSION

An ELISA for *trans*-3-hydroxycotinine was developed that detected this major urinary metabolite of nicotine with an apparent I-50 of about 3.0 ng/ml. This test was relatively specific for *trans*-3-hydroxycotinine in that it has a 10 fold higher apparent affinity for *trans*-3-hydroxycotinine than for cotinine or *cis*-3-hydroxycotinine; in human urine the *trans* form predominates over the *cis* form (>98%). This test is essentially unreactive with nicotine and its other metabolites since this antibody has 1,000 times less affinity for these agents than *trans*-3-hydroxycotinine.

In addition to its sensitivity, this test is relatively resistant to interfering materials in biological samples. When this test was run in the presence of 20 μl of human saliva, the apparent I-50 for *trans*-3-hydroxycotinine was not significantly affected; when the test was run in the presence of human urine, the I-50 was reduced about 10-fold. Urine samples of many species affectively contain substances that cause some background interference. It has been our experience with other ELISA's that these background effects are best controlled by sample dilution.

This apparent resistance to matrix effects or interfering substances in matrix is a useful characteristic of this ELISA. No immunoassay based test is entirely free of matrix effects, and the utility of an immunoassay is determined largely by its sensitivity for the analyte of choice, and its ability to distinguish between the analyte and extraneous material. This is especially true for tests such as a *trans*-3-hydroxycotinine ELISA, which may be required to detect very low levels of *trans*-3-hydroxycotinine as in small experimental animal (mouse) models or in epidemiological studies on environmental tobacco smoke.

The ELISA results from the whole body smoked-exposed rat urine samples (6 smoked and 2 control) showed low levels of *trans*-3-hydroxycotinine and high levels of cotinine. In humans, the *trans*-3-hydroxycotinine metabolite has been suggested as a better biomarker of tobacco smoke exposure because it is more abundant in smokers than the cotinine metabolite, due to the production in humans of a *trans*-3-hydroxycotinine glucuronide. In rats, however, there are two other metabolites that are longer lived than cotinine, cotinine-N-oxide and 2'-hydroxydemethylcotinine (Kyerematen et. al. 1991). Our results are

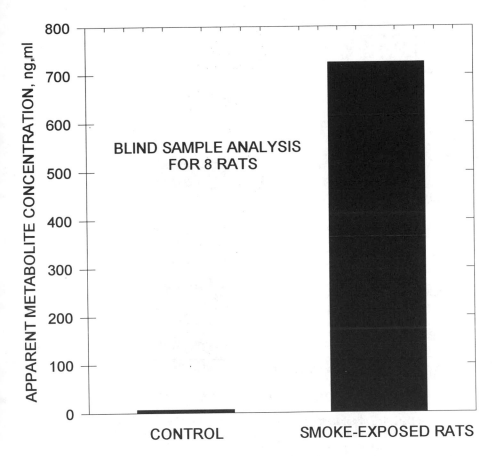

Figure 4: Detection of apparent *trans*-3-hydroxycotinine metabolite from rat urine specimens using the *trans*-3-hydroxycotinine ELISA. The right hand bar indicates the apparent urine levels of *trans*-3-hydroxycotinine in six smoke-exposed rats, while the left hand bar indicates the apparent urine levels in two control rats.

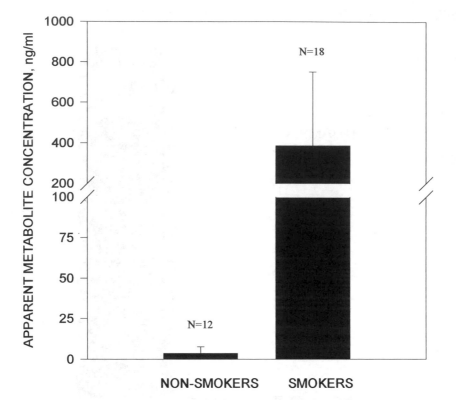

Figure 5: Detection of apparent *trans*-3-hydroxycotinine from human saliva specimens using the *trans*-3-hydroxycotinine ELISA. The left hand bar shows the apparent saliva levels of *trans*-3-hydroxycotinine in nonsmokers, while the right hand bar shows the apparent saliva levels in smokers. The errror bars represent the standard error of the mean.

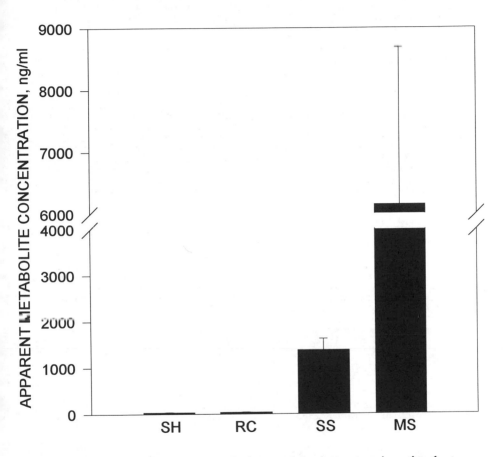

Figure 6: Detection of apparent *trans*-3-hydroxycotinine in mouse urine using the *trans*-3-hydroxycotinine ELISA. The bars indicate (from right to left) the route of administration of smoke to four groups of five rats per group e.g. main-stream(MS), side-stream(SS), or control (sham and room) mice. The error bars indicate the standard error of the mean.

consistent with those of Kyerematen in that they also found less *trans*-3-hydroxycotinine than cotinine in the rats after tobacco smoke exposure.

Also, from an analytical standpoint there have been reports indicating procedural problems when extracting the *trans*-3-hydroxycotinine metabolite due to its high water solubility making the detection of *trans*-3-hydroxycotinine difficult by HPLC or GC/MS. This problem may be resolved by using this ELISA assay which requires no extraction procedure.

Experiments using smoked-exposed mice further established the sensitivity and utility of this *trans*-3-hydroxycotinine ELISA. To our knowledge this is the first study which suggests that there is a *trans*-3-hydroxycotinine metabolite produced in mice. After analysis with both the cotinine and *trans*-3-hydroxycotinine ELISA's, we found that the apparent levels of *trans*-3-hydroxycotinine were higher than those of cotinine. In this case, cotinine may have artificially raised the *trans*-3-hydroxycotinine levels due to cross-reaction; however, because *trans*-3-hydroxycotinine was found in greater amounts compared to cotinine, our work strongly suggests that this metabolite exists in mice exposed to tobacco smoke. We were also impressed by the assay's ability to discern between the two routes of administration of the smoke e.g. mainstream smoke exposure and sidestream smoke exposure. These data clearly suggest the potential for application of this assay when assessing animal models for tobacco smoke exposure.

Finally, the ability of this test to detect *trans*-3-hydroxycotinine in saliva samples from human smokers and nonsmokers was evaluated. This test appeared to be remarkably sensitive when it was used to distinguish between salivary samples from self-declared smokers and non-smokers. As shown in Figure 6, the saliva levels of *trans*-3-hydroxycotinine in samples from about 30 smokers averaged 386.9 ng/ml of apparent *trans*-3-hydroxycotinine, while those from non-smokers averaged about 3.6 ng/ml, close to a one hundred fold difference in apparent *trans*-3-hydroxycotinine levels.

The very low backgrounds found in salivary samples and the relative ease and non-invasiveness of collection of this sample makes salivary sampling a very attractive testing mode. Beyond this, recent opinion in this field suggests that saliva or serum are likely to yield the most useful data concerning relative exposure to nicotine (Watts et al., 1990). In this regard, the problem with urine is that volume, pH, urine flow and renal function are unpredictable variables (Watts et al., 1990) and correcting for creatine content, a suggested maneuver (Hoffmann and Brunemann, 1983), is only a partial solution; this is because creatine excretion rates are quite variable between individuals.

These data are entirely consistent with what is known of the metabolism and disposition of *trans*-3-hydroxycotinine in man (Bjercke et al., 1986; Kyerematen et al., 1990; Watts et al., 1990). *trans*-3-Hydroxycotinine is the major metabolite found in plasma and its plasma half-life, at approximately 6 hours, is relatively long. *trans*-3-Hydroxycotinine is therefore a highly effective biological marker of nicotine exposure. Because of the very low matrix or background effect in urine and saliva when using this ELISA, both of these biological fluids provide excellent means to distinguish between smokers and non-smokers when using *trans*-3-hydroxycotinine as a biological marker. An additional useful feature of this assay concerns the difficult extraction procedure currently used in isolating the *trans*-3-hydroxycotinine metabolite from biological fluids. Simply stated ELISA's

need no sample preparation which allow for quick and easy metabolite
identification. We also have raised questions regarding the production
of the *trans*-3-hydroxycotinine metabolite in mouse, and we hope to
pursue this issue in the future utilizing the high sensitivity of this
ELISA.

REFERENCES

Benkirane, S., A. Nicolas, M.-M. Galteau, and G. Siest. 1991. Highly
sensitive immuno-assays for the determination of cotinine in serum and
saliva: Comparison between RIA and an avidin-biotin ELISA. *Eur J Clin
Chem Clin Biochem*. 29.405-410.

Benowitz, N.L. 1983. *The use of biologic fluid samples in assessing
tobacco smoke consumption. Measurement in analysis and treatment of
smoking behavior*. Eds. J. Grabowski and C.S. Bell. NIDA Research
Monograph #48. U.S. Government Printing Office, Washington, D.C.

Bjercke, R., G. Cook, N. Rychlik, H. Gjika, H. Van Vunakis, and J.
Langone. 1986. Stereospecific monoclonal antibodies to nicotine and
cotinine and their use in enzyme-linked immunosorbent assay. *J Immunol
Meth*. 90:203-213.

Bridges, R.B., J.G. Combs, J.W. Humble, J.A. Turbek, S.R. Rehm, and
N.J. Haley. 1990. Population characterisitcs and cigarette yield as
determinants of smoke exposure. *Pharmacol Biochem Behav*. 37(1):17-28.

Dange E. and Castagnoli N., (1972) Structure of hydroxycoyinine. a
nicotine metabolite *J. Med. Chem*., 15, 356-360.

Gairola, C.G. 1986. Free lung cell response of mice and rats to
mainstream cigarette smoke exposure. *Toxicaol Appl Pharmacol*. 84:567-
575.

Hoffmann, D., and K.D. Brunemann. 1983. Endogenous formation of N-
nitrosoproline in cigarette smokers. *Cancer Res*. 43:5570-5574.

Kyerematen, G.A., M.L. Morgan, B. Chattopadhyay, J.D. deBethizy, and
E.S. Vesell. 1990. Disposition of nicotine and eight metabolites in
smokers and nonsmokers: Identification in smokers of two metatolites
that are longer lived than cotinine. *Clin Pharm Therap*. 48(6):641-651.

Kyerematen, G.A., E.S. Vesell. 1991. Metabolism of Nicotine. *Drug
Metabolism Reviews*. 23(1&2): 3-41.

Langone, J.J., H.B. Gjika, and H. Van Vunakis. 1973. Nicotine and its
metabolites. Radioimmunoassays for nicotine and cotinine. *Biochem*.
12(24):5025-5030.

Neurath, G.B., M. Dunger, O. Krenz, and F.G. Pein. 1988. trans-3'-
Hydroxycotinine: A main metabolite in smokers. *Klin Wochenschr*. 66(Suppl
XI): 2-4.

Noland, M.P., R.J. Kryscio, R.S. Riggs, L.H. Linville, L.J. Perritt, and
T.C. Tucker. 1988. Saliva cotinine and thiocyanate: Chemical indicators
of smokeless tobacco and cigarette use in adolescents. *J Behav Med*.
11(5):423-433.

Noland, M.P., R.J. Kryscio, R.S. Riggs, L.H. Linville, L.J. Perritt, and
T.C. Tucker. 1990. Use of snuff, chewing tobacco, and cigarettes among
adolescents in a tobacco-producing area. *Addict Behav*. 15(6):517-530.

Rosa, M., R. Pacifici, I. Altieri, S. Pichini, G. Ottaviani, P. Zuccaro. 1992. How the steady-state cotinine concentration in cigarette smokers is directly related to nicotine intake. *Clin Pharmacol Therap.* 52:324-329.

Stanley, S.D. 1992. Development and validation of immunoassay-based tests for environmental tobacco smoke exposure. Ph.D. diss., University of Kentucky, Lexington.

Stanley, S.D., A. Jeganathan, T. Wood, P. Henry, S. Turner, W.E. Woods, M.L. Green, H-H. Tai, D. Watt, J. Blake, and T. Tobin. 1991. Morphine and etorphine: Detection by ELISA in equine urine. *J Anal Tox.* 15:305-310.

Voller, A., D.W. Bidwell, and A. Bartlett. 1976. The enzyme linked immunosorbent assay (ELISA). *Bull Wld Health Organ.* 53:55-56.

Watts, R., J.J. Langone, G. Knight, and J. Lewtas. 1990. Cotinine analytical workshop report: Consideration on analytical methods for determining cotinine in human body fluids as a measure of passive exposure to tobacco smoke. *Envir Hlth Persp.* 84:173-182.

Wenkert,E., Dave, K.G., Dainis, I., Reynolds, G.D. (1970) General methods of synthesis of indole alkaloids, VII. Attempted approach to the Iboga-Voacanoga series. *Austral. J. Chem.*, 23, 73.

Wie, S., and B.D. Hammock. 1982. The use enzyme linked immunosobent assay (ELISA) for the determination of Triton-X nonionic detergents. *Anal Biochem.* 125:168-176.

Robert W. Gensemer[1,4], Lisha Ren[2], Kristin E. Day[1,3], Keith R. Solomon[1], and Bruce M. Greenberg[2]

FLUORESCENCE INDUCTION AS A BIOMARKER OF CREOSOTE PHOTOTOXICITY TO THE AQUATIC MACROPHYTE *LEMNA GIBBA*

REFERENCE: Gensemer, R. W., Ren, L., Day, K. E., Solomon, K. R., and Greenberg, B. M., "Fluorescence Induction as a Biomarker of Creosote Phototoxicity to the Aquatic Macrophyte *Lemna gibba*," *Environmental Toxicology and Risk Assessment: Biomarkers and Risk Assessment—Fifth Volume, ASTM STP 1306,* David A. Bengtson and Diane S. Henshel, Eds., American Society for Testing and Materials, 1996.

ABSTRACT: Biomarkers of polycyclic aromatic hydrocarbon (PAH) toxicity to aquatic plants were developed using the wood preservative creosote. We tested physiological indicators of photosynthetic performance in cultures of the floating aquatic macrophyte *Lemna gibba* (G3). Creosote was applied at concentrations ranging from 1-300 ppm, and plants were grown under laboratory lighting that mimics the relative levels of UV radiation found in natural sunlight (simulated solar radiation; SSR). Population growth bioassays demonstrated that similar to individual PAHs, creosote exhibited UV-enhanced phototoxicity. Chlorophyll content and chlorophyll fluorescence induction parameters were also diminished by creosote, and closely corresponded to functional responses of population growth by the end of each experiment. Fluorescence induction thus is a validated biomarker assay that is closely and functionally related to population growth inhibition in aquatic plants.

KEYWORDS: Creosote, biomarkers, photosynthesis, population growth, duckweed, *Lemna gibba*, phototoxicity, fluorescence induction

[1]Centre for Toxicology, University of Guelph, Guelph, Ontario, N1G 1Y4, Canada

[2]Department of Biology, University of Waterloo, Waterloo, Ontario, N2L 3G1, Canada

[3]Canada Centre for Inland Waters, P.O. Box 5050, Burlington, Ontario, L7R 4A6, Canada

[4]Corresponding author, and present address: Department of Biology, Boston University, 5 Cummington Street, Boston, MA, 02215, U.S.A.

There is a strong need for suborganismal endpoints in aquatic toxicity testing and risk assessment.   These types of endpoints are often referred to as 'biomarkers' (or 'bioindicators') and are most commonly defined as biochemical, physiological, or histological indicators of contaminant exposure or effect at the suborganismal or organismal level (McCarthy and Shugart 1990, Benson and DiGiulio 1992, Huggett et al. 1992). Because biomarker assays usually represent biochemical aspects of toxicant modes of action (e.g. membrane damage, enzyme dysfunction, DNA mutation, etc.), they may provide rapid and direct indications of whether contaminants are impacting biological systems.   Although tremendous advances have been made in the development and application of biomarkers in recent years, less information is available concerning the ability of biomarkers to predict or describe ecological events at the population, community, or ecosystem levels (Huggett et al. 1992). Validation of direct and mechanistic links between biomarker responses to endpoints representing higher levels of ecological organization thus is necessary to realize the full predictive and explanatory potential of these sensitive and rapid assays.

Numerous biomarkers have been developed for the polycyclic aromatic hydrocarbons (PAHs; Benson and DiGiulio 1992). A unique property of PAHs is that ultraviolet (UV) radiation in sunlight enhances their toxicity to aquatic animals (Bowling et al. 1983, Oris and Giesy 1985, Holst and Giesy 1989) and aquatic plants (Gala and Giesy 1992, Greenberg et al. 1993, Huang et al. 1993). PAH phototoxicity results either from photomodification (e.g. oxidation) of the PAH parent compounds to more active species (Huang et al. 1993) or from photosensitization reactions (Newsted and Giesy 1987), or more likely a combination of both processes (Greenberg et al. 1993).

Even though these studies have described the phenomenon of PAH phototoxicity, most employed only individual or population-level endpoints (e.g. growth, mortality, reproduction). Several biological processes could be exploited for use as PAH biomarkers (e.g. enzymatic dysfunction, genotoxicity, membrane damage, etc., Benson and DiGiulio 1992). For plants, probably the most basic and important suborganismal process that can be inhibited by chemical contaminants is photosynthesis (Simpson et al. 1988, Judy et al. 1990). Many assays have been developed that measure photosynthetic performance, of which one of the most sensitive is a chlorophyll fluorescence induction assay of photosynthetic quantum efficiency (Hipkins and Baker 1986, Büchel and Wilhelm 1993). Fluorescence induction is indicative of environmental stress to both higher plants and aquatic algae (Greene et al. 1992, Klinkovsky and Naus 1994), but the assay has not been applied widely with respect to chemical contaminants in aquatic ecosystems. Therefore, we investigated the validity of fluorescence induction as a toxicity biomarker in the aquatic plant *L. gibba*, using the wood preservative creosote as a mixed source of PAHs (Environment Canada 1993).   Our objectives were to examine how the suborganismal-level fluorescence induction assay responded to creosote exposure, and to quantify its functional relationship to a standard population-level toxicity bioassay.

MATERIALS AND METHODS

Culture Conditions and Experimental Design

Cultures of *Lemna gibba* L. G-3 were maintained aseptically on half-strength Hutner's medium and grown under 50 μmol·m^{-2}·s^{-1} of continuous cool-white fluorescent light at 24 °C (Greenberg et al. 1992). To examine the phototoxicity of creosote, plants were incubated under an artificial lighting system designed to mimic the spectral quality of natural sunlight (Greenberg et al. 1995). This simulated solar radiation (SSR) source was produced by a combination of 2 cool-white fluorescent bulbs plus a 350 nm photoreactor lamp and a 300 nm photoreactor lamp (Southern New England Ultraviolet Company). The lamps were arranged such that relative fluence rates of visible:UV-A:UV-B radiation was 100:10:1, approximating that of terrestrial sunlight (Henderson 1977, Greenberg et al. 1995). Total visible fluence rate was 100 μmol·m^{-2}·s^{-1}. Fluence rates and spectral quality were periodically confirmed using a calibrated spectroradiometer (Oriel Instruments, Stratford, CT) and a quantum light meter (LiCor, Lincoln, NE). Plants exposed to SSR were protected from UV-C exposure by covering experiment dishes with polystyrene petri dish tops (Phoenix Biomedical, Baxter-Canlab, Missisauga, Ontario). In visible light controls, plants were exposed to creosote under cool-white fluorescent bulbs.

Plants were exposed to creosote in 10 ml of half-strength Hutner's medium placed in 5cm polystyrene petri dishes. Creosote (100% creosote, Stella Jones, Inc., Vancouver, British Columbia), was taken from the same batch as that being used in a related study of creosote toxicity in artificial aquatic ecosystems (Robinson and Gensemer 1994). Prior to use, creosote was artificially 'weathered' to remove some of the more volatile, low molecular weight chemical constituents (e.g. benzene, naphthalene) that would not persist normally in natural environments (Environment Canada 1993). A single batch of liquid creosote thus was added to beakers and stirred continuously for 48 hr with a magnetic stirrer in a darkened fume hood to prevent photooxidation prior to use in all experiments. Working creosote solutions were then prepared by dilution with a dimethyl sulfoxide (DMSO) delivery solvent to ensure exposure of all PAHs contained in the creosote. The final DMSO concentration (0.1% v/v) does not significantly affect plant growth compared to DMSO-free controls (Huang et al. 1991). In the present experiments, identical DMSO concentrations were added to all control and creosote addition treatments.

Creosote was applied in a logarithmic series of final target doses including: 0, 1, 3, 10, 30, 100, and 300 ppm nominal creosote (μL·L^{-1}, v/v). All treatments were performed in triplicate, with the entire experiment (including all treatment levels and replicates) being repeated at least once. Complete sets of creosote exposures were performed under both visible light and SSR, but only growth rate data from the visible light exposures will be presented here (see Gensemer et al. in prep for additional details). Least-squares linear regression (SyStat, SPSS Inc, Evanston, IL) was used to quantify the relationship between the response of each endpoint (converted to percent of control) as a function of log-transformed creosote concentration. These linear models were also used to estimate EC50s as the creosote concentration at which endpoint performance was reduced 50% compared to controls.

Toxicity Testing (population-level and suborganismal-level endpoints)

Toxicity tests using *L. gibba* were performed after simultaneous exposure to creosote and SSR. Two sets of endpoints were used to encompass both population-level, and suborganismal-level responses (i.e. 'biomarkers') to creosote. Population-level responses were assayed using a standard 8-day static-renewal test for growth rate as measured by increases in leaf numbers. For these assays, growth media and creosote were replaced every 48 hours to minimize depletion of ambient nutrient and creosote concentrations over time. Leaf numbers were recorded prior to each media replacement, and used to calculate growth rates expressed as a doubling frequency (see Greenberg et al. 1992 for details).

Fluorescence Induction Kinetics

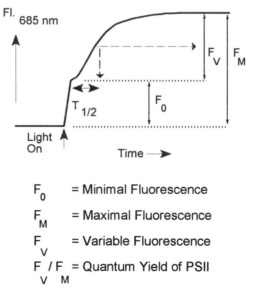

F_0 = Minimal Fluorescence

F_M = Maximal Fluorescence

F_V = Variable Fluorescence

F_V / F_M = Quantum Yield of PSII

Figure 1: Diagrammatic representation of chlorophyll fluorescence induction kinetics.

Suborganismal-level responses were assayed using changes in total plant chlorophyll content (Greenberg et al. 1992) and the quantum efficiency of photosynthesis. The photosynthetic assay was based on the 'Kautsky' induction kinetics of *in vivo* chlorophyll fluorescence induction (Hipkins and Baker 1986, Büchel and Wilhelm 1993). First, plants were dark-adapted for at least 10-20 minutes to ensure that all photosynthetic electron acceptors were fully oxidized. A plant sample was then placed in a spectrofluorometer (Photon Technology International, New Brunswick, NJ) fitted with a photon-counting photomultiplier. A mechanical camera shutter then opened to emit a single, saturating beam of actinic light (435 nm) to the plants, after which fluorescence was detected at an emission wavelength of 695 nm. Relative fluorescence intensity (counts·sec^{-1}) was then recorded for 8-10 seconds, with the resulting fluorescence trace being saved for microcomputer analysis of chlorophyll fluorescence induction parameters: F_o, F_m, F_v/F_m, and $t_{1/2}$ (Fig. 1). F_o is the initial fluorescence level of the fully oxidized chlorophylls in the absence of actinic light. After exposure to actinic light for a few seconds, fluorescence rises to a maximum (F_m) as electrons begin to reduce the electron acceptors of photosytem II (PSII). Variable fluorescence (F_v) represents the mathematical difference between F_o and F_m, from which F_v/F_m is calculated and represents the quantum efficiency or photochemical yield of PSII (Hipkins and Baker 1986, Büchel and Wilhelm 1993). The time it takes for fluorescence to reach a level halfway between F_o and F_m is termed $t_{1/2}$, and is a measure of the size and accessability of the plastoquinone pool which accept electrons from PSII (Judy et al. 1990, Simpson et al. 1988). The inhibiting effects of xenobiotics on PSII reaction centers or any process downstream of PSII would be expressed as diminished values for F_v/F_m and $t_{1/2}$.

Results from suborganismal endpoints were recorded from two identical sets of plants from each treatment, one set being sacrificed at 48 hours, the other set being sacrificed at the end of the 8-day toxicity test from which population growth rate calculations were made. The 48 hour time interval was chosen to determine whether chlorosis and fluorescence induction were early indicators of stress because they often need only short periods to respond to contaminant insults (Gensemer, Dixon, and Greenberg, in prep.). Two complete sets of creosote additions (with replication and repeats as already described) were performed simultaneously with plants for 1) 48 hour, and 2) 8-day endpoint determinations. Enough plants were removed from each petri dish for a single chlorophyll determination, and two sets of fluorescence induction measurements. Fluorescence could not be measured reliably from severely chlorotic plants, so these were treated as missing data.

RESULTS AND DISCUSSION

Relationships Among Endpoints at Different Levels of Organization

One of the difficulties in comparing physiological with population-level assays are the different units and scales over which these data are collected. While abundant data exist based on endpoints at single levels of biological organization, comparatively little attention has been paid to extrapolating quantitatively from suborganismal to population and higher-level endpoints (Huggett et al. 1992, Suter 1995). Simply ranking the differential sensitivity of various endpoints (usually derived as single point estimates, e.g. EC50) is not adequate because this does little to suggest mechanistic or causal relationships between them.

Another approach is to directly compare the entire functional response of each bioassay endpoint after normalizing the data to the same scale (Fig. 2). With this approach,

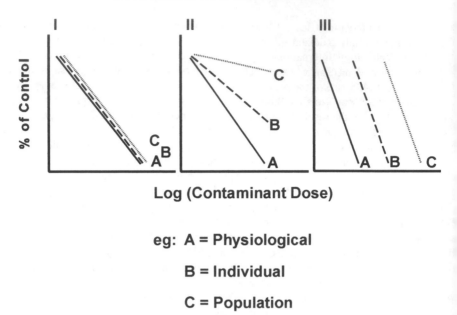

Log (Contaminant Dose)

eg: A = Physiological

B = Individual

C = Population

Figure 2: Hypothetical relationships among bioassay endpoints. See text for explanation.

empirical relationships that might exist among endpoints can be used to generate hypotheses to test: 1) whether biomarkers are predictive of higher-level endpoint responses, and 2) whether functional or mechanistic relationships might exist that explain these empirical patterns.   For example, situation I represents perfect correspondence between three hypothetical endpoints at various levels of organization and the chemical dose applied, implying that close mechanistic relationships might exist between the physiological and higher-level parameters.   Situations II and III both represent differential sensitivity of each endpoint to the contaminant, and would provide similar rankings of EC50 values estimated from each bioassay.   However, the mechanistic or functional relationships between the endpoints could be quite different depending on which situation applied.   For situation II, endpoints respond over the same concentration range, but with differential sensitivity to the chemical dose applied.   In this example, the physiological endpoint is certainly predictive of the higher level ecological events, but with much greater sensitivity.   This would implicate different modes of action of the contaminant at each level of organization, the presence of compensatory factors at higher levels, etc.   For situation III, all endpoints respond with the same relative sensitivity (e.g. have the same slopes), but respond over entirely different concentration ranges.   In such a case, it is less clear to what extent the response of the physiological endpoint at low concentrations is predictive of higher-level responses at higher

concentrations The endpoints respond to the contaminant over entirely different concentration ranges, thus mechanistic relationships are less clearly identified, if indeed they exist at all.
In all these examples (Fig. 2), linear dose-responses are assumed, but other models could also
be used.

Creosote Toxicity to *L. gibba*

Based on population growth rates, creosote was highly phototoxic to *L. gibba*, with
EC50 values exhibiting a 5-fold decrease when plants were incubated under SSR lighting
relative to visible light controls (Table 1). This confirmed our expectations that a contaminant
largely consisting of PAHs would also exhibit significant phototoxicity, even when present
as a complex mixture containing small amounts of organic contaminants other than PAHs
(Environment Canada 1993). Creosote toxicity to *L. gibba* was similar to that of individual
PAHs which typically exhibit growth EC50 values of 1-20 ppm grown under SSR (Huang et
al. 1993, Ren et al. 1993). Creosote also inhibited strongly both the quantum efficiency of
PSII and associated electron transport processes when plants were grown under SSR. In a
typical example, variable fluorescence ($F_m - F_o$) was reduced significantly in the presence of
10 ppm creosote (Fig. 3), with much less time being required to reach half of the variable

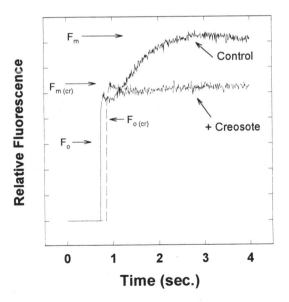

Figure 3: Fluorescence induction traces from *L. gibba* after exposure to 10 ppm creosote
and SSR.

fluorescence ($t_{1/2}$) compared to controls. As with population growth rates, all three physiological endpoints indicated that creosote toxicity was enhanced when grown under SSR vs. visible light controls (Gensemer et al. in prep).

When incubated under SSR, the effects of creosote on plant chlorophyll content and photosynthetic endpoints recorded on day 8 were strikingly similar to population growth (Fig. 4B; see Table 2 for control data). All endpoints taken on day 8 exhibited similar EC50 values, and slopes of regressions between endpoint response (as % control) and creosote concentration were within each other's 95% confidence limits (Table 1). Photosynthetic endpoints and chlorophyll contents from plants sampled after 2 days also imply that creosote negatively affected the plants. However, the fluorescence data recorded on day 2 responded somewhat less sensitively to creosote than did population growth or any of the day 8 endpoints (Fig. 4A). EC50 values for day 2 endpoints were ca. 5-fold higher than their day 8 counterparts, and regression slopes were ca. 50% lower for $t_{1/2}$ and F_v/F_m , and moderately lower for chlorophyll (Table 1). Furthermore, regressions for the day 2 photosynthetic endpoints usually explained less variance as predictors of creosote toxicity than their day 8 counterparts (Table 1) with the exception of $t_{1/2}$. The later exhibited greater variability as a predictor of toxicity than any of the other endpoints, even though mean values still corresponded well to the performance of other endpoints.

TABLE 1--Linear regressions describing bioassay endpoint responses (% controls) as a function of the logarithm of creosote dose (ppm). N/C denotes 'not calculable'.

	Slope (SE)	Intercept (SE)	r^2	p value	N	EC_{50} (ppm)
Growth Rate:						
Visible	−38.5 (2.5)	115.3 (3.5)	0.885	<0.0001	32	49.7
SSR	−45.0 (3.4)	96.3 (4.8)	0.872	<0.0001	28	10.7
Day 2 (SSR):						
Chlorophyll	−38.5 (9.5)	114.7 (11.3)	0.494	0.0008	19	47.9
$t_{1/2}$	−21.1 (5.6)	41.6 (7.0)	0.302	0.0008	34	N/C
F_v/F_m	−23.5 (6.7)	91.6 (8.4)	0.276	0.0014	34	58.9
Day 8 (SSR):						
Chlorophyll	−45.1 (7.5)	106.8 (9.8)	0.591	<0.0001	27	18.2
$t_{1/2}$	−46.8 (27.5)	99.9 (21.4)	0.146	0.1062	19	11.6
F_v/F_m	−48.5 (13.2)	109.2 (10.3)	0.443	0.0018	19	16.6

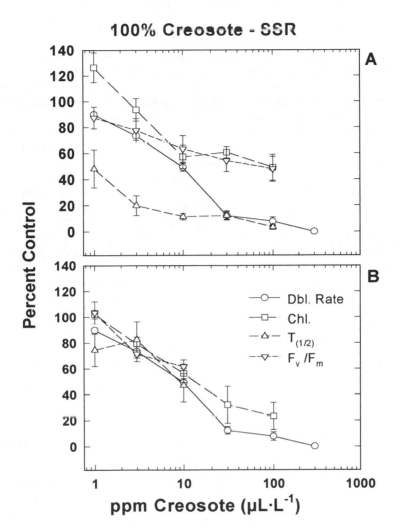

Figure 4: Responses of suborganismal (chlorophyll content and fluorescence induction) and population-level (doubling rates) assays to creosote when grown under SSR, and recorded on A) 2 days, and B) 8 days after experiment initiation. Data are represented as percents of control (= no added creosote), and error bars represent 1 S.E. about each treatment mean. Control data are presented in Table 2. Missing data represent severely chlorotic plants from which fluorescence data were not obtainable.

Implications for Fluorescence Induction as a Biomarker for Creosote Toxicity

Functional responses of fluorescence induction parameters to creosote were closely related to those of chlorosis and population growth, thereby making them potentially useful as biomarkers of creosote toxicity in *L. gibba*. These relationships were particularly good when data were recorded at the end of each experiment rather than 48 hours after exposure. Given sufficient time for inhibition of photosynthesis and chlorosis, therefore, these suborganismal endpoints hold great promise as accurate and useful indicators of creosote impacts in aquatic plants. Relative to the hypothetical endpoint relationships outlined in Fig. 1, fluorescence induction parameters generally exhibited a Type I response that implies close correspondence between physiological (photosynthesis) and population-level (growth) responses. This is not surprising considering the crucial role photosynthesis plays in energy production for plant cells. Decreases in photosynthetic energy production should result directly in diminished cell division rates and, hence, plant growth rates. In addition, inhibition of photosynthesis should subsequently result in lower rates of primary productivity. In fact, some fluorescence induction parameters quantitatively relate to C-fixation rates (Büchel and Wilhem 1993, Hofstraat 1994), thus fluorescence induction also may be predictive of contaminant impacts at the ecosystem level (e.g. productivity). However, further experimentation mechanistically linking the effects of contaminants on photosynthesis to those of population and higher-level impacts will be required to fully validate these relationships.

Table 2 -- Raw data for control treatments expressed as means (± S.E.).

	Day 2	Day 8
Doubling Rate (dbl·day^{-1})	N/A	0.49 (0.02)
N =		6
Chlorophyll (µg·mg^{-1})	0.59 (0.03)	0.48 (0.03)
N =	6	6
$t_{1/2}$ (sec.)	0.330 (0.043)	0.331 (0.026)
N =	6	8
F_v/F_m	0.55 (0.05)	0.59 (0.03)
N =	6	8

Fluorescence induction parameters occasionally exhibited differential sensitivity to creosote when compared to population growth rates (Type II response), but this usually occurred after only 2 days of exposure (Table 1; Fig. 4). This implies that creosote toxicity may be incompletely expressed in *L. gibba* after only two days. This has also been observed in similar experiments using single PAHs (Greenberg, unpublished data), and appears to result from short-term acclimation of plants to changes in laboratory lighting soon after movement from culture maintenance (visible) to experimental (SSR) lighting conditions. This would not be a problem for field-based applications of fluorescence induction assays, because natural populations are already acclimated to their particular combined exposures of contaminants and light.

CONCLUSIONS

In summary, fluorescence induction holds much promise as a plant biomarker that accurately and mechanistically corresponds to population growth inhibition in aquatic plants. The present study demonstrates that these bioassays are accurate predictors of population growth inhibition after simultaneous exposure to creosote and SSR in lab populations of *L. gibba*. However, much remains to be developed with regards to the application of these assays as biomarkers of plant toxicity in nature. Understanding the mechanistic relationships between photosynthetic inhibition (as detected by fluorescence induction) and population growth is critical to correctly interpreting and applying these bioassays as descriptors of contaminant toxicity. In particular, the potentially confounding influences of external environmental factors such as nutrient stress, light, and temperature (Greene et al. 1992, Hofstraat et al. 1994, Klinkovsky and Naus 1994) need to be assessed relative to the performance of fluorescence induction as a toxicity bioassay. Finally, the methodological utility of fluorescence induction assays in field populations is largely unexplored, and will be required to assess the full application of these methods for environmental assessments outside of the laboratory. Preliminary experiments using creosote in outdoor mesocosms (Robinson and Gensemer 1994) have demonstrated that fluorescence induction results correlate closely with population growth and biomass inhibition in rooted macrophytes (Marwood, Gensemer, and Greenberg, unpublished data). Therefore, the first step in validating the performance of photosynthetic biomarkers in the field suggests that this approach will achieve excellent utility in assessing contaminant impacts to natural populations of aquatic plants.

ACKNOWLEDGMENTS

We thank Chris Marwood for technical assistance with the fluorescence induction assays, J. McCann, K. Munro, and R.D. Robinson for their input and advice, and Stella Jones, Inc. for supplying the creosote. This study was supported by Environment Canada through the Canadian Network of Toxicology Centres, and by the Natural Sciences and Engineering Council of Canada.

REFERENCES

Benson, W.H., and DiGiulio, R.T., 1992. "Biomarkers in hazard assessments of contaminated sediments", In Sediment toxicity assessment, Burton, G.A., Jr., Ed., Lewis Publishers, Boca Raton, FL, pp. 241-265.

Bowling, J.W., Leversee, G.J., Landrum, P.F., and Giesy, J.P., 1983, "Acute mortality of anthracene-contaminated fish exposed to sunlight", Aquatic Toxicology, Vol. 3, pp. 79-90.

Büchel, C., and Wilhelm, C., 1993, "*In vivo* analysis of slow chlorophyll fluorescence induction kinetics in algae: progress, problems and perspectives", Photochemistry and Photobiology, Vol. 58, pp. 137-148.

Cook, R.H., Pierce, R.C., Eaton, P.B., Payne, J.F., Lao, R.C., Vavasour, E., and Onuska, F.I., 1983, "Polycyclic aromatic hydrocarbons in the aquatic environment: Formation, sources, fate, and effects on aquatic biota", NRC associate committee on scientific criteria for environmental quality. Publication No. NRCC 18981, National Research Council of Canada, Ottawa, Ontario.

Environment Canada, 1993, CEPA Priority Substances List Assessment Report: Creosote-impregnated waste materials, Catelog Number En 40-215/13E, Environment Canada, Ottawa, Ontario.

Gala, W.R., and Giesy, J.P., 1992, " Photo-induced toxicity of anthracene to the green alga, *Selenastrum capricornutum*", Archives of Environmental Contamination and Toxicology, Vol. 23, pp. 316-323.

Greenberg, B.M., Huang, X.-D., and Dixon, D.G., 1992, "Applications of the aquatic higher plant *Lemna gibba* for ecotoxicological assessment", Journal of Aquatic Ecosystem Health, Vol. 1, pp.147-155.

Greenberg, B.M., Huang, X.-D., Dixon, D.G., Ren, L., McConkey, B.J., and Duxbury, C.L., 1993, "Quantitative structure activity relationships for the photoinduced toxicity of polycyclic aromatic hydrocarbons to duckweed - a preliminary model", In Environmental toxicology and risk assessment: 2nd volume, ASTM STP 1216, Dwyer, F.J., Ingersoll, C.G., and La Point, T.W., Eds., American Society for Testing and Materials, Philadelphia, PA, pp. 369-378.

Greenberg, B.M., Dixon, D.G., Wilson, M.I., Huang, X.-D., McConkey, B.J., Duxbury, C.L., Gerhardt, K., and Gensemer, R.W., 1995, "Use of artificial lighting in environmental assessment studies", In Environmental Toxicology and Risk Assessment: 4th Volume, ASTM STP 1262, LaPoint, T.W., Price, F.T., and Little, E.E., Eds., American Society for Testing and Materials, Philadelphia, PA, 1995.

Greene, R.M., Geider, R.J., Kolber, Z., and Falkowski, P.G., 1992, "Iron-induced changes in light harvesting and photochemical energy conversion processes in eukaryotic marine algae", Plant Physiology, Vol. 100, pp. 565-575.

Henderson, S.T., 1977, Daylight and its Spectrum, Adam Hilger, Bristol, U.K.

Hipkins, M.F., and Baker, N.R., 1986, "Spectroscopy", In Photosynthesis energy transduction: A practical approach, Hipkins, M.F., and Baker, N.R., Eds., IRL Press, Oxford, England, pp. 51-101.

Hofstraat, J.W., Peeters, J.C.H., Snel, J.F.H., and Geel, C., 1994, "Simple determination of photosynthetic efficiency and photoinhibition of *Dunaliella tertiolecta* by saturating pulse fluorescence measurements", Marine Ecology Progress Series, Vol. 103, pp.187-196.

Huang, X.-D., Dixon, D.G., and Greenberg, B.M., 1991, "Photoinduced toxicity of polycyclic aromatic hydrocarbons to the higher plant *Lemna gibba* L. G-3", In Plants for toxicity assessment: Second volume, ASTM STP 1115, Gorsuch, J.W., Lower, W.R., Wang, W., and Lewis, M.A., Eds., American Society for Testing and Materials, Philadelphia, PA, pp. 209-216.

Huang, X.-D., Dixon, D.G., and Greenberg, B.M., 1993, "Impacts of ultraviolet radiation and photomodification on the toxicity of polycyclic aromatic hydrocarbons to the higher plant *Lemna gibba* G-3 (Duckweed)", Environmental Toxicology and Chemistry, Vol. 12, pp. 1067-1077.

Hugget, R.J., Kimerle, R.A., Mehrle, P.M. Jr., and Bergman, H.L., 1992, Biomarkers. Biochemical, physiological and histological markers of anthropogenic stress, SETAC Special publication series. Lewis Publishers, Boca Raton, FL.

Judy, B.M., Lower, W.R., Miles, C.D., Thomas, M.W., and Krause, G.F., 1990, "Chlorophyll fluorescence of a higher plant as an assay for toxicity assessment of soil and water", In Plants for Toxicity Assessment, ASTM STP 1091, Wang, W.W., Gorsuch, J.W., and Lower, W.R., Eds., American Society for Testing and Materials, Philadelphia, PA, pp. 308-318.

Klinkovsky, T., and Naus, J., 1994, "Sensitivity of the relative F_{pl} level of chlorophyll fluorescence induction in leaves to the heat stress", Photosynthesis Research, Vol. 39, pp. 201-204.

McCarthy, J.F., and Shugart, L.R., 1990, Biomarkers of environmental contamination, Lewis Publishers, Boca Raton, FL.

Neff, J.M., 1979, Polycyclic aromatic hydrocarbons in the aquatic environment: Sources, fates and biological effects, Applied Science Publishers, London.

Newsted, J.L., and Giesy, J.P., 1987, "Predictive models for photoinduced acute toxicity of polycyclic aromatic hydrocarbons to *Daphnia magna*, Strauss (Cladocera, crustacea)", Environmental Toxicology and Chemistry, Vol. 6, pp. 445-461.

Oris, J.T., and Giesy, J.P., 1987, "The photoenhanced toxicity of anthracene to juvenile sunfish (*Lepomis* spp.)", Aquatic Toxicology, Vol. 6, pp. 133-146.

Ren, L., Huang, X.-D., McConkey, B.M., Dixon, D.G., and Greenberg, B.M., 1993, "Photoinduced toxicity of three polycyclic aromatic hydrocarbons (fluoranthene, pyrene and Naphthalene) to the duckweed *Lemna gibba* L. G-3", Ecotoxicology and Environmental Safety, Vol. 28, pp. 160-171.

Robinson, R.D., and Gensemer, R.W., 1994, CNTC Validated Bioindicators Project Mesocosm Study: Standardized Procedures Manual, Centre for Toxicology, University of Guelph, Guelph, Ontario.

Simpson, G., Morissette, J.C., and Popvic, R., 1988, " Copper quenching of the variable fluorescence in *Dunaliella tertiolecta*. New evidence for a copper inhibition effect on PSII photochemistry", Photochemistry and Photobiology, Vol. 48, pp. 329-332.

Suter, G.W., 1995, "Endpoints of interest at different levels of biological organization", In Ecological Toxicity Testing: Scale, Complexity, and Relevance, Cairns, J., and Niederlehner, B.R., Eds., Lewis Publishers, Boca Raton, FL, pp. 35-48.

Douglas J. Fort[1], Enos L. Stover[1], Sterling L. Burks[1], Randall A. Atherton[1], and James T. Blankemeyer[2]

UTILIZING BIOMARKER TECHNIQUES: CELLULAR MEMBRANE POTENTIAL AS A BIOMARKER OF SUBCHRONIC TOXICITY

REFERENCE: Fort, D. J., Stover, E. L., Burks, S. L., Atherton, R. A., and Blankemeyer, J. T., "Utilizing Biomarker Techniques: Cellular Membrane Potential as a Biomarker of Subchronic Toxicity," *Environmental Toxicology and Risk Assessment: Biomarkers and Risk Assessment—Fifth Volume, ASTM STP 1306*, David A. Bengtson and Diane S. Henshel, Eds., American Society for Testing and Materials, 1996.

ABSTRACT: A biomarker assay designed to monitor the health of *Daphnia sp.* as well as evaluate sites of toxicant action was used to study the toxic effects of copper, diazinon, and polyacrylamide. The assay used the uptake of a fluorescent cellular membrane-bound dye and corresponding fluorescence measurement as an early indicator of change in cellular membrane potential. This change in the membrane potential is an indicator of potential cellular stress. Following short-term exposure to the electrochromic dye, di-4-ANEPPS, and the toxicants, fluorescence readings were collected, stored in a database management system, and output for graphical display and statistical analysis. Median inhibitory concentrations (IC50), No Observed Effect Concentrations (NOEC), and Lowest Observed Effect Concentrations (LOEC) values for copper were approximately 52.6, 35.0, and 50.0 μg/L. The approximate IC50, NOEC, LOEC values for diazinon and polyacrylamide were 0.45, 0.25, and 0.50 μg/L; and 350.0, 300.0, and 500.0 μg/L, respectively. Fluorescence microscopy indicated that copper primarily affected the mouth parts (orofacial) and digestive tract. Diazinon, however, primarily caused an effect on the anterior portion of the nervous system. Polyacrylamide appeared to induce toxicity throughout the entire epithelial layer of the *Daphnia*. These results suggested this assay may be effectively used to monitor for organism stress or toxicity as well as evaluate potential sites of toxic action.

KEYWORDS: *Daphnia*, membrane potential, sites of action, di-4-ANEPPS, copper, diazinon, polyacrylamide

Recent emphasis on integrated ecological hazard assessment has necessitated the development and validation of alternative tools for estimating ecological impairment, such as biomarker-based assays. The utility and versatility of these biomarker-based assays must be considered in the development of new model systems. Models which are capable of monitoring organism stress or toxicity as well as able to enhance evaluation of potential mechanisms of action are especially attractive. These alternative

[1]Vice President; President; Vice President; and Assistant Project Manager, respectively, THE STOVER GROUP, P.O. Box 2056, Stillwater, OK 74076
[2]Professor of Zoology, Oklahoma State University, Stillwater, OK 74078

assay systems may be used to monitor the potential ecological hazard of effluents, manufactured products, hazardous waste site soils/sediments, and regulated chemicals. DaphniaQuant™ (Oklahoma State University, Stillwater, OK 74074) is an assay designed to detect the health of *Daphnia sp.* at the cellular level (Blankemeyer et al. 1993a). This biomarker system assay uses the uptake of fluorescent dye and corresponding fluorescent measurement as an early indicator of toxicity. Following short-term exposure to a test chemical or mixture, fluorescence readings are collected, stored in a customized database system, and output for graphical observation or statistical analysis. Validation studies conducted with ten different reference toxicants, as well as over twenty five complex environmental mixtures (Fort et al. 1994a; Fort et al. 1994b; Fort et al. 1995) comparing results of the cell membrane potential-based bioassay to results from standard acute whole organism toxicity tests with daphnids were encouraging in that a high degree of correlation ($r^2 > 0.85$) was observed. However, only recently has the ability of this system to evaluate possibilities of toxic action been studied. In this report, the toxicities and general sites of action of copper, diazinon, and polyacrylamide in *Daphnia* are discussed.

EXPERIMENTAL METHOD

Materials

Reagent grade copper sulfate and polyacrylamide were obtained from Sigma Chemical Company (St. Louis, MO). Optimum grade diazinon was obtained from the Fluka Chemical Corporation (Ronkonkoma, NY).

General Description of System

The DaphniaQuant™ instrument effectively measures the electrical activity of cellular membranes as an alternative bioindicator of the sublethal effects of aqueous contaminants (Blankemeyer 1995). In this biomarker system, changes in cellular membrane potential of live, free-swimming *D. magna* were recorded following exposure to a given toxicant or complex mixture. The resultant membrane potential was compared to an unexposed control (Fort et al. 1993). Changes in the cellular membrane potential were measured by the intensity of fluorescence of an electrochromic, membrane-bound dye, dialkylaminostryl pyridiniumsulfonate (di-4-ANEPPS). Di-4-ANEPPS was spiked into the test solution and passively absorbed into the lipophilic portions of daphnid membranes within minutes of exposure. Exposure to contaminants which affect membrane transport kinetics or simply open membrane channels causes rapid changes in intracellular ion concentrations. These changes resulted in a corresponding change in fluorescence of the dye. A schematic layout of the instrument portion of the DaphniaQuant™ machine is illustrated in Appendix 1. In terms of the spectrofluorometer, a quartz-halogen lamp delivered a light output to a chopper wheel which is turned by a stepper motor. The stepper motor was controlled by an embedded computer. On opposite sides of the chopper wheel were interference filters that pass selected wavelengths of light, one at 480 nm and the other at 580 nm. The light periods were thus divided into two specific wavelengths by the filters mounted on the chopper wheel.

The light, composed of two temporally separate color bursts, passed through the chopper and struck a collection lens. The collection lens was focused on a glass cuvette mounted in a sample chamber. At a 90 degree angle to the sample chamber was another collection lens and an interference filter with a center wavelength of 630 nm. Only the emission at the appropriate wavelength passed the emission interference filter and was focused on the photomultiplier tube. The count of photons striking the photomultiplier tube was synchronized to the appropriate filter in the chopper wheel by the embedded computer. Thus, each emission count of photons was associated with a specific excitation wavelength. The photon count was then acquired by a photon counting circuit that stores the data in the memory of the embedded computer. After about twenty seconds, the acquired data was analyzed to determine the fluorescence of the organsisms in the cuvette.

The purpose of the two excitation wavelengths was to provide a measurement of membrane potential via the blue (480 nm) wavelength and a measure of how much dye and how many daphnids were in the cuvette via the yellow (580 nm) excitation. The ratio of the emissions from the two excitation wavelengths provided a membrane potential measurement independent of how many daphnids were present and how much dye was loaded in the daphnids.

DaphniaQuant™ Test Procedure

D. magna were cultured in accordance with standard EPA methodology (Weber 1991). Twenty organisms were placed in each of six beakers containing hard reconstituted water [prepared as described by Weber et al. (1989)] and increasing concentrations of toxicant for 30 min. Di-4-ANEPPS in methanol (1 x 10^{-6}M) was then added to the exposure vessels, allowed to diffuse through the sample chamber, and load into the organisms. Following 30 minutes of dye loading, the 20 exposed organisms were transferred into each of four cuvettes containing five organisms each and fluorescence readings were collected. Because changes in the toxicant exposure time alters the results obtained, 30 minute exposure periods were strictly maintained through this study. Although dye exposure time does not appreciably alter fluorescence measurements up to three hours (Fort et al. 1993; Fort et al. 1994a; Fort et al. 1994b; Fort et al. 1995), dye loading was limited to 30 min. for consistency throughout the study. The hard reconstituted water treatment served as the control. None of the test compounds altered or interfered with the fluorescence of the dye or the loading of the dye. One range-finding and three definitive DaphniaQuant™ tests were conducted with each chemical. Fluorescence ratios, as described above, were determined for each control and/or treatment replicate and stored in a database for statistical analysis.

Fluorescence Microscopy

Following evaluation and quantification of fluorescence intensity, organisms were mounted whole for fluorescence microscopy using a Nikon Labophot fluorescence microscope equipped with a dichroic mirror (excitation filter) with a cut-off of 500 nm (low pass), a Schott glass emission filter with a 580 nm cut-off (long pass), and a Nikon FX-35 35 mm camera. Observation followed by photographic documentation of five randomly selected *D. magna* out of 20 were recorded per beaker.

Data Interpretation and Statistical Analysis

No Observed Effect Concentration (NOEC) and Lowest Observed Effect Concentration (LOEC) values were calculated using either Dunnett's test (parametric) or Steel's Many-One Rank test (non-parametric) [$P=0.05$ for both] via Toxstat software, version 3.3 (University of Wyoming, Laramie, WY). Chronic Values were determined for each test by calculating the geometric mean of the NOEC and LOEC values (Weber et al. 1989).

Fluorescence ratios of each replicate electronically stored in a software database were output for statistical analysis, as described above. Median inhibitory concentration (IC50) values were derived from the concentration-response curves using the Trimmed Spearman-Karber method (Hamilton et al. 1977). Results of exemplary experiments with each reference toxicant are provided in the Results Section.

RESULTS

Copper

Table 1 presents the results of the cellular membrane potential alteration in *D. magna* as the results of short-term exposure to copper. The effect of increasing concentrations of copper on the alteration of cellular membrane potential is illustrated in Figure 1. The mean IC50, NOEC, LOEC and Chronic Values of the three replicate experiments were 52.6, 30.0, 50.0, and 38.7 µg/L, respectively. Intense fluorescence occurred primarily in the orofacial region and the gastrointestinal tract and was concentration-dependent. On a whole organism level, the increased fluorescence intensity resulting from the alteration of the cellular membrane was concentration-dependent (Figure 1).

Diazinon

Table 2 presents results of cellular membrane potential alteration in *D. magna* as the result of short-term exposure to diazinon. The effect of increasing concentrations of diazinon on the alteration of cellular membrane potential is given in Figure 2. The mean IC50, NOEC, LOEC, and Chronic Values of the three replicate experiments were 0.45, 0.23, 0.37, and 0.29 µg/L, respectively. Fluorescence microscopic evaluation indicated that the most intense fluorescence emittance was noted in the anterior portion of the nervous system and was dependent on the concentration of diazinon. Each of the three lobes of the primitive brain region fluoresced with nearly equal intensity and were substantially more intense than the remainder of the organism. The concentration-response relationship illustrated in Figure 2 indicates that the extent of cellular membrane potential alteration, as noted by increased fluorescence intensity, was dependent upon the exposure concentration of diazinon.

Polyacrylamide

Table 3 presents the results of cellular membrane potential alteration in *D. magna* as the result of short-term exposure to polyacrylamide. Figure 3 illustrates the effect of increasing concentration of polyacrylamide on the alteration of cellular membrane potential. The mean IC50, NOEC, LOEC, and Chronic Values of the three replicate experiments were 350, 250, 300, 270.4 µg/L, respectively. Fluorescence microscopic evaluation of the exposed *D. magna* indicated that the most intense fluorescence was located around the periphery of the organism in the epithelial cells. Very little, if any, fluorescence was found to be internalized within the organisms with the exception of the anterior lobe of the brain. As with the other test compounds, the increased fluorescence intensity resulting from alteration of the cellular membranes was dependent upon the exposure concentration of polyacrylamide.

DISCUSSIONS

Several studies conducted with different classes of toxicants have indicated that the membrane potential-based bioassays may be suitable bioindicators of environmental contamination and organism stress (Blankemeyer et al. 1993a; Blankemeyer and Hefler 1990; Blankemeyer and Bowerman 1992; Stringer and Blankemeyer 1993; Blankemeyer et al. 1992; Blankemeyer et al. 1993b). Early studies indicated that narcotizing compounds including oil, petroleum-derived solvents, and chlorinated solvents induced changes in cellular membrane potential as the result of perturbation of membrane pumps or ion channels. These effects were used to explain the mechanism

TABLE 1--Effect of Copper on the Alteration of Cellular Membrane Potential in *Daphnia magna*.

TEST	IC50[1] (µg/L)	NOEC[2] (µg/L)	LOEC[3] (µg/L)	Chronic Value[4] (µg/L)
1	48.7 (45.7-51.7)	30.0	50.0	38.7
2	56.4 (48.4-64.4)	30.0	50.0	38.7
3	52.7 (50.5-54.9)	30.0	50.0	38.7

[1] Median effective concentration with 95% fiducial interval in parenthesis.
[2] No Observed Effect Concentration, (P=0.05).
[3] Lowest Observed Effect Concentration (P=0.05).
[4] Geometric mean of NOEC and LOEC values.

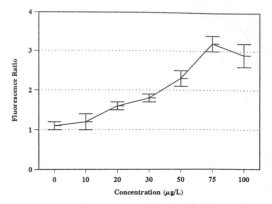

Figure 1--Concentration - response relationship of cellular membrane potential in *Daphnia magna* following copper exposure

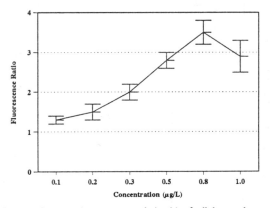

Figure 2--Concentration - response relationship of cellular membrane potential in *Daphnia magna* following diazinon exposure

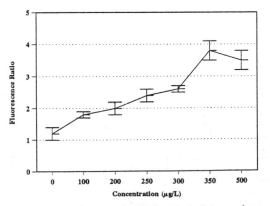

Figure 3--Concentration - response relationship of cellular membrane potential in *Daphnia magna* following polyacrylamide exposure

TABLE 2--Effect of Diazinon on the Alteration of Cellular Membrane Potential in *Daphnia magna*.

TEST	IC50[1] (μg/L)	NOEC[2] (μg/L)	LOEC[3] (μg/L)	Chronic Value[4] (μg/L)
1	0.62 (0.58-0.66)	0.30	0.50	0.39
2	0.31 (0.28-0.34)	0.20	0.30	0.25
3	0.42 (0.40-0.44)	0.20	0.30	0.25

[1] Median effective concentration with 95% fiducial interval in parenthesis.
[2] No Observed Effect Concentration, (P=0.05).
[3] Lowest Observed Effect Concentration (P=0.05).
[4] Geometric mean of NOEC and LOEC values.

TABLE 3--Effect of Polyacrylamide on the Alteration of Cellular Membrane Potential in *Daphnia magna*.

TEST	IC50[1] (μg/L)	NOEC[2] (μg/L)	LOEC[3] (μg/L)	Chronic Value[4] (μg/L)
1	280.0 (200.0-360.0)	200.0	250.0	223.6
2	470.0 (420.0-520.0)	300.0	350.0	324.0
3	300.0 (250.0-350.0)	250.0	300.0	273.9

[1] Median effective concentration with 95% fiducial interval in parenthesis.
[2] No Observed Effect Concentration, (P=0.05).
[3] Lowest Observed Effect Concentration (P=0.05).
[4] Geometric mean of NOEC and LOEC values.

of action of this class of chemicals (narcotizing) at the cellular level. Subsequent studies with naturally occurring plant glycoalkaloids commonly found in potatoes determined that alpha-chaconine and alpha-solanine substantially increased di-4-ANEPPS fluorescence up to 1600 and 400 percent of the control fluorescence in albino *Xenopus* embryos. These results suggested that these plant toxins exerted a strongly toxic effect. Interestingly, the adverse effect of these compounds correlated well with conventional whole-organism bioassays conducted concurrently with the membrane fluorescence assays. Solanadine which had no effect on membrane fluorescence, likewise was not found to be highly toxic in the traditional whole organism test systems.

More recently, the DaphniaQuant™ system was used to correlate the toxic effects of eight benchmark reference toxicants and over fifteen complex environmental samples with the results of 48-h *D. pulex* and 7-d conventional *C. dubia* bioassay results (Fort et al. 1994a; Fort et al. 1994b; Fort et al. 1995). The 48-h LC50 values of copper, diazinon, and polyacrylamide in *D. magna* were found to be 58.7 mg/L, 0.4 μg/L, and 0.4 mg/L which were consistent with the EC50 values determined from this biomarker test system.

Likewise, the 7-d chronic values for survival in *C. dubia* for copper, diazinon, and polyacrylamide were 37.5 mg/L, 0.2 μg/L, and 0.2 mg/L which were also consistent with the chronic values estimated from this biomarker test system. Results from the studies indicated that this system was capable of producing similar quantitative results as the traditional acute and subchronic cladoceran assays. Since the sensitivity of the DaphniaQuant™ assay will likely vary with the class of compounds being evaluated, increased validation is warranted with representative compounds from a wide array of chemical classes. Although the sensitivity of this assay may differ for specific chemical classes, the speed, precision, and versatility of this new system are significantly important attributes.

Results from the studies indicated that not only is this biomarker system capable of monitoring organismal toxicity, but it also provides a preliminary means of evaluating sites of toxic action. Copper appeared to cause its primary effects on the mouth and gastrointestinal tract. Diazinon seemed to exert its effect primarily on the brain region. Since the primary mode of action of this organophosphate insecticide is acetylcholinesterase inhibition, action on the center of the daphnid nervous system is not necessarily unexpected. However, the significance at membrane potential alteration, biotransformation, and toxicokinetics have not been fully elucidated to date and require further study. Polyacrylamide seemed to have its primary effect on daphnid epithelial cell layer, but also caused a secondary response in the anterior portion of the brain. Effects on the epithelial layer may be the result of polyacrylamide cross linking (polymerization) since a rosette of physically-attached *Daphnia* was observed following exposure to polyacrylamide. Increased fluorescence associated with the anterior lobe of the brain also suggests that a nervous system-linked effect may exist which is consistent with the finding that polyacrylamide is capable of cross-linking intermediate filaments of the nervous system and inducing axonopathy (Anthony and Graham 1991).

In the future, the cellular membrane potential biomarker assay will continue to be used to evaluate toxic action of pure chemicals and complex toxicant mixtures, such as industrial process waters, effluents, surface waters, groundwater, sediments, and soil extracts. Preliminary studies have been conducted using this cellular membrane biomarker system with other species, including larval fathead minnow (*Pimephales promelas*), the saltwater mysid *Mysidopsis bahia*, and albino *Xenopus laevis* (frog) embryos. Results collected so far indicate that this technology can be used to evaluate ecological hazard using a complete battery of test organisms.

Results from the studies presented in this report indicated that this biomarker model system was capable of producing rapid, quantitative, toxicity data with copper, diazinon, and polyacrylamide, as well as rapidly evaluating sites of toxicant action on a preliminary basis. However, additional work with a variety of toxicants known to hyperpolarize and/or depolarize cellular membranes, as well as with established sites of ratios will need to be performed to determine the validity of this approach. The need for routine toxicity screening as a means of assessing and establishing water quality criteria warrant further work with this novel toxicity monitoring system. Ultimately, this toxicity monitoring assay will provide the scientific community with a rapid means of evaluating potential ecological impact, as well as assistance in evaluating sites of toxic action.

ACKNOWLEDGEMENTS

DaphniaQuant™ is a proprietary product of STOVER ENVIRONMENTAL PRODUCTS, INC. and protected by patents held by Oklahoma State University. STOVER ENVIRONMENTAL PRODUCTS, INC. holds an exclusive licensing agreement to make, use, sell, lease, or further license this technology under a Technology Joint Development Agreement effective September 8, 1992. Foreign patents are pending. The authors would like to thank Mr. Larry Moore and Ms. Mollie Jackson for their technical assistance during this project. This work was supported in part by a grant from the Oklahoma Center for the Advancement of Science and Technology (OCAST) [AR4-074]. The authors also express their gratitude to Ms. Kyla Reedy and Mrs. Penny Stover for their help in preparing this manuscript.

REFERENCES

Anthony, D.C. and Graham, D.G., "Toxic Responses of the Nervous System," In: Casarett and Doull's Toxicology - The Basic Science of Poisons, 4th Ed., Amdur, M.O., Doull, J., and Klaassen, C.D., Ed. MacGraw-Hill, NY, 1991, pp. 407-429.

Blankemeyer, J.T., "Apparatus for Rapid Toxicity Testing of a Liquid," U.S. Patent No. 5,459,070, Oklahoma State University, Stillwater, OK, 1995.

Blankemeyer, J.T., "Method for Rapid Toxicity Testing of a Liquid," U.S. Patent No. 5,416,005, Oklahoma State University, Stillwater, OK, 1995.

Blankemeyer, J.T. and Bowerman, M, "Effect of Cyclic Organics on Active Transport of Sodium in Frog Skin," Bulletin of Environmental Contamination and Toxicology, Vol. 50, 1992, pp 132-137.

Blankemeyer, J.T. and Hefler, C.R, "Effect of Naphthalene on Short-Circuit Current in Frog Skin," Bulletin of Environmental Contamination and Toxicology, Vol 45, 1990, pp 627-632.

Blankemeyer, J.T., Stringer, B.K., Bantle, J.A., Friedman, M., "DaphniaQuant™ - A Rapid Daphnia Assay Using Membrane Potential as a Bioindicator," Third Symposium on Environmental Risk Assessment, J. Gorsuch, G. Lindeman, C. Ingersoll, and T. LaPointe, Eds., American Society for Testing and Materials, Special Technical Publication #1218-In Vitro Toxicology, Philadelphia, PA, 1993a.

Blankemeyer, J.T., Stringer, B.K., Rayburn, J.R., Friedman, M. and Bantle, J.A., "Effect of Potato Glycoalkaloids on the Membrane Potential of Frog Embryos," Journal of Agricultural Food Chemistry, Vol. 40, 1992, pp 2022-2026.

Blankemeyer, J.T., Stringer, B.K., Bantle, J.A., and Friedman, M., "Correlation of a Cellular Assay - CHAWQ - with FETAX," Second Symposium on Environmental Risk Assessment, J. Gorsuch, G. Lindeman, C. Ingersoll, and T. LaPointe, Eds., American Society for Testing and Materials, Special Technical Publication #1173-In Vitro Toxicology, Philadelphia, PA, 1993b.

Fort, D.J., Stover E.L., and Atherton, R.A., "DaphniaQuant™ Users Manual, Version 1.0," STOVER ENVIRONMENTAL PRODUCTS, INC., Stillwater, OK, 1993.

Fort D.J., Stover, E.L., Atherton, R.A., Blankemeyer, J.T., and Burks, S.L., "Development and Preliminary Validation of the Rapid Toxicity Quantification System, DaphniaQuant™. In: Proceedings of the 49th Annual Purdue Industrial Waste Conference, West Lafayette, IN, 1994a.

Fort D.J., Stover, E.L., Atherton, R.A., Blankemeyer, J.T., and Burks, S.L., "DaphniaQuant™ - A Rapid Toxicity Test System for the Food Processing Industry. In: Proceedings of the Food Industry Environment Conference, Atlanta, GA, 1994b.

Fort D.J., Stover, E.L., Atherton, R.A., Blankemeyer, J.T., and Burks, S.L., "Versatility of the New, Rapid, Toxicity Monitoring System, DaphniaQuant™. In: Proceedings of Toxic Substances in the Environment, Water Environmental Federation Specialty Conference, Chicago, IL, 1995.

Hamilton, M.A., Russo, R.C., and Thurston, R.V., "Trimmed Spearman-Karber Method of Estimating Median Lethal Concentration in Toxicity Bioassays," Environmental Science and Technology, Vol. 11, 1977, pp 714-719.

Stringer, B.K. and Blankemeyer, J.T., "Effect of 6-aminonicotinamide on Membrane Potential of Frog Embryos," Bulletin of Environmental Contamination and Toxicology, Vol. 57, 1993, pp 557-563.

Weber, C.I., "Methods for Testing the Acute Toxicity of Effluents and Receiving Waters to Freshwater and Maine Organisms," EPA/600/3-88/036, Duluth, MN, 1991.

Weber, C.I., Peltier, W.H., Norberg-King, T.J., Horning, W.B., Kessler, F.A., Merkedick, J.K., Neiheisel, T.W., Lewis, P.A., Klemm, D.J., Pickering, Q.H., Robinson, E.L., Lazorchak, J.M., Wymer, L.J., and Freyberg, R.W., "Short-term methods for estimating the chronic toxicity of effluents and receiving waters to freshwater organisms-second edition, "EPA/600/4-89/001, Cincinnati, OK, 1989.

Douglas J. Fort[1] and Enos L. Stover[1]

EFFECT OF LOW-LEVEL COPPER AND PENTACHLOROPHENOL EXPOSURE ON VARIOUS EARLY LIFE STAGES OF *XENOPUS LAEVIS*

REFERENCE: Fort, D. J. and Stover, E. L., "Effect of Low-Level Copper and Pentachlorophenol Exposure on Various Early Life Stages of *Xenopus laevis,*" *Environmental Toxicology and Risk Assessment: Biomarkers and Risk Assessment—Fifth Volume, ASTM STP 1306,* David A. Bengtson and Diane S. Henshel, Eds., American Society for Testing and Materials, 1996.

ABSTRACT: An evaluation of the effects of low-level copper and pentachlorophenol exposure on various early life stages of the South African clawed frog, *Xenopus laevis*, was performed using stage-specific and long-term continuous exposures. Stage-specific exposure experiments were conducted such that separate subsets of embryos and larvae from the same clutch were exposed to two toxicants, copper and pentachlorophenol, from 0 d to 4 d (standard Frog Embryo Teratogenesis Assay - *Xenopus* [FETAX]), 4 d to 8 d, 8 d to 12 d, and 12 d to 16 d. Results from two separate concentration-response experiments indicated that sensitivity to either toxicant increased in each successive time period. Longer-term exposure studies conducted for 60 to 75 days indicated that copper, but not pentachlorophenol induced reduction deficiency malformations of the hind limb at concentrations as low as 0.05 mg/L. Pentachlorophenol concentrations as low as 0.5 μg/L inhibited tail resorption. However, copper did not adversely affect the process of tail resorption. These results indicated that studies evaluating longer-term developmental processes are important in ecological hazard evaluation.

KEYWORDS: *X. laevis*, FETAX, copper, pentachlorophenol, limb deficits, tail resorption

The sensitivity of a given species to toxicant stress may vary significantly during different early life stages. However, very few, if any, standardized amphibian toxicity test systems are capable of evaluating differential effects during early life stages. No amphibian-based bioassays currently monitor longer-term developmental processes, such as limb development and metamorphosis. Several investigators evaluated stage-specific toxicity in amphibians (Berrill et al. 1993; Berrill et al. 1994; and Freda 1986). Several studies have demonstrated stage-specific differences in toxicity whereas, others have failed to show a causal relationship between developmental stage and toxic response. Variations in stage-specific responses have been suggested to be the results of inherent species differences, as well as differences in the toxicants studied. However, each investigator suggested the importance of complete early life stage studies of specific target species in the process of assessing ecological hazard. Results from stage-specific toxicity tests of copper and pentachloropenol in *X. laevis*, and longer-term exposure experiments designed to evaluate limb development and

---

[1] Vice President and President, respectively, THE STOVER GROUP, P.O. Box 2056, Stillwater, OK 74076

tail resorption (metamorphosis) processes are presented in this report. Copper and pentachlorophenol were selected as candidate compounds for this study based on previous studies in FETAX indicating that copper induced severe skeletal abnormalities, whereas pentachlorophenol caused significant reduction in larval growth. Thus, the objectives of the study were to determine if the longer-term assay could indicate whether copper was capable of interfering with normal limb development and pentachlorophenol could inhibit the process of tail resorption.

EXPERIMENTAL METHOD

Materials

ACS-grade copper sulfate, 6-aminonicotinamide (6-AN) (Sigma Chemical Company, St. Louis, MO) and pentachlorophenol (Fluka Chemical Corporation, Ronkonkoma, NY) were used throughout the experimental program. Verification of stock solution concentrations was performed using atomic absorption spectroscopy and gas chromatography-mass spectroscopy (GC-MS) for copper and pentachlorophenol analyses, respectively.

X. laevis Assay Protocol

Animal Care & Breeding--X. laevis adult care, breeding and embryo collection were performed as described in ASTM Standard E1439-91 (ASTM 1991).

Stage-Specific Exposure Studies--Embryo-larval stage-specific exposure experiments were performed under the general guidance of the ASTM Standard E1439-91 (ASTM 1991). A summary of the early life stage exposure periods and endpoints monitored is provided in Table 1. For each set of tests performed with each toxicant, 0 d to 4 d, 4 d to 8 d, 8 d to 12 d, and 12 d to 16 d exposure periods were used to evaluate stage-specific changes in sensitivity. Zero d to 4 d (Standard FETAX) tests were initiated using blastula stage embryos (stage 8). Embryos not used in this initial exposure period were then cultured in FETAX Solution, a reconstituted water medium suitable for the culture of X. laevis embryos and larvae (Dawson and Bantle 1987), until needed for the subsequent exposure periods. FETAX Solution consisted of 625 mg NaCl, 96 mg $NaHCO_3$, 75 mg $MgSO_4$, 60 mg $CaSO_4 \cdot H_2O$, 30 mg KCl, and 15 mg $CaCl_2$ per L of solution. Larvae were fed Tetramin fish food for live bearers (Tetra Werke, Melle, Germany) starting at 4 d at a rate of approximately 1 mg/larva/day. Dissolved oxygen and pH were monitored daily.

Sets of 20 embryos or larvae were placed in 60-mm covered plastic Petri dishes with varying concentrations of either copper or pentachlorophenol dissolved in FETAX solution. For each compound six (range-finder experiments) to eight (definitive concentration-response experiments) concentrations were tested in duplicate (Table 2). Four sets of control dishes of 20 X. laevis embryos or larvae were exposed to FETAX Solution alone and designated negative controls. For each experiment conducted, four separate dishes of 20 X. laevis embryos or larvae were exposed to 6-AN [FETAX positive control], two sets at 2,500 mg/L (approximate LC50) and two sets at 5.5 mg/L (approximate EC50 [malformation]). All control and treatment vessels contained a total of 8 mL of solution. One range test and two definitive tests were performed with each compound. The pH of the test compounds ranged from 7.0-7.5. Embryos and larvae were cultured at 24 ± 0.5°C throughout the tests and culturing processes. Little

TABLE 1--Summary of Early Life Stage Exposure Periods and Endpoints Monitored.

Stage or Developmental Process	Time Period[1]	Endpoints
Early Embryo-Larval	0-4 (8-45)	Survival, Malformation, Growth
Larval	4-8 (45-48.5)	Survival, Malformation, Growth
Larval	8-12 (48.5-49)	Survival, Malformation, Growth
Larval	12-16 (49-50.5)	Survival, Malformation, Growth
Limb Development	0-60 (8-60)	Malformation
Metamorphosis	0-75 (8-66)	Tail Resorption

[1] Expressed as d with stage denoted in parenthesis (Nieuwkoop and Faber 1994).

TABLE 2--Concentration Series Range Tested in Stage-Specific Exposure Studies.

Time Period[2]	Test Concentration Range[1]	
	Copper	Pentachlorophenol
0-4 (8-45)	0.75, 0.85, 0.95, 1.00, 1.10, 1.15, 1.25, 1.50	0.05, 0.10, 0.15, 0.18, 0.25, 0.33, 0.66, 0.75
4-8 (45-48.5)	0.50, 0.67, 0.75, 1.00, 1.05, 1.10, 1.15, 1.20	0.01, 0.05, 0.06, 0.07, 0.08, 0.10, 0.25, 0.50
8-12 (48.5-49)	0.15, 0.20, 0.25, 0.30, 0.50, 0.65, 0.70, 0.75	0.005, 0.01, 0.015, 0.02, 0.1, 0.15, 0.20, 0.25
12-16 (49-50.5)	0.04, 0.045, 0.05, 0.055, 0.10, 0.20, 0.30, 0.40	0.001, 0.002, 0.003, 0.004, 0.01, 0.033, 0.066, 0.10

[1] Expressed as mg/L.
[2] Expressed as d with developmental stage in parenthesis.

difference in the toxicities of pentachlorophenol and copper were noted providing the pII did not deviate from this range.

All solutions were renewed every 24 h of the tests, dead embryos/larvae were removed and recorded, and fresh solutions added during each of the tests conducted. Following exposure, the larvae were fixed in 3 % formalin, pH 7.0, and the number of live malformed organisms determined by external morphological evaluation aided by a dissecting microscope (Nieuwkoop and Faber 1994). Head-tail length (growth) was measured using an IBM compatible computer equipped with digitizing software (Jandell Scientific, Corte Madera, CA).

Long-Term Exposure Studies--Long-term exposure studies were also conducted in general accordance with the methods cited in ASTM E1439-91 (ASTM 1991). Experiments designed to evaluate hind limb development were conducted for approximately 60 d, whereas experiments performed to evaluate effects of toxicant exposure on tail resorption were performed for approximately 75 d. Sets of 20 blastula stage embryos were placed in 500 mL Pyrex glass bowls containing 0.05 and 0.01 mg/L copper and 2.5 and 0.5 μg/L pentachlorophenol. These concentrations represented 0.5 and 0.1 times the lowest respective EC50 (malformation) from the stage-specific sensitivity studies. Dilutions were prepared in FETAX Solution. Two separate bowls of 20 embryos were exposed to FETAX solution alone. Treatment and control dishes contained a total of 200 mL of solution. The pH of the test solutions was maintained between 7.0-8.0. As with the short-term studies, little difference in toxicity was noted within this pH range with either compound. However, since future test compound toxicity may be affected by pH, modifications have been made recently to decrease pH fluctuation during testing. Embryos and larvae were cultured at 24 $\pm$ 0.5°C. Two separate experiments were performed with each test chemical.

To minimize stress on the developing larvae, test solutions were only renewed if the dissolved oxygen dropped below 6.0 mg/L (Fort et al. 1995). Fresh solutions were added to replace evaporation losses. Toxicant concentrations were measured weekly throughout the exposure period. Fresh toxicant was spiked into the replacement solution. Embryo-larval staging was performed during the renewal process. Tests were terminated once the larvae reached stage 60 (approximately 60 d) and stage 66 (approximately 75 d) for the evaluation of hind limb development and tail resorption (metamorphosis) assessment. At the completion of the exposure, larvae were fixed in 3 % formalin, pH=7.0, and the gross effects on limb development and tail resorption noted. Limb defects assessment was aided by the use of a dissecting microscope.

Data Analysis--For the stage-specific sensitivity tests, mortality and malformation rates for each test concentration were determined, as well as for the control treatments. For the definitive tests, probit analysis was used to determine the 96-h median lethal concentration, median teratogenic concentration, and the respective 95% fiducial intervals. A Mortality/Malformation Index (MMI) which has been useful in evaluating potential teratogenic hazard (Courchesne and Bantle 1985; Dawson and Bantle 1987; Dawson et al. 1989) was also determined. Statistical differences in MMI values were determined by the method of Finney (1971). For each definitive test, the minimum concentration to inhibit growth (MCIG) was calculated using the t-test for grouped observations (P < 0.05).

For the longer-term exposure studies evaluating effects on limb development the type and rate of hind limb malformations of the control and exposed larvae were determined (Nieuwkoop and Faber 1994). Statistical comparisons of the control treatment to the exposure concentrations were performed using Dunnett's test ($P=0.05$) via Toxstat, ver. 3.3 (University of Wyoming, Laramie, WY).

For the continuous exposure studies evaluating effects on tail resorption, video images were captured using an 8 mm video camera (Foster et al. 1994). A 386/16 MHZ computer with ZIP IMAGE processing software and High Resolution Technologies (HRT) video frame grabber were used to digitize the tail length at developmental stages 63-66. A ruler video taped with the larvae was used to correct for image distortion and calibrate the length measuring program to ensure accurate measurements of the larvae. Tail lengths were measured with HRTlib, an image processing/support library for HRT512-8 video frame grabber. Statistical comparisons of the control and exposure treatments were performed using the t-test for grouped observations, $P < 0.05$.

RESULTS

Control Data

During the stage-specific exposure experiments, the FETAX Solution control mortality and malformation rates, in the 0 d to 4 d tests were 8 of 320 (2.5%) and 12 of the 312 surviving larvae (4.0%), respectively; in the 4 d to 8 d tests were 5 of 320 (1.6%) and 11 of the surviving 315 surviving larvae (3.6%); in the 8 d to 12 d tests were 3 of 320 (0.3%) and 7 of the remaining 317 (2.3%); and in the 12 d to 16 d exposure tests were 1 of 320 (0.03%) and 5 of the remaining 319 survivors (1.6%). The 2,500 mg/L 6-AN control induced mortality rates of 65%, 70%, 75%, and 82.5% (N=160) in the 0 d to 4 d, 4 d to 8 d, 8 d to 12 d, and 12 d to 16 d exposure studies. The malformation rates in each of the tests with 2,500 mg/L 6-AN were 100%. The 5.5 mg/L 6-AN control induced mortality rates of 0%, 0%, 2.5%, and 0% (N=160) in the 0 d to 4 d, 4 d to 8 d, 8 d to 12 d, and 12 d to 16 d exposure experiments, respectively. The malformation rates were 60%, 62.5%, 55%, and 50%, respectively.

The FETAX Solution control mortality and malformation rates for the continuous exposure experiments designed to monitor limb development were 12 of 320 (3.8%) and 10 of the surviving 308 larvae (3.3%), respectively. Exposure to 2,500 mg/L and 5.5 mg/L 6-AN induced mortality rates of 100% and 17.5% (N=160 for both), respectively. Exposure to 5.5 mg/L 6-AN induced a malformation rate of 55.3% (N=123). Of these malformed larvae, each had defective limb development. The FETAX Solution control mortality and malformation rates for the continuous exposure treatments designed to monitor tail resorption were 23 of 320 (7.2%) and 19 surviving 297 larvae (6.4%), respectively.

Stage-Specific *X. laevis* Assay Results

LC50 Endpoint--Stage-specific lethal responses in *X. laevis* exposed to copper and pentachlorophenol from each of the respective time periods are presented in Table 3. The LC50 values for both copper and pentachlorophenol decreased from approximately 1.32 mg/L and 0.54 mg/L in the 0 d to 4 d exposure to 0.2 mg/L and 0.06 mg/L in the 12 d to 16 d exposure period, respectively. A step-wise increasing sensitivity to both toxicants was noted with increasing developmental stage.

EC50 (malformation) Endpoint--Stage-specific embryo-larval malformation responses in *X. laevis* are presented in Table 4. As observed with the lethal response, a similar pattern of increasing sensitivity was noted with increasing developmental stage.

TABLE 3--Stage-Specific Lethal Response to Copper and Pentachlorophenol Exposure in *X. laevis.*

Time Period[2]	Copper Test 1	Copper Test 2	Pentachlorophenol Test 1	Pentachlorophenol Test 2
		LC50[1]		
0-4 (8-45)	1.25 (1.20-1.30)	1.38 (1.35-1.41)	0.52 (0.50-0.54)	0.56 (0.55-0.57)
4-8 (45-48.5)	1.08 (1.02-1.14)	1.15 (1.10-1.20)	0.35 (0.33-0.37)	0.42 (0.39-0.45)
8-12 (48.5-49)	0.42 (0.40-0.44)	0.65 (0.60-0.70)	0.12 (0.08-0.16)	0.15 (0.13-0.17)
12-16 (49-50.5)	0.15 (0.10-0.20)	0.24 (0.22-0.26)	0.05 (0.02-0.08)	0.06 (0.04-0.08)

[1] Median 96-h lethal effect concentration expressed as mg/L, with 95% fiducial interval in parentheses.
[2] Expressed as d with developmental stage in parenthesis.

TABLE 4--Stage-Specific Malformation Response to Copper and Pentachlorophenol Exposure in *X. laevis.*

Time Period[2]	Copper Test 1	Copper Test 2	Pentachlorophenol Test 1	Pentachlorophenol Test 2
		EC50[1]		
0-4 (8-45)	0.95 (0.90-1.0)	0.99 (0.98-1.00)	0.07 (0.05-0.09)	0.10 (0.09-0.11)
4-8 (45-48.5)	0.92 (0.90-0.94)	0.89 (0.87-0.91)	0.05 (0.03-0.07)	0.07 (0.05-0.09)
8-12 (48.5-49)	0.38 (0.35-0.41)	0.42 (0.40-0.44)	0.01 (0.008-0.012)	0.03 (0.01-0.05)
12-16 (49-50.5)	0.10 (0.08-0.12)	0.15 (0.12-0.18)	0.006 (0.005-0.007)	0.008 (0.007-0.009)

[1] Median 96-h teratogenic concentration expressed as mg/L, with 95% fiducial interval in parentheses.
[2] Expressed as d with developmental stage in parentheses.

The EC50 (malformation) values for both copper and pentachlorophenol decreased from approximately 0.97 mg/L and 0.09 mg/L in the 0 d to 4 d exposure period to 0.13 mg/L and 0.007 mg/L in the 12 d to 16 d exposure period, respectively.

Mortality/Malformation Index (MMI) Endpoint--Stage-specific changes in the MMI values of copper and pentachlorophenol are given in Table 5. For copper, MMI changed insignificantly (P >0.05) through each of the four exposure periods. MMI values for copper ranged from 1.11, recorded in test 1 of the 8 d to 12 d exposure, to 1.60, noted in test 2 of the 12 d to 16 d exposure experiment. A similar trend was observed for pentachlorophenol. MMI values for test 1 of the 8 d to 12 d exposure were significantly greater (P ≤0.05) than the other MMI values determined for pentachlorophenol. The remaining pentachlorophenol MMI results ranged insignificantly (P >0.05) from 5.60 recorded in test 2 of the 0 d to 4 d exposure to 8.33 calculated for test 1 of the 12 d to 16 d exposure period experiment.

Growth Inhibition Endpoint--Stage-specific growth inhibiting effects of copper and pentachlorophenol increased with each exposure period, and thus developmental stage (Table 6). Embryos exposed to copper from 0 d to 4 d demonstrated inhibited growth (MCIG) at approximate concentrations of 1.13 mg/L which equated to nearly 85.6% of the respective LC50 values for this exposure period. Larvae exposed to copper from 12 d to 16 d showed growth inhibition at approximate concentrations of 0.048 mg/L which equated to nearly 25.5% of the respective LC50 values for this exposure period. Growth inhibition in embryos exposed to pentachlorophenol from 0 d to 4 d was observed at concentrations of approximately 0.17 mg/L which relates to nearly 30.8% of the respective LC50 values for this exposure period. However, the growth inhibiting effects of pentachlorophenol for the 12 d to 16 d exposure period were observed at approximately 0.004 mg/L which equated to nearly 6.3% of the respective LC50 values for this exposure period.

Long-Term Exposure Results

Limb Development--Copper, but not pentachlorophenol, induced substantial malformation of the hind limbs. Eighty-five percent of larvae exposed to 0.05 mg/L copper through stage 60 demonstrated severely abnormal hind limb development. Hind limb malformations induced by copper were primarily characterized as being reduction deficiencies in which the femur developed normally, but remaining distal assemblages including the tibia, fibula, and metatarsals failed to develop leaving a stump. Only 2.5% of the embryos exposed to 0.01 mg/L copper showed this type of deficit and developed normally. Defects noted as the result of copper exposure were different from hind limb malformations induced by 6-AN, which also caused reduction deficits, however in the form of adactyly.

Tail Resorption--The effects of 0.01 mg/L and 0.05 mg/L copper on tail resorption in *X. laevis* are presented in Table 7. Based on data collected at developmental stages 63 through 66, neither copper concentration inhibited tail resorption when compared to the FETAX Solution control [grouped t-test, P<0.05]. This finding was substantiated at the conclusion of the exposure (stage 66). Normally metamorphosing *X. laevis* showed little or no remaining tail at stage 66. However, the majority of larvae exposed to 0.5 µg/L pentachlorophenol reaching stage 66 had a remaining tail bud (mean length=1.9 ± 0.5 mm) (Table 8). Tail resorption inhibition

TABLE 5--Stage-Specific Changes in the *X. laevis* Mortality/Malformation Index (MMI) of Copper and Pentachlorophenol.

Time Period[2]	MMI[1]			
	Copper		Pentachlorophenol	
	Test 1	Test 2	Test 1	Test 2
0-4 (8-45)	1.32	1.39	7.43	5.60
4-8 (45-48.5)	1.17	1.29	7.00	6.00
8-12 (48.5-49)	1.11	1.55	12.00[3,4,5]	5.00
12-16 (49-50.5)	1.50	1.60	8.33	7.50

[1] Ratio of the respective 96-h LC50 and EC50 (malformation) values.
[2] Expressed as day with developmental stage in parentheses.
[3] Significantly greater than 0-4 d exposure period at P=0.05 (Finney 1971).
[4] Significantly greater than 4-8 d exposure period at P=0.05 (Finney 1971).
[5] Significantly greater than 12-16 d exposure period at P=0.05 (Finney 1971).

TABLE 6--Stage-Specific Growth Inhibiting Effects of Copper and Pentachlorophenol in *X. laevis.*

Time Period[2]	Copper Test 1	MCIG[1] Test 2	Pentachlorophenol Test 1	Test 2
0-4 (8-45)	1.10 (88.0)	1.15 (83.3)	0.15 (29.5)	0.18 (32.1)
4-8 (45-48.5)	0.67[3] (62.3)	0.67[3] (58.3)	0.07[3] (21.2)	0.08[3] (16.7)
8-12 (48.5-49)	0.20[3,4] (62.3)	0.25[3,4] (59.5)	0.015[3,4] (21.2)	0.020[3,4] (13.3)
12-16 (49-50.5)	0.045[3,4,5] (30.2)	0.05[3,4,5] (20.8)	0.003[3,4,5] (5.6)	0.004[3,4,5] (6.7)

[1] Mimimum concentration to inhibit growth (P<0.05) expressed as mg/L and percent of 96-h LC50 in parenthesis.
[2] Expressed as day with developmental stage in parentheses.
[3] Significantly less than 0-4 d exposure (t-test [grouped], P<0.05).
[4] Significantly less than 4-8 d exposure (t-test [grouped], P<0.05).
[5] Significantly less than 8-12 d exposure (t-test [grouped], P<0.05).

TABLE 7--Effect of Sublethal Concentrations of Copper on Tail Resorption in X. laevis.

Concentration[1]	Developmental Stage[2]	Tail Length[3]	
		Test 1	Test 2
Control[4]	63	43.2 ± 2.8	45.6 ± 3.4
	64	12.6 ± 1.5	15.3 ± 1.8
	65	1.9 ± 0.6	2.7 ± 0.5
	66	ND	ND
0.05	63	44.5 ± 3.5	46.3 ± 2.9
	64	15.4 ± 2.6	15.6 ± 3.1
	65	2.3 ± 1.2	2.5 ± 0.8
	66	ND	ND
0.01	63	41.5 ± 1.9	43.1 ± 5.2
	64	13.6 ± 0.8	16.1 ± 2.6
	65	3.2 ± 1.7	3.1 ± 1.5
	66	ND	ND

[1] Expressed as mg/L. Concentrations selected represent 0.5 and 0.1 times the EC50 value for the most sensitive development stage.
[2] Based on staging from Nieuwkoop and Faber 1994.
[3] Mean length in mm ± standard error, N=20.
[4] FETAX Solution.

TABLE 8--<u>Effect of Sublethal Concentrations of Pentachlorophenol on Tail Resorption</u> in <u>X. laevis.</u>

Concentration[1]	Developmental Stage[2]	Tail Length[3]	
		Test 1	Test 2
Control[4]	63	42.8 ± 1.7	44.5 ± 2.1
	64	15.3 ± 0.9	17.3 ± 1.8
	65	0.8 ± 0.3	0.4 ± 0.4
	66	ND	ND
2.5	63	47.5 ± 2.5[5]	45.3 ± 1.8
	64	38.6 ± 1.8[5]	33.5 ± 1.9[5]
	65	25.2 ± 3.5[5]	26.3 ± 4.1[5]
	66	19.5 ± 1.6[5]	19.8 ± 1.2[5]
0.5	63	45.3 ± 2.8	44.6 ± 1.8
	64	21.2 ± 3.1[5]	26.1 ± 2.1[5]
	65	7.2 ± 1.1[5]	10.1 ± 1.8[5]
	66	1.9 ± 0.5[5]	2.2 ± 1.1[5]

[1] Expressed as $\mu g/L$. Concentrations selected represent 0.5 and 0.1 times the EC50 value for the most sensitive development stage.
[2] Based on staging from Nieuwkoop and Faber 1994.
[3] Mean length in mm ± standard error, N=20.
[4] FETAX Solution.
[5] Statistically different from control, grouped t-test, $P > 0.05$.

was even more dramatic following exposure to 2.5 μg/L pentachlorophenol with a mean remaining tail length of 19.5 ± 1.6 mm.

DISCUSSIONS

Results from these studies indicated that the toxicity of copper and pentachlorophenol is stage specific in *X. laevis* with the latter stages of early development (through stage 50) being more sensitive than the early stages of organogenesis (through stage 45).

Results from the longer-term exposure studies suggested that, in general, measurement of adverse effects on limb development and developmental events associated with metamorphosis are important in assessing potential hazards to amphibian populations. The results presented indicated that copper was capable of inducing limb reduction/deficit malformations at low concentrations, whereas low-levels of pentachlorophenol inhibited the process of tail resorption during metamorphosis.

Since sensitivity to copper and pentachlorophenol appeared to be dependent on developmental stage with sensitivity increasing with each subsequent set of stages, the ability to predict the ultimate hazard using short-term tests may be somewhat limiting and should be evaluated with the proper perspective. The 0 d to 4 d FETAX developmental toxicity test is capable of providing developmental toxicity information on processes of organogenesis. However, the ability of the FETAX test to determine potential effects on longer-term processes, such as limb development and events associated with metamorphosis, have not been thoroughly explored. Preliminary attempts to correlate skeletal defects noted in the FETAX test to limb malformations in *X. laevis* have been encouraging. Several compounds in addition to copper have shown this general response, including t-retinoic acid, 6-aminonicotinamide, semicarbizide, and thiosemicarbizide. The relationship between skeletal abnormalities induced in 4 d larvae and limb defects observed later in development is currently being further investigated. The correlation between skeletal defects observed in FETAX and limb defects reported in mammalian literature is fairly strong (Fort et al. 1988; Fort et al. 1989; Fort et al. 1991; Fort et al. 1992; Fort et al. 1993; Fort et al. 1995). The ability to predict effects on metamorphosis will be more difficult, as no easily accessible measurement from 0 d to 4 d has been capable of consistently predicting inhibition of the events associated with metamorphosis. Postembryonic physiological and molecular biomarkers have been exploited as a means of evaluating the process of metamorphosis, including assays for triiodothyronine activation of vitellogenin gene activity by estradiol (Rabelo et al. 1994; Kawahara et al. 1989). However, a significant amount of attention is now being placed on evaluating any measurable links between early embryo development and inhibition of metamorphosis. If successful, these assays, in combination with the FETAX test, could effectively provide a short-term prediction of potential longer-term effects.

Similar effects of copper on skeletal and limb development have been observed in *X. laevis* (Luo et al. 1993 and Bantle et al. in press) and higher vertebrate species (Kaye et al. 1976; Rest 1976; Heller et al. 1978; Allen et al. 1982). Stage-specific sensitivity of amphibian species to anthropogenic contaminants have also been documented by previous investigators (Freda 1986; Berrill et al. 1993; Berrill et al. 1994). Explanation for differences include differential developmental trajectories, selective gene expression, and pharmacodynamic advances in the larvae as the result of development. All three explanations may have merit in terms of explaining stage-specific responses in *X. laevis*. Based on the results of the longer-term studies, both copper and pentachlorophenol could affect biochemical and molecular processes active in later stages of development. However, toxicodynamic differences in the processes of adsorption, distribution, metabolism, and excretion may also account for stage-specific differences in sensitivity. Furthermore, increases in copper toxicity with developmental stage may be due to increased absorption into and distribution through the organism as the circulatory system becomes more advanced. Since copper is not biotransformed it is unlikely that this process is increasing the toxicity of copper. Anatomical advances in target organ development may also have played a factor. Increases in pentachlorophenol toxicity may be explained by each of the four aforementioned disposition processes. However, increased biotransformation capacity developed in post-4 d larvae may account for the majority of the increased toxicity wit developmental stage. Similar responses have been observed with several other bioactivated or bioinactivated toxicants (Fort et al. 1988; Fort et al. 1989). However, the present study only evaluated early embryo development through 16 d of development. Sensitivity trends for later development have not yet been studied in *X. laevis*. Thus, it is possible that changes in sensitivity (robustness) may be reversed in more advanced developmental stages (i.e., metamorphosis).

Based on the results from these studies, it may be possible to predict mechanisms of toxicant action on limb development and tail resorption. Copper cause: a reduction deficit which resulted in no formation of the assemblages distal to the femur. Since the current model for vertebrate limb development suggests that the apical ectodermal ridge (AER) of the limb bud primordia is responsible for progressive differentiation in the distal direction (Loomis 1986), copper may be affecting the function of the AER. 6-AN, on the contrary, causes adactyly (lack of formation of the digits). Because a second pattern forming region, the zone of polarizing activity (ZPA is thought to be responsible for anterior-posterior differentiation of the limbs, it is plausible that 6-AN exerts its activity on this region of the developing limb. The limb development assay may prove to be a suitable alternative assay for evaluating mechanism of action of toxicants affecting limb development.

Since the process of metamorphosis is so complex, identifying a specific mode of action is difficult. Additional studies are currently being performed to evaluate the xenoestrogenic activity of pentachlorophenol in *X. laevis* and how it may alter the processes of metamorphosis. However, since pentachlorophenol is considered to be a potent uncoupler of oxidative phosphorylation and thus affects bioenergetics, the result may be due to compromised energy production during metamorphosis.

Overall, the results from these studies verified the importance of evaluating long-term effects of toxicants on critical developmental processes in amphibians. Future studies will be performed to further standardize and validate these testing processes so that they can be widely used in ecological hazard assessment.

ACKNOWLEDGMENTS

The authors would like to thank Ms. M. Jackson for her technical assistance on this project. Gratitude is also expressed to Ms. K. Reedy and Mrs. P. Stover for their help in preparing this manuscript. This work was supported in part by a grant (AR5-002) from the Oklahoma Center for the Advancement of Science & Technology (OCAST).

REFERENCES

Allen, T.M., Manoli, A. and LaMont, R.L., "Skeletal Changes Associated with Copper Deficiency," Clinical Orthopathy, Vol. 168, 1982, pp 206-210.

American Society for Testing and Materials, "Standard Guide for Conducting the Frog Embryo Teratogenesis Assay - Xenopus (FETAX)," Standard E1439-91, American Society for Testing and Materials, Philadelphia, PA, 1991.

Bantle, J.A., Finch, R.A., Burton, D.T., Fort, D.J., Dawson, D.A., Linder, G., Rayburn, J.R., Hull, M., Kumsher-King, M., Gaudet-Hull, A.M., Turley, S.D. and Stover, E.L., "FETAX Interlaboratory Validation Study: Phase III Testing," Journal of Applied Toxicology, 1996, in press.

Berrill, M., Bertram, S., McGillivray, L., Kolohon, M., and Pauli, B., "Effects of Low Concentrations of Forest-Use Pesticides on Frog Embryos and Tadpoles," Environmental Toxicology and Chemistry, Vol. 13, 1994, pp 657-664.

Berrill, M., Bertram, S., Wilson, A. Louis, S., Brigham, D., and Stromberg, C., "Lethal and Sublethal Impacts of Pyrethroid Insectides on Amphibian Embryos and Tadpoles," Environmental Toxicology and Chemistry, Vol. 12, 1993, pp 525-539.

Courchesne, C.L. and Bantle, J.A., "Analysis of the Activity of DNA, RNA, and Protein Synthesis Inhibitors on Xenopus Embryo Development," Teratogenesis, Carcinogenesis, and Mutagenesis, Vol. 5, 1985, pp 177-193.

Dawson, D.A. and Bantle, J.A., "Development of a Reconstituted Water Medium and Initial Validation of FETAX," Journal of Applied Toxicology, Vol. 7, 1987, pp 237-244.

Dawson, D.A., Fort, D.J., Newell, D.L., and Bantle, J.A., Developmental Toxicity Testing with FETAX: Evaluation of Five Validation Compounds," Drug and Chemical Toxicology, Vol. 9, 1989, pp 377-388.

Finney D.J., Statistical Methods in Biological Assay, 2nd Ed., Griffin, London, 1971.

Fort, D.J., Dawson, D.A., and Bantle, J.A., "Development of a Metabolic Activation System for the Frog Embryo Teratogenesis Assay - Xenopus (FETAX)," Teratogenesis, Carcinogenesis, and Mutagenesis, Vol. 8, 1988, pp 251-263.

Fort, D.J., James, B.L., and Bantle, J.A., "Evaluation of the Developmental Toxicity of Five Compounds with the Frog Embryo Teratogenesis Assay: Xenopus (FETAX)," Journal of Applied Toxicology, Vol. 9, 1989, pp 377-388.

Fort, D.J., Rayburn, J.R., and Bantle, J.A., "Evaluation of Acetaminophen-Induced Developmental Toxicity using FETAX," Drug and Chemical Toxicology, Vol. 15, 1992, pp 329-350.

Fort, D.J., Rayburn, J.R., DeYoung, D.J., and Bantle, J.A., "Assessing the Efficacy of an Aroclor 1254-Induced Exogenous Metabolic Activation System for FETAX," Drug and Chemical Toxicology, Vol. 14, 1991, pp 143-160.

Fort, D.J., Stover, E.L.and Norton, D., "Ecological Hazard Assessment of Aqueous Soil Extracts using FETAX," Journal of Applied Toxicology, Vol. 15, 1995, pp 183-191.

Fort, D.J., Stover, E.L., Rayburn, J.R., Hull, M.A., and Bantle, J.A., "Evaluation of the Developmental Toxicity of Trichloroethylene and Detoxification Metabolites using Xenopus," Teratogenesis, Carcinogenesis, and Mutagenesis, Vol. 13, 1993, pp 35-45.

Foster, S.C., Burks, S.L., Fort, D.J., Stover, E.L., and Matlock, M.D., "Development and Evaluation of a Nondestructive measure of Fish Growth for Sublethal Toxicity Assessment, Bulletin of Environmental Contamination and Toxicology, Vol. 53, 1994, pp 85-90.

Freda, J., "The Influence of Acidic Pond Water on Amphibians: A Review," Water, Air, and Soil Pollution, Vol. 30, 1986, pp 439-450.

Heller, R.M., Kirchner, S.G., O'Neill, J.A., Hough, A.J., Howard, L., Kramer, S.S., and Green, H.L., "Skeletal Changes of Copper Deficiency in Infants Receiving Prolonged Total Parenteral Nutrition," Journal of Pediatrics, Vol. 92, 1978, pp 947-949.

Kawahara, A., Kohora, S., and Amano, M., "Thyroid Hormone Directly Induces Hepatocyte Competence for Estrogen-Dependent Vitellogenin Synthesis During Metamorphosis of Xenopus laevis, Developmental Biology, Vol. 132, 1989, pp 73-80.

Kaye, C.I., Fisher, D.E., and Esterly, N.B., "Cutis laxa, Skeletal Anomalies, and Ambiguous Genitalia," American Journal of Diseases of Children, Vol. 127, 1974, pp 115-117.

Loomis, W.H., Developmental Biology, MacMillan, New York, 1986.

Luo, S.Q., Plowman, M.C., Hopfer, S.M., and Sunderman, F.W., "Embryotoxicity and Teratogenicity of Cu2+ and Zn2+ for Xenopus laevis, Assayed by the FETAX Procedure," Annals of Clinical and Laboratory Science, Vol. 23, 1993, pp 111-120.

Nieuwkoop, P.D. and Faber, J., Normal Table of Xenopus Laevis (Daudin), Garland Publishing, Inc., New York, 1994.

Rabelo, E.M., Baker, B.S., and Tata, J.R., "Interplay Between Thyroid Hormone and Estrogen in Modulating Expression of their Receptor and and Vitellogenin Genes During Xenopus Metamorphosis," Mechanisms of Development, Vol. 45, 1994, pp 49-57.

Rest, J.R., "The Histological Effects of Copper and Zinc on Chick Embryo Skeletal Tissue in Organ Culture," British Journal of Nutrition, Vol. 36, 1976, pp 243-254.

Richard L. Dickerson[1,] Julie A. Hoover[2], Margie M. Peden-Adams[2], Whitney E. Mashburn[2], Catherine A. Allen[3], and Diane S. Henshel[4]

ALTERATIONS IN CHICKEN EMBRYONIC DEVELOPMENT AS A SENSITIVE INDICATOR OF 2,3,7,8-TETRACHLORODIBENZO-P-DIOXIN EXPOSURE

REFERENCE: Dickerson, R. L., Hoover, J. A., Peden-Adams, M. M., Mashburn, W. E., Allen, C. A., and Henshel, D. S., "**Alterations in Chicken Embryonic Development as a Sensitive Indicator of 2,3,7,8-Tetrachlorodibenzo-P-Dioxin Exposure,**" *Environmental Toxicology and Risk Assessment: Biomarkers and Risk Assessment—Fifth Volume, ASTM STP 1306*, David A. Bengtson and Diane S. Henshel, Eds., American Society for Testing and Materials, 1996.

ABSTRACT: 2,3,7,8-Tetrachlorodibenzo-p-dioxin (2,3,7,8-TCDD) exposure may be detected by chemical analysis or by its biological effects on *in vivo* or *in vitro* systems. Chemical analysis is expensive and does not give indications of the bioavailability of the material to an organism. Dosing an *in vitro* system with an extract obtained from an environmental sample has numerous advantages. This method is relatively cheap, quite sensitive, and can be used to generate quantitative dose response relationships as well as quantitative structure activity relationships. One method that is currently being used in our laboratories and others is a whole embryo model which consists of fertile hen's eggs injected on day 0. The eggs are incubated for either 48 or 96 hours and the embryos removed and examined for malformations. In addition, alterations in the

---

[1] Assistant Professor and Section Leader, and [2]Graduate Students, Biochemical and Behavioral Toxicology, Department of Environmental Toxicology and The Institute of Wildlife and Environmental Toxicology, Clemson University, Pendleton, SC 29670, Dr. Dickerson is the corresponding author.

[3] Undergraduate Student and [4]Assistant Professor, School of Public and Environmental Affairs, Indiana University, Bloomington, IN 47405

vitelline vasculature are examined in the 96 hour embryos. This model is able to detect significant 2,3,7,8-TCDD effects at levels of 2 - 20 pg/g egg (ppt), depending on the endpoint. The results of this study were compared to results of the H4IIE assay based on EROD induction. Although the H4IIE assay is more sensitive, the egg injection method provides more data on effects.

KEYWORDS: developmental effects, 2,3,7,8-TCDD, dioxin, Times Beach, bird, in ovo exposure, H4IIE.

    2,3,7,8-TCDD or "dioxin' is the most toxic member of a class of compounds referred to as halogenated aromatic hydrocarbons (HAHs). Other members of this class of compounds include the polychlorinated biphenyls (PCBs), the polybrominated biphenyls (PBBs), the polychlorinated diphenyl ethers (PCDEs) and polychlorinated dibenzofurans (PCDFs). The PCBs, PBBs, and PCDEs were manufactured commercially while the PCDDs and PCDFs are formed in undesirable side reactions during the production of chlorinated phenolic compounds and during combustion of phenyl compounds in the presence of halogens. Currently, the major sources of 2,3,7,8-TCDD in the environment are incineration of municipal and industrial waste and kraft pulp and paper production (Gough 1991). However, 2,3,7,8-TCDD has also entered the environment through the spraying of herbicides contaminated with 2,3,7,8-TCDD (Agents Orange, Purple and White, 2,4,5-T), industrial plant mishaps (Seveso, Italy), and inappropriate use of waste oil (Times Beach, Missouri).

    Exposure of vertebrates to 2,3,7,8-TCDD results in a wide spectrum of toxic and biochemical effects. These include a progressive loss of weight referred to as the wasting syndrome, dermal effects such as alopecia and chloracne, cancer, endocrine effects, thymic involution and other immunotoxic effects, enzyme induction and teratogenesis (Poland and Knutson 1982, Malaby et al. 1991). Most of the research into the effects of 2,3,7,8-TCDD has been confined to rodent models and *in vitro* systems. However, limited research indicates that piscivorous birds consuming fish contaminated with 2,3,7,8-TCDD and related compounds have reduced reproductive success and the offspring, when present, demonstrate a number of malformations including crossed beaks and brain asymmetry (Elliott et al. 1989, Hart et al. 1991, Henshel et al. 1995, Hoffman et al. 1996).

    The effects of 2,3,7,8-TCDD on development in avian species include cardiac malformations, edema of the pericardium and rump, beak malformations, and skeletal abnormalities (Cheung et al. 1981, Henshel et al. 1993, Peterson et al. 1993, White et al. 1993, Hoffman et al. 1996). This chemical and other dioxins may also cause edema, decreased body weight, and increased liver weight when fed to young chicks (Cecil et al. 1974, Nosek et al 1993, Hoffman et al. 1996).

Embryonic day 2 (E2) abnormalities caused by 2,3,7,8-TCDD exposure include embryo mortality, asymmetrical somites, abnormal curvature of the heart, and delayed brain and head curvature. 2,3,7,8-TCDD exposure results in delayed and abnormal tail and limb bud development, abnormal visceral arches, and decreased vitelline vasculature development at embryonic day 3 (E3) (Henshel et al. 1993). At embryonic day 4 (E4), embryos exposed to 2,3,7,8-TCDD exhibited delays in developmental indicators such as abnormal limbs and visceral arches, a small or missing maxillary process, a high length to width ratio of the limb buds and a decreased vitelline vasculature development (Henshel et al. 1993).

The presence of 2,3,7,8-TCDD and similar HAHs at uncontrolled waste sites may be detected by chemical analysis of environmental samples, the observation of dioxin-induced effects in wildlife inhabiting the site or by administering extracts of environmental samples to an *in vivo* or *in vitro* system. Chemical analysis, although sensitive and highly specific, is expensive and does not give indications of the bioavailability of the material to an organism. Likewise, measuring dioxin-induced effects in wildlife gives direct information on bioavailability and risk; however, insufficient specimens may be present for meaningful statistics. Dosing an *in vitro* system with an extract obtained from an environmental sample has numerous advantages. This method is relatively cheap, quite sensitive, and can be used to generate quantitative dose response relationships as well as quantitative structure activity relationships. One method that is currently being used in our laboratory and others is to dose the H4IIE rat hepatoma cell line or the MCF-7 breast cancer cell line and measure CYP1A1 induction (both), estrogen receptor binding activity (MCF-7) and proliferation (MCF-7). These methods can detect 2,3,7,8-TCDD concentrations of approximately 10^{-13} M (0.03 pg/g). In this study we compare the use of transformed cell lines to a whole embryo system to determine which method gives a greater sensitivity for detection of 2,3,7,8-TCDD in environmental samples. This whole embryo model consists of fertile hen's eggs injected on day 0. The eggs are incubated for either 48 or 96 hours and the embryos removed and examined for malformations. In addition, alterations in the vitelline vasculature are examined. The results for injecting pure 2,3,7,8-TCDD into the eggs as compared to dosing the cell lines indicate the two methods differ by an order of magnitude in sensitivity.

EXPERIMENTAL METHODS

Chemicals and Biochemicals

The 2,3,7,8-TCDD used in this study was obtained from Cambridge Isotopes (Boston, MA). The olive oil (Bertolli™) used as a vehicle was extra-light and obtained from a local grocery store. It was checked for the presence of organochlorine and organophosphate contamination before use. 7-ethoxyresorufin and 7-pentoxyresorufin were purchased from Molecular Probes (Eugene, OR). The remainder of the chemicals and expendables were obtained from Sigma (St. Louis, MO) as were all of the media requirements for cell cultures, with the exception of the non-essential amino acid solution which was purchased from Biowhitaker (Walkersville, MD).

Egg Source and Storage

White Leghorn (*Gallus domesticus*) eggs from the Clemson University Poultry Center were used. The eggs were stored at 10°C until used in the study and no eggs were stored for more than 14 days.

Egg Injection and Incubation

Three hundred White Leghorn eggs were randomly sorted into six treatment groups (50 eggs per group). The eggs were labeled as to treatment group and number, weighed to the nearest 0.01 gram, and washed with Betadine™. The average weight of the eggs was 60 ± 1 gram and this was used to fix the injection volume. Each egg was candled to locate the air sac and its boundary was marked on the egg shell in pencil. The egg tops were wiped with 70% ethanol and a Dremel™ tool equipped with a 1/16" burr was used to perforate the shell inside of the air sac line. A sterile Hamilton syringe was used to inject six µl of either 0, 20 pg/ml, 200 pg/ml, 2 ng/ml, 20 ng/ml, or 200 ng/ml TCDD in olive oil. The injection hole was sealed with melted paraffin. Following injection, the eggs were placed in egg flats, incubated at 100°F at 60% relative humidity, and rotated every two hours. The incubator, fabricated entirely of stainless steel at Clemson University for 2,3,7,8-TCDD work, was equipped with high and low temperature alarms and maintained the set temperature to within 0.5 °F.

Egg Analysis and Hatchling Treatment

Ten eggs per treatment were removed at 48 hours and at 96 hours. On days 5, 9, 14, and 18, the 30 remaining eggs per group were candled to determine viability. Those eggs determined to be non-viable were opened and the embryo placed in phosphate buffered formaldehyde (pH 7.5) for later analysis of staging and developmental abnormalities. On the 18th day of incubation, the surviving eggs were placed in hatching baskets in the hatchery at 99°F and 60% humidity until hatching or the end of 24 days. All unhatched eggs were preserved in 10% buffered formalin for later embryological study and staging. Hatchlings were raised in the brooder and fed Purina Starter™ for 14 days. The hatchlings were sacrificed on posthatching day 14 for biochemical analysis.

Analysis of 48 Hour Embryos

Ten eggs were used for E2 analysis. The embryos were removed and placed in 10% phosphate buffered formalin for later analysis. For analysis, the embryos were placed in glass petri dishes containing phosphate buffered saline and examined with a Wild M8 stereomicroscope equipped with a Leitz camera. Heart morphology, body curvature, head fold, and somites were classified as abnormal or normal compared to the overall stage. The overall staging of the 48 hour embryos was based on the number of somites present according to the methods of Hamburger and Hamilton (1951).

Analysis of 96 Hour Embryos

Five eggs were used for E4 analysis. The egg shell was carefully removed from the air sac area. Egg white was removed and more egg shell was dissected away. This process was continued until the entire vitelline vasculature could be visualized. The vasculature was photographed using a Nikon 9009 camera with a Nikkor 60 mm macro lens and Kodak Tmax™ 100 film. The embryo was removed, placed in 10% phosphate buffered saline, and stored at room temperature for later analysis. For analysis, the embryos were examined using a camera-equipped stereomicroscope. The visceral arches, allantois, heart, limb buds, and curvature were examined and classified as normal or abnormal according to stage. The eyes were also examined and measured. The embryos were staged using the curvature primarily or the stage of the most recent consistent indicators if the curvature was grossly delayed (Hamburger and Hamilton 1951). The photographs of the vitelline vasculature were analyzed for vascular shape, size, and condition and for rating vasculature parameters such as vessel kinking, vascular ring size, ring periphery hemolysis, and vasculature hemisphere fusion. The parameters measured were recorded as normal, abnormal, or grossly abnormal.

Biochemical Analysis

Fourteen-day-old hatchlings were weighed and examined for gross external abnormalities. The hatchlings were anesthetized with a saturated CO_2 atmosphere until unconscious. Blood was then collected by cardiac puncture until death occurred. The blood was collected into heparinized and non-heparinized tubes for hemagglutination and hormone analysis, respectively (Hoover 1994, Peden 1996, Alonso 1996). The thymus and spleen were collected and stored in RPMI-1640 for CD4/CD8 ratios and T/B cell proliferation, respectively (Hoover 1994, Peden 1996). It was more feasible to look at B cell function from the spleen because of the large amounts of tissues to be processed; therefore, the bursa was not harvested. The livers were also collected from chicks of each group and stored at -80°C until CYPIA1/2 and CYPIIB1/2 analysis could be performed as described below. Liver microsomes were prepared as described by Gard (1995). Ethoxyresorufin-O-deethylase (EROD) and pentoxyresorufin-O-dealkylase (PROD) assays were performed on the microsomes. Activity was determined by the methods of Prough et al. (1978) and Burke et al. (1985) respectively, which were modified for use in a 96-well fluorometric plate reader as reported by Gard (1995). Slight species specific modifications were made. Microsomes were diluted 20 fold for both EROD and PROD analysis and samples were run in triplicate. The final concentrations ([FC]) of 7- ethoxyresorufin and 7-pentoxyresorufin were 4 x 10^{-6} and 2 x 10^{-5}, respectively. The final well volume was 180 μl (20 μl diluted microsome sample, 25 μl substrate, 125 μl Buffer B (0.1M Tris buffer + 1.6 mg/ml BSA: 800 mg

BSA, 500 ml Buffer A), and 10 μl NADPH or Buffer A). NADPH (0.1M) was used to initiate the reaction. Blanks were prepared with Buffer A (0.1M Tris buffer: 11.26g Tris HCL, 3.51g Tris Base, 1L ddH$_2$O, pH 7.8) instead of NADPH. Fluorescence was read using a Perkin-Elmer LS 50 Luminescence Spectrometer that read each plate five times to obtain a kinetic determination of the reaction rate. The excitation wavelength was 530 nm and the emission wavelength was 585 nm. Protein concentration was determined using the bicinchoninic acid (BCA) technique of Smith et al. (1985), modified for use with a 96-well plate reader. The total well volume was 210 μl (10 μl diluted microsome sample and 200 μl BCA solution; 50:1 / V:V / BCA : Copper (II) Sulfate Pentahydrate). Enzyme activities were expressed as picomoles of substrate dealkylated per mg protein per minute.

Cell Culture and Dosing

The rat hepatoma cell line H4IIE was obtained from American Type Culture Collection. The H4IIE cells were maintained in 75 cm^2 flasks in Dulbecco's Modified Essential Medium supplemented with 10% fetal calf serum, penicillin - streptomycin mixture, non-essential amino acids (NEAA), and sodium bicarbonate as reported in Mashburn (1995). The cells were incubated to 90% of confluence in an incubator kept at 100% relative humidity, 5% CO$_2$ and 37°C. The cells were then subcultured to additional flasks by the addition of trypsin-EDTA to remove the monolayer of cells and resuspended in fresh media.

The cells were exposed to 2,3,7,8-TCDD in 48-well plates. The wells each contained 1,000 cells and were allowed to grow 48 hours prior to dosing. The concentrations of 2,3,7,8-TCDD used were from 10^{-12} molar (M) to 10^{-8} molar (M) and three wells were used per concentration. The plates containing the H4IIE cells were incubated for 48 hours. At the end of the incubation period, the medium was removed from the plates containing the H4IIE cells and the plates were frozen at -80°C until EROD analysis could be performed. This analysis was performed using a modification of the assay described above for the liver and kidney microsomes as reported in Mashburn (1995). EROD [FC]= 1.7 x 10^{-5} M and a 48-well flat bottom cell culture plate was used.

RESULTS AND DISCUSSION

Table 1 lists mortality by dose group at each of the candling intervals and at hatch. The slightly lower survival of the control group may be because they were the first group injected. The majority of the embryonic deaths occurred prior to the embryonic day 14 candling. In general, these data show a dose-dependent increase in mortality. Figure 1 shows the mortality as a function of embryonic staging. For this portion of the study, all embryos that had an injection site near the blastocyst were excluded. Note that only those stages at which mortality occurred are listed on the

X-axis. Mortality appeared to cluster either early in embryonic development or just prior to hatch. Approximately 60% of the mortality occurred within 6 days of incubation (stage 28 or less). The second peak in mortality occurred between days 19 and 21 of incubation (stage 45). This peak accounted for approximately 20% of the overall embryonic mortality. Analysis of the data by treatment group shows that in the controls both mortality peaks were of similar size whereas with treatment the first mortality peak increased in number with increasing 2,3,7,8-TCDD dose. The mortality rate for the controls was relatively high. We believe this may have been due to egg storage prior to incubation longer than one week. Nonetheless, it is clear that embryo mortality is significantly increased at 200 ppt, 2 ppb (2000 ppt), and 20 ppb (20,000 ppt) TCDD.

Overall staging was determined as per Hamburger and Hamilton (1951), and 48 and 96 hour embryos were specifically staged as described above. Note that the staging of the day 2 embryos was based on the number of somites counted on a stereo microscope as described by Hamburger and Hamilton (1951). Because the staging compromised a range of 3 somites between integral stage numbers, some day 2 embryos received a non-integral stage number. The results of this analysis are shown in Figure 2. The average stage number decreased with increasing concentrations of 2,3,7,8-TCDD. In addition, the range between minimum and maximum stage at any given 2,3,7,8-TCDD concentration was increased compared to control values.

TABLE 1--Mortality (%) following 2,3,7,8-TCDD injection into chicken eggs

TCDD Concentration	Embryonic Day 5	Embryonic Day 9	Embryonic Day 14	Embryonic Day 18	Day of Hatch
0 ppt	3.3	36.7	40.0	43.3	63.3
2 ppt	6.7	10.0	20.0	23.3	53.3
20 ppt	10.0	26.7	36.7	36.7	46.7
200 ppt	6.7	36.7	63.3*	66.7*	93.3*
2 ppb	6.7	73.3*	100.0*	100.0*	100.0*
20 ppb	3.3	30	96.7*	96.7*	100.0*

* significant at $p < 0.05$, n=30 eggs for each group, 100%=30 eggs

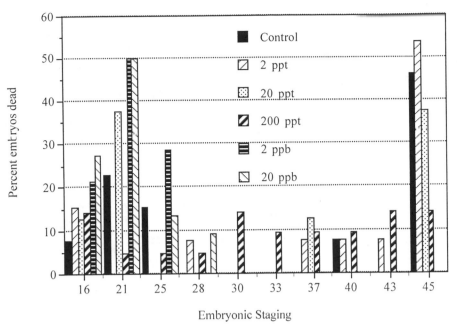

FIGURE 1--Mortality as a function of embryo staging

Table 2 contains the data from the analysis of day 4 embryo staging. The staging of day 4 embryos was based on the degree of body curvature of the embryos and are listed as mean ± SEM. Note that the embryos receiving intermediate doses of 2,3,7,8-TCDD (20 ppt and 200 ppt) were developmentally younger, on the average than those receiving no, low or high doses of this compound. Moreover, the range of observed stages was also greatest for those embryos receiving the intermediate doses of 2,3,7,8-TCDD (20, 200 ppt and 2 ppb) as compared to those embryos receiving no, low or high doses of 2,3,7,8-TCDD; however, this was not found to be significantly different.

Treatment with 2,3,7,8-TCDD also resulted in changes in the vitelline vasculature of the day 4 embryos. These data are listed in Table 3. These changes were categorized as severe kinking, hemolysis and qualitative increases in the density of the vasculature. At dose levels below 20 ppt, peripheral ring vasculature hemolysis was not evident but showed a dose-dependent increase at the higher concentrations of 2,3,7,8-TCDD. Severe kinking of the vasculature was evident at the lowest treatment level and showed a dose-dependent increase. The density of the vasculature was markedly increased at all 2,3,7,8-TCDD concentrations, but this change was not dose-dependent.

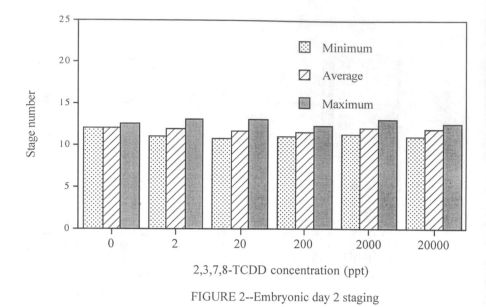

FIGURE 2--Embryonic day 2 staging

In the day 4 embryos morphological abnormalities were observed. These included heart malformations, alterations from normal body curvature, and abnormalities in the visceral arches. The rate of occurrence of these abnormalities as a function of 2,3,7,8-TCDD exposure is listed in Table 4. Heart malformations began to appear at doses of 20 ppt and showed a dose-dependent increase. In these embryos, the hearts may have been abnormally thin (underdeveloped) or not folded properly. The control embryos had an incidence rate of abnormal body twist of approximately 10% and this rate was found to increase with increasing 2,3,7,8-TCDD exposure. In addition, a dose-dependent increase in visceral arch abnormalities was found. No significant increase was observed in eye abnormalities as compared to control embryos.

TABLE 2-- Embryonic day 4 staging

TCDD Concentration	Average Stage	Range
0 ppt	20.889 ± 2.111	20-22
2 ppt	20.556 ± 1.444	19-22
20 ppt	19.778 ± 2.000	16-23
200 ppt	19.667 ± 2.000	16-22
2 ppb	20.333 ± 2.000	18-22
20 ppb	21.500 ± 1.667	21-23

* not significant at p < 0.05, n= 10 for all groups

Rump edema, a common finding in 2,3,7,8-TCDD exposed avian species, increased in a dose-dependent manner in stage 40 to 45 embryos. In addition, a dose dependent increase in beak malformation and total abnormalities were observed and these are listed in Table 5.   Neither the 2 nor the 20 ppb treatment groups survived to this stage of development. Numerous other abnormalities were observed but did not show a dose-dependency. These, however, were included in the total abnormalities. Neck edema, alterations in beak position, head shape and position, curved spine, enlarged hatch muscle, external intestines and backward bent legs were among the abnormalities observed.

TABLE 3--2,3,7,8-TCDD-induced changes in E4 vasculature

TCDD Concentration	Severe Kinking (Percent)	Hemolysis (Percent)	Dense Vasculature (Percent)
0 ppt	0	0	18
2 ppt	18	0	80*
20 ppt	0	0	68*
200 ppt	35	50*	70*
2 ppb	70*	70*	100*
20 ppb	70*	90*	90*

* significant at p < 0.05, n=10 for all groups

TABLE 4--Morphological abnormalities in E4 embryos

TCDD Concentration	Heart Malformations (%)	Abnormalities in Body Twist (%)	Abnormalities in Visceral Arches (%)
0 ppt	0	10	0
2 ppt	0	20	20
20 ppt	20	20	30
200 ppt	11	45*	35*
2 ppb	32*	22	90*
20 ppb	23	35*	80*

* significant at $p < 0.05$, n=10 for all groups

A dose-dependent increase in EROD and PROD activity was present in the hatchlings euthanized 14 days after hatch and this is shown in Figure 3. It is not clear whether the PROD activity is the result of cytochrome 2B1/2 activity or due to substrate cross-reactivity of the cytochrome P450 1A1/2 gene products in this species. The increases in activity seen were significant at the $p < 0.01$ level for all 2,3,7,8-TCDD exposure levels as compared to controls.

Figure 4 shows the dose-response induction of EROD activity by 2,3,7,8-TCDD in the H4IIE cell line. Note that the EC_{50} for induction is approximately 10^{-12} M and this corresponds to approximately 0.3 ppt. In contrast, the EC_{50} for EROD induction in the chicken embryo liver is approximately 2 ppt, almost an order of magnitude higher.

TABLE 5--Abnormalities observed in embryos near hatching

TCDD Concentration	n	Rump Edema (%)	Beak Malformation (%)	Any Abnormality (%)
0 ppt	7	0	14	55
2 ppt	9	23	45*	88*
20 ppt	3	66*	66*	100*
200 ppt	8	40*	50*	100*

* significant at $p < 0.05$

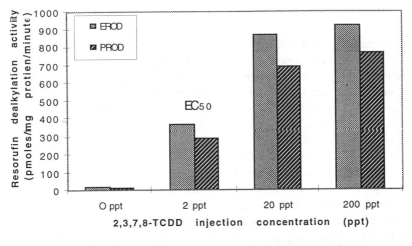

Figure 3--EROD and PROD induction in hatchlings.

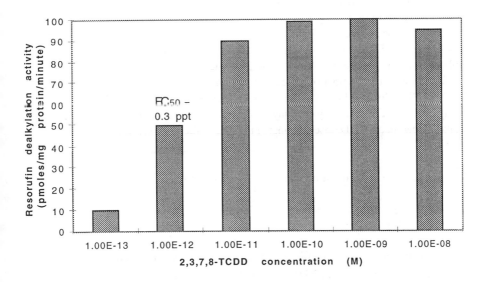

Figure 4 --EROD induction in the H4IIE cell line.

CONCLUSIONS

EROD induction in the H4IIE rat hepatoma cell line is a more sensitive indicator of 2,3,7,8-TCDD exposure than most of the endpoints measured in the chicken embryo. The most sensitive endpoints in the early chicken embryo are: the range of developmental stages (E2 embryos); vitelline vasculature; and visceral arch abnormalities (E4 embryos). The egg injection model, therefore, offers significant advantages as a tool for ecological risk assessments and other effects assessments. First, although EROD induction in a cell line can be considered a biomarker of exposure, it does not provide a measure of effect in an intact or developing organism. Second, the use of the chicken egg injection model allows for the determination of what population effects may be produced by exposure to either soil extracts or extracts prepared from food sources. Third, the egg injection model requires approximately equal equipment investment but provides more useful information.

In addition, the following specific conclusions may be drawn from this study. First, E2 embryos were generally staged younger with increased concentrations of 2,3,7,8-TCDD and the width of the range between minimum and maximum stage was more variable. Also, the most dose-dependent E2 abnormalities were in visceral arches, the heart, and body twist of the embryos.

A variation in staging was seen with increasing 2,3,7,8-TCDD dose; however, the dose response curve was found to be "U" shaped. In this age of embryos, the most dose-dependent E4 abnormality was an alteration in visceral arches. For the older embryos, dose-related near-hatch abnormalities included rump edema and beak malformations. The number of embryos containing abnormalities increased with 2,3,7,8-TCDD dose. After hatching, no weight difference between 2,3,7,8-TCDD groups was observed for day 0 or day 14 chicks. However, both EROD and PROD were induced in a TCDD dose responsive manner in the chicken embryo liver.

This research was supported by grants from the NIEHS and the US F&WS.

REFERENCES

Alonso, K.R., "2,3,7,8-TCDD Induced Alterations in Parental (P$_0$) Exposed Chickens and First Filial (F$_1$) Generation Reproductive Endpoints, Endocrine levels, and Receptor Function," Thesis, Clemson University, August 1996.

Burke, M.D., Thompson, S., Elcombe, C.R., Halpert, J., Haaparanta, T., and Mayer, R.T., "Ethoxy-,Pentoxy-, and Benzyloxyphenoxazones and homologes: A series of substrates to distinguish between different induced cytochromes P450," Biochem. Pharmacol, Vol 34, pp.3337-3345, 1985.

Cecil, H. C., Bitman, J., Lillie, R. J., Fries, G. F., and Verrett, J.,
"Embryotoxicity and Teratogenic Effects in Unhatched Fertile Eggs from Hens
Fed Polychlorinated Biphenyls (PCBs)," Bulletin of Environmental
Contamination and Toxicology, Vol. 11, No. 6, pp 489-495, 1974.

Cheung, M.O., Gilbert, E.F., and Peterson, R.E., "Cardiovascular Teratogenicity of
2,3,7,8-Tetracholrodibenzo-p-Dioxin in the Chick Embryo" Toxicology and
Applied Pharmacology, Vol 61, pp. 197-204, 1981.

Elliot, J. E., Butler, R. W., Norstrom, R. J., and Whitehead, P. F.,
"Environmental Contaminants and Reproductive Success of Great Blue Herons
Ardea herodias in British Columbia, 1986-1987," Environmental Pollution,
Vol. 59, pp. 91-114, 1989.

Gard, N.W., "Induction of Immunotxicity and Mixed-Function Oxygenase Activity as
Biomarkers of Exposure to Enviromental Contaminates in the Deer Mouse
(Peromyscus maniculatus)," Dissertaion, Clemson University, December 1995.

Gough, M., "Human Exposures from Dioxin in the Soil-A Meeting Report,"
Journal of Toxicology and Environmental Health, Vol. 32, pp. 205-245, 1991.

Hamburger, V., and Hamilton, H. L., "A series of Normal Stages in the
Development of the Chick Embryo," Journal of Morphology, Vol. 88,
pp. 49-92, 1951.

Hart, L. E., Cheng K.M., Whitehead, P.E., Shah, R.M., Lewis, R.J., Ruschkowski,
S.R., Blair, R.W., Bellward G.D., and Bandiera S.M., "Effects of Dioxin
Contamination on the Growth and Development of Great Blue Heron
embryos," Journal of Toxicology and Environmental Health, Vol. 32, pp. 331-
344, 1991.

Henshel, D. S., Hehn, B. M., Vo, M. T., and Steeves, J. D., "A Short Term Test
for Dioxin Teratogenicity Used in Chicken Embryos," In: Environmental
Toxicology and Risk Assessment: ASTP STP 1216, J.W. Gorsuch, F. J.
Dwyer, C. J. Ingersol and T. W. LaPoint, eds., American Society for Testing
and Materials: Philadelphia, PA, pp. 159-174, 1993.Henshel, D.S., Martin,
J.W., Norstrom R., Whithead P., Steeves, J.D., and
Cheng, K.M., "Morphometric Abnormalities in Brains of Great Blue Heron
Hatchlings Exposed in the Wild to PCDDs," Environmental Health
Perspectives, Vol 103, Sup 4, pp. 61-66, 1995.

Hoffman, D.J., Rice, C.P., Kubiak, T.J., "PCBs and Dioxins in Birds," In:
Environmental Contaminates in Wildlife, W.N. Beyer, G.H. Heinz, and A.W.
Redmon, eds., SETAC Publication Lewis Publishers, CRC Press, Boca Raton,
Fl, Chap. 7, pp. 167-209, 1996.

Hoover, J.A., "The effect of 2,3,7,8-TCDD on Chicken Embronic Developement and
Hatchling Survival," Thesis, Clemson University, December 1994.

Malaby, T.A., Moore, R. W., et al., "The Male Reproductive System is Highly
    Sensitive to In Utero and Lactaional 2,3,7,8-Terachlorodibenzo-p-Dioxin
    Expousre," Banbury Report 35, Biological risk Assessments of Dioxins and
    Related Compounds, M.A. Gallo, R.J. Scheplain and V.D. Heijden eds., Cold
    Spring Harbor, New York, Cold Spring Harbor Laboratory Press, 1991.
Mashburn, W.E., "Use of an In Vitro Bioassay to Assess PCB Contamination,"
    Thesis, Clemson University, December 1995.
Nosek, J.A., Sulivan, J.R., Craven, S.R., Gendron-Fitzpatrick, A., and Peterson R.E.,
    "Embryotoxicity of 2,3,7,8-Tertachlorodibenzo-p-Dioxin in the Ring-Necked
    Pheasant," Environmental Toxicology and Chemistry,Vol 12, pp. 1215-1222,
    1993.
Peden, M.M., "2,3,7,8-TCDD Induced Alterations in Adult and Hatchling Chicken
    Immune Function and CYPIAI Activity," Thesis, Clemson University,
    May 1996.
Peterson, R. E., Theobald, H. M., and Kimmel, G. L., " Developmental and
    Reproductive Toxicity of Dioxins and Related Compounds: Cross Species
    Comparisons," Critical Reviews in Toxicology, Vol. 22, No. 3, pp. 283-33,
    1993.
Poland, A., and Knutson, J C., "2,3,7,8-Tetrachlorodibenzo-p-Dioxin and
    Related Halogenated Aromatic Hydrocarbons: Examination of the Mechanism
    of Toxicity," Annual Review of Pharmacology and Toxicology, Vol. 22,
    pp. 517-554, 1982.
Prough, R.A., Burke, M.D., and Mayer, R.T., "Direct Flourometric Methods for
    Measuring Mixed-Function Oxidase Activity," Methods Enzymol.,
    Vol 52(C), pp.372-377, 1978.
Smith, P.K., Krohn, R.I., et al., "Measurement of Protein Using Bicinchoninic Acid,"
    Analytical Biochemistry, Vol 150, pp. 76-85, 1985.
White, D.H., and Hoffman, D.J., "Effects of Poychloinated Dibenzo-p-dioxins and
    Dibenzofurans on Nesting Wood Ducks (Aix Sponsa) at Bayou Meto,
    Arkansas," Environmental Health Perspectives, Vol 103, Suppl 4, pp. 37-39,
    1995.

Diane S. Henshel[1]

AN ARGUMENT FOR THE CHICKEN EMBRYO AS A MODEL FOR THE DEVELOPMENTAL
TOXICOLOGICAL EFFECTS OF THE POLYHALOGENATED AROMATIC HYDROCARBONS
(PHAHS)

REFERENCE: Henshel, D. S., "An Argument for the Chicken Embryo as a Model for the
Developmental Toxicological Effects of the Polyhalogenated Aromatic Hydrocarbons (PHAHs),"
*Environmental Toxicology and Risk Assessment: Biomarkers and Risk Assessment—Fifth Volume,
ASTM STP 1306*, David A. Bengtson and Diane S. Henshel, Eds., American Society for Testing and
Materials, 1996.

ABSTRACT: The choice of an animal model is ultimately crucial to
toxicological testing. If one does not use the appropriate model for
the chemical and endpoint being studied, then the test results may not
really provide the appropriate toxicological information. There are
three basic types of animal models: sentinel models, screening models,
and mechanistic models. Each of these models has specific needs and
requirements, some of which overlap, some of which are distinctly
different. Therefore, some animal models are more appropriate for
evaluating the effects of some chemicals than are other animal models.
This article will present the argument that the chicken embryo is
especially appropriate as an animal model for studying the mechanism of
the developmental toxicological effects of the polyhalogenated aromatic
hydrocarbons (PHAHs).
   The PHAHs are a group of toxicologically related compounds
including, in part, the polychlorinated dibenzodioxins, dibenzofurans
and biphenyls. The chicken (*Gallus gallus*) embryo is relatively
sensitive to the toxicological effects of the PHAHs being approximately
two orders of magnitude more sensitive than the mature bird. The
chicken embryo has been used to demonstrate general toxicological
effects (i.e. the LD50), immunotoxicity, cardiovascular toxicity,
teratogenicity, hepatotoxicity and neurotoxicity. Many of these
effects, or analogous effects, have also been observed in mammals and
fish. Thus, most animals appear to respond to the PHAHs with a similar
toxicological profile, indicating that many of the biomarkers used for
the PHAHs are valid across a number of species, including the chicken.
Furthermore, the chicken embryo is relatively inexpensive to use for
toxicity testing. In addition, all effects detected are due to direct
effects on the embryo and are not complicated by maternal interactions.
In short, for sensitivity, ease of use, cost and applicability of
results to other animals, the chicken embryo is an excellent animal
model for evaluation of the mechanism underlying the developmental
toxicological effects of the PHAHs.

KEYWORDS: TCDD, PCB, bird, development, teratogen, heart, brain, embryo

----

[1]Indiana University, School of Public and Environmental Affairs,
Bloomington, IN 47405

Animal Models
    A major focus in toxicology today is biomarkers, the uses of
biomarkers and when and how one uses biomarkers in risk assessment. But
before choosing a biomarker to use, it is important to realize that each
biomarker may be specific to the animal in which it is measured. Thus
the choice of an animal model is just as important as the choice of the
biomarker that is used. Although there has been much discussion in the
literature about animal models for toxicity, there seems to be some
differences of opinion about which animals are appropriate models for
toxicological assessment. Some of these apparent contradictions stem
from the fact that authors may have different intended meanings when
they use the term "animal model" (Hill and Hoffman 1984, Hood 1990).
There are three basic types of animal models which are used within
toxicology, and especially environmental toxicology: Sentinel species,
animals used for toxicological screening, and animals used to study the
mechanism of toxic action.

    A sentinel model species is an animal which warns us of potential
toxic effects. These species may be used purposely, as warning systems
in a potentially dangerous situation; or they may be the animals in
which a toxic effect is first noticed. A sentinel model species needs
to be as sensitive or more sensitive than the most sensitive individual
in the population or species of interest. For ecotoxicology, a sentinel
species must be equally or more sensitive than the other species in the
ecosystem of concern. If the animal model is not sufficiently sensitive,
then it will not provide a sufficient warning when contaminants have
reached potentially toxic levels. The expectation is, of course, that
the mechanism of toxic action is similar in both the animal model and
the population of interest. However, this is not absolutely essential.
The classic example of the use of a sentinel animal model entailed the
use of canaries in underground mines as early warning systems for
changes in air quality, generally due to the accumulation of the
odorless carbon monoxide[2]. More recent examples of this include the
Great Lakes Bald Eagle and Herring Gull which, in the 1950s and 1960s,
began having problems reproducing successfully due (at least in large
part) to the levels of organochlorines accumulating in the aquatic food
chain (Colburn, 1991; Gilbertson, 1988; Mineau et al, 1984). More
recent evidence on a large number of animals have indicated that these
chemicals do indeed affect the endocrine and reproductive systems, and
that these chemicals in the Great Lakes food chain may now have
affected a large number of animals, including humans (Colburn et al,
1993).
    Chickens have also been valuable as a sentinel species. In the
late 1950s chicks consumed feed contaminated with a "toxic fatty
material" which turned out to contain polychlorinated dibenzodioxins
(PCDDs), the most potent of which was 2,3,7,8-tetrachlorodibenzo-p-
dioxin (TCDD). These chicks developed what became known as "Chick Edema
Disease", a group of syndromes which included decreased weight gain,
problems with gait, a general "unthriftiness" in appearance, and sudden
death. Upon necropsy these birds were found to have pericardial,
subcutaneous and/or abdominal edema, adrenal hemorrhage and kidney
degeneration (Schmittle et al, 1958; Sanger et al, 1958). This
"disease", once the puzzle of the causative factor was solved, was one
of the first indications scientists had that PCDDs and the related
polychlorinated biphenyls (PCBs) were highly toxic.

    Traditional toxicological testing utilizes screening models.
These animals are used to evaluate the likelihood that a given chemical

---

[2]Methane gas also accumulates in mines, and while it is less toxic than
carbon monoxide, it is explosive and therefore dangerous. Methane,
however, has a smell which provides some warning.

will have a specific type of toxicological effect (death, tumor-induction, reproductive impairment, teratogenicity). The screening models should respond to the chemical via the same toxic mechanism of action as does the population of concern. Depending on the endpoint measured, the response of the screening model will probably be chemical-specific in that the sensitivity of the response and resultant benchmark doses (i.e. LD50 or LD10, ED50 or ED10), may vary with both the animal and the chemical. Further, a model species to be used for pre-screening of toxic effects needs to be approximately as sensitive as the most sensitive individuals in the population of interest. If the model species is <u>too</u> sensitive, too many chemicals will falsely test positive, that is too many chemicals will be toxic to the model species, but nontoxic to the species of interest. Industry is especially concerned that the toxicological screening models are only as sensitive as needed to protect the species of interest. Any chemical that tests positive in the initial screening tests have to go through the full toxicological battery, which adds to the cost and time of bringing a chemical or process to market. On the other hand, if the model species is not sensitive enough, it will be ineffective for pre-screening and chemicals will be assessed as non-toxic that indeed have an adverse effect on the population of concern. Ideal animal models for toxicological screening are just sensitive enough, but not too sensitive, a situation where the line is often unclear. As a result, certain standard models (rats, mice, rabbits, dogs) are used most of the time, regardless of how appropriate the animal model is for each chemical and each endpoint.

Studies evaluating the best animal model for teratogenicity testing emphasize the point that the more sensitive animal models may also produce the most false positives. When monkeys (non-human primates, the closest family of testing animals to humans) and humans were compared regarding teratogenic sensitivity to 38 chemicals known to be, or suspected to be teratogenic in humans, monkeys only tested positive to 30% (n = 11) of the chemicals. When 165 chemicals that have not been shown to be teratogenic to humans were evaluated, monkeys tested negative to 80% (n = 132) of the chemicals, a positive to negative ratio of 0.375. Monkeys appear to be relatively insensitive, and thus using monkey testing results exclusively would underprotect humans. By comparison, rats, which have a high sensitivity (80% co-positives), have a relatively low specificity rate (50% co-negatives), a ratio of 1.6. This ratio indicates that rats are overly sensitive compared to humans. By this evaluation method, rabbits seemed to be the best model of all, having 60% co-positives and 70% co-negatives (Frankos, 1985), a ratio of 0.857, the closest ratio to one with a reasonably high sensitivity and specificity. Despite these results, rats are the most common animal used for teratogenicity testing, although rabbits are often the second animal tested when more than one animal model is used (IRI, 1990a)

Another classic screening model is the rabbit-based Draize test, which is used to assess chemically-induced dermal and ocular irritation (Klaassen and Eaton, 1991). This test has been controversial, and was perceived by Animal Rights activists to cause unnecessary pain. As a result, it has been modified, but not abandoned. Other traditional uses of animal models in toxicological screening tests include the rodent carcinogenicity test (rats and mice) and the rodent chronic toxicity test (primarily rats). The rodents have been chosen as the preferred model because of their relatively short life span, their susceptibility to tumor induction, and the established database on their physiological and pathological responses to a wide variety of chemicals (IRI 1990b).

Not all of the most appropriate screening models are rodents, lagomorphs, or even mammals. Adult chickens are the best animal model found so far for organophosphate - induced delayed neuropathy (OPIDN), a syndrome that occurs in humans as well. Chickens have been shown to be excellent models for a number of neurotoxicants, including solvents (Abou-Donia, 1992).

Mechanistic animal models are animals which are used to evaluate
the mechanism of action which underlies an observed toxic effect. For
mechanistic models, the relative sensitivity of the animal model is not
that important. What is most important is that the mechanism of toxic
action is identical for a given chemical and a given endpoint between
the animal model and the population of interest. This is critical
because a mechanistic model is used to evaluate not just the mechanism
of action, but the control of that mechanism so that the effects of that
toxic action may be protected against or corrected once an exposure has
occurred.   In this case, the relative sensitivity of the species of
concern compared to the model species must be determined, but there is a
wider latitude for difference in relative sensitivity so long as the
underlying mechanisms are similar in the two systems.
     The classic example for the mechanistic animal model used to study
(human-related) reproductive, developmental, endocrine and even
behavioral effects has been the monkey, which (of the animal models
used) has a reproductive system which is the closest to human.   The
monkey is an expensive animal to maintain and use, and they are more
difficult to obtain now.   Furthermore, any laboratory that uses
primates is prone to being a target for Animal Rights groups. Thus,
initial testing is usually carried out in rodents or other non-primate
animals.   However, for final testing of mechanisms (especially those
related to the effects listed above), it is generally believed that
primates are the best model for humans.

     Thus the choice of an animal model must first depend on what type
of animal model is needed, sentinel, screening or mechanistic.   The
second question to address is whether the testing will be used to
evaluate human or ecological health impacts. For example, if the
potential effects of an aquatic pollutant on the health of an ecosystem
needs to be assessed, fish, amphibians, aquatic reptiles, piscivorous
birds and piscivorous mammals may all be animal populations of interest.
Any or all of these type of animals might be used to examine the
potential effect of the pollutant on the ecosystem in question.
Potential food chain effects (bioaccumulation, biomagnification) might
also have to be considered, depending on the types of pollutants
present.   If, however, the test will be used to evaluate the health and
side effects of a potential food additive before it is put on the
market, the population of interest is human.   In this situation, the
most appropriate animal model may be decided by the regulations, rather
than by biology.   If the testing will be used to satisfy regulatory
requirements, the "most appropriate animal model" for given types of
effects are recommended by the Environmental Protection Agency and the
Food and Drug Administration (IRI, 1990b; FDA, 1993).   For example, as
far as the EPA and the FDA are concerned, for most chemicals to be
tested the appropriate model to use for toxicological testing is going
to be a mammal.   Considering developmental toxicity, the rationale for
this is that mammals have placentas, as do we (equally mammalian)
humans.   And it is important to know whether the disposition of the
chemical within the mother will affect the toxicity of the chemical for
the developing embryo.   This is especially important for chemicals which
are either detoxified or bioactivated by the mother.
     If, however, the question is what are the direct effects of the
chemical on the embryo, such a placental bias should not be as
important.   In fact, early animal development (and animal development in
general) is similar throughout the vertebrates, and is very similar for
birds and mammals, both of which are at the high end of their part of
the evolutionary tree.   This similarity holds especially well when
considering the factors that control embryonic development such as
hormones, growth factors and oncogenes.   When evaluating the mechanisms
that control the developmental toxicity of a chemical, it is beneficial
to be able to evaluate the process of development.   Thus, animal models
which are accessible in their natural environment throughout the period
of development are preferable for the evaluation of early embryonic
toxicological effects.

The next factor that needs to be considered when choosing an animal model is how appropriate each animal is for the chemical and endpoint that needs to be studied. For example, if the need is to evaluate the potential teratogenic effects of TCDD-like compounds cleft palate would be an appropriate endpoint. In this case, the most appropriate animal model is the C57BL/6 mouse. which is relatively sensitive to TCDD-like effects and in which cleft palate appears at non-fetotoxic (i.e. lethal) concentrations (Birnbaum, 1991). However, in other mammalian models, such as the rat, the fetotoxicity appears before cleft palate, even though in both animals the receptor controlling cleft palate formation, and presumably fetotoxicity as well, is the aryl hydrocarbon (Ah) receptor (Poland and Glover, 1980; Hassoun et al. 1984).

Two other series of factors that need to be considered when choosing a developmental animal model include convenience factors and analytical factors (Hood, 1990). The convenience factors include:

▸   Cost - It is best if the animal is as cheap as possible to buy and maintain since toxicity testing in general requires a large number of assays with a reasonable sample size to enhance the statistical significance of the results.

▸   The availability of the animals - If the animals are not readily available when needed, it can cause both scheduling complications, and (if a second supplier is needed) can mean using two sub-strains of animals which can affect the consistency of the results;

▸   Ease of handling - Docile animals cause fewer complications for the animal care workers. Difficult to handle animals may also be more costly and less efficient to maintain. For example, the control rate of mortality may be higher, which will then affect the results of any testing, and will decrease the number of healthy animals available for use;

▸   Ease of breeding - Animals that are difficult to breed, or have a low fertility rate can cause scheduling complications if viable embryos are not available when needed.
   A short gestation/incubation time is also preferable, especially if evaluating an endpoint at or near the end of incubation/gestation. The shorter the gestation time, the shorter the time required for maintaining the animals (mothers, for mammals, or eggs, for non-mammalian species). The shorter gestation times also allow for carrying out more tests in a given period of time.
   The clutch and litter size also make a difference since the larger the clutch or litter size, the larger the sample size, and the fewer number of mothers that will be needed.

▸   Accessibility of the embryo - Embryo accessibility is mainly important if one evaluates early endpoints, or studies the mechanisms of developmental toxicity.

Analytical factors include:

■   Ease of determining mating or egg laying - For mammalian species it is critical to know when gestation began, especially if the application of the chemical is time dependent (i.e. at a known time after the start of embryonic development). This is also important if evaluating the embryo at a known age before the end of gestation.
   For domestic avian species, egg laying is obvious. But when evaluating wild species in their natural environment, being able to determine when the eggs are laid can be an important factor, especially for birds which nest in inaccessible locations (Great

Blue Herons, for example).

■   A large knowledge base - Whether studying the mechanism of action, or just doing developmental toxicological screening it helps the evaluation if specifics about the development of the species are known. A large literature base allows the comparison of results when evaluating toxicological effects. This helps to confirm whether the control results were as expected. This also provides a measure of how well the laboratory is running the tests and maintaining the animals. In addition, if carrying out an analysis of the mechanism of action it helps to understand how specific developmental processes are controlled in that animal in order to be able to evaluate whether the test chemical had any effect on the process being examined.

■   Probe availability - If studying the mechanism of action, or using a molecular or biochemical biomarker to screen for toxicity, it is useful to use a species in which a large number of molecular or biochemical probes (cDNA, antibodies, enzymes) are available. (The alternative, of course, is to prepare the probes in one's own laboratory which can be a very time-consuming process.)

The Chicken Embryo as a Model for TCDD-Like PHAH Developmental Toxicity

The chicken embryo is very sensitive to the effects of TCDD and related compounds. By comparison to the adult chicken, which has an LD50 of 25 - 50 ppb for TCDD, the chicken embryo has an LD50 of about 250 ppt, a difference of 100 fold (Greig et al, 1973; Allred and Strange, 1977; Henshel, 1993a). By comparison, the LD50 for adult rats (Sprague-Dawley, Sherman, Spartan) is similar to the LD50 for adult chickens (Beatty et al, 1978; Schwetz et al, 1973), yet the cumulative maternal dose that induces an LD41 in the Sprague-Dawley embryos is only 5 to 10 fold less than the dose associated with the LD50 in the adults (Beatty et al, 1978). This does not indicate that the rat embryos are actually absorbing that entire dose. In mice, for example, embryonic target tissue (the palate and the urinary tract) only take up approximately 0.0005% of the total maternal dose (Abbott et al, 1989). This results in a target tissue concentration which is 0.033 - 0.05% of the maternal whole body concentration. Clearly, the mammalian embryo is not necessarily exposed to the entire maternal dose. Thus, the mammalian embryo may be more sensitive than is at first indicated by considering only the cumulative maternal dose which yields an embryonic LD50.

By the end of incubation, chick embryos exposed *in ovo* to TCDD or PCBs exhibit a dose-related increase in mortality and decrease in hatch and bursa weight (Brunstrom and Darnerud, 1983; Nikolaidis et al, 1988; Henshel, 1993a). Whereas increased embryonic mortality is seen in all animals so far, not all animals have a decreased weight at hatch/birth. Decreased birth weight in response to developmental exposure to TCDD-like compounds has been reported in rats, hamsters and humans, but not mice, which respond with an increased birth weight. (Couture et al, 1990; Yamashita and Hayashi, 1985). A number of other pathologies have been reported in chicken after *in ovo* exposure to TCDD and related compounds. These include pericardial, abdominal and subcutaneous edema, liver, heart and limb anomalies, thymic hypoplasia, microophthalmia, beak and visceral arch deformities, effects on vascularization, and abnormal nervous system development (Cheung et al, 1981; Brunstrom and Darnerud, 1983; Rifkind et al, 1985; Nikolaidis et al, 1988a, Brunstrom and Lund, 1988; Summer, 1992; Henshel, 1993a,b,c). Some of these are similar to pathologies seen in other animals, including other birds (Hoffman et al, 1996). The palate, which is a sensitive target tissue in mice (see above), is a visceral arch derivative, as is the beak. Fish exposed to TCDD and related compounds are also reported to develop heart and vasculature anomalies (Walker et al, 1991). Edema and thymic hypoplasia or atrophy is reported in many animals (edema: fish, mouse, hamster, monkey, human; thymic hypoplasia/atrophy: mouse, rat, guinea pig, hamster, monkey)(Vos et al, 1973; Allen et al, 1977; Moore et al, 1979; Henck et al, 1981; Yamashita and Hayashi, 1985; Walker et al, 1991).

Congener analysis indicates that at least the increased chicken embryo mortality is linked in some way to the activation of the Ah receptor mechanism (Brunstrom, 1989), although not all developmental effects of TCDD-like compounds on the chicken embryo have been shown to be mediated by the Ah receptor. Certainly, the Ah receptor is present in the chicken embryo at least as early as the third day of incubation (Denison et al, 1986).

How good then is the chicken embryo as a developmental model for TCDD-related PHAH toxicity? As a sentinel model, the chicken embryo needs to be relatively sensitive to the effects of TCDD-like compounds. The chicken embryo is very sensitive to TCDD. The LD50 of 250 ppt makes it one of the more sensitive embryo models, and certainly one of the more sensitive avian embryos (Martin et al, 1989; Nosek et al, 1989; Hoffman et al, 1996). However, it is not clear specifically how much TCDD (or PCB) is taken up by the mammalian embryos. Thus, the LD50 comparison is less clear when comparing the relative sensitivity of the chicken and mammalian embryos.

The chicken embryo responds to the TCDD-like PHAHs in a characteristic manner, which makes it appropriate to use for toxicological screening. Furthermore, there is a suite of toxicological endpoints which can be evaluated in the early chicken embryo on incubation days 2,3, and 4 (Henshel et al, 1993c). Using this suite of toxicological endpoints (the Early Avian Embryo Assay) a teratogenic screening assay can be carried out in approximately one week. In addition, chickens can be placed in a constructed setting (such as a Superfund site), or enticed to eat exotic foods (fish, soil) in order to evaluate the bioavailability of chemicals of concern and their effects on reproduction (Petreas et al, 1991; Summer, 1992). Further, at least some of the chicken embryo responses to TCDD-like compounds are likely to be mediated by the Ah receptor, which seems to be true across a large number of species. As a screening model, then, the chicken embryo is a sensitive species, in which the toxicity is mediated by a mechanism common to many vertebrates and in which teratogenicity can be assessed in a relatively short period of time. The chicken embryo may, however, be overly sensitive to TCDD-like compounds compared to all the other embryonic animal models, which would result in an excess of false positives when testing unknown related compounds.

As a mechanistic animal model, the relative sensitivity of the chicken embryo is not as critical. The chicken embryo, as mentioned above, manifests many of its toxicological responses to the TCDD-like PHAHs via the Ah receptor mechanism, in common with many vertebrates including humans. The chicken embryo also manifests many of the suite of developmental toxicological effects seen in other animals, including some (such as heart malformations) not yet reported in mammals. This versatility means that the chicken embryo could be used to study the effects of TCDD-like compounds on a large number of developing organ systems. And, because the chicken develops by itself in the egg, there are no maternal interactions to complicate the interpretation of how the chemical is afffecting the developing embryo.

Chicken embryo development, especially early development, is similar to all vertebrate embryonic development, especially mammalian. Thus, effects seen in the chicken embryo are likely to be parallel to effects seen in the mammalian embryonic models. The chicken embryo has been a standard model for embryonic development for over a century, and thus its developmental control mechanisms are well understood. There are a considerable number of chicken probes (cDNA, antibodies) available which are directed against developmental control factors (hormones, growth factors, oncogenes, homeobox genes). Chicken embryos are therefore very useful animal models for studying the mechanisms controlling the developmental toxicological effects of chemicals that affect the process of development, as TCDD-like compounds do.

     In conclusion, the chicken embryo is a good developmental animal
model, especially a mechanistic model, for TCDD-like PHAH toxicity for
following reasons:
1) It is relatively sensitive to the effects of the PHAHs, and as such
is a good species to use for biomonitoring purposes (in a constructed
situation).
2) At least some of the effects of the TCDD-like PHAHs on the chicken
embryo appears to be mediated by the same mechanisms (i.e. the Ah
receptor) that mediates many of the manifestations of TCDD-like toxicity
in other embryos.
3) It is a classic model for embryological studies, and thus details of
the chicken's embryological development, and the mechanisms controlling
that development, are relatively well understood. Thus, a large
literature database about the details of chicken embryonic development
has been established.
4) Since the chicken embryo is such a well-established model for
embryonic development, there are a large number of molecular and
biochemical probes available for studying developmental control
mechanisms.
5) Embryological development of the chicken, and control thereof, is
similar to that of mammalian species. Thus, the results of studies
evaluating the mechanism of PHAH developmental toxicity are likely to be
directly applicable to mammalian species.
6) Each egg can be individually dosed to a known concentration of the
toxicant;
7) Using a bird as a model species enables one to study the direct
effect of the toxicant on the embryo, avoiding maternal complications;
8) The chicken embryo is a relatively inexpensive developmental test
species compared to using mammalian embryological animal models.

REFERENCES

Abbott, B.D., Diliberto, J.J., and Birnbaum, L.S., 1989, "2,3,7,8-
Tetrachlorodibenzo-p-Dioxin Alters Embryonic Palatial Medial Epithelial
Cell Differentiation in Vitro," Toxicology and Applied Pharmacology,
Vol. 100, pp. 119 - 131.

Abou-Donia, M.B., 1992, "Principles and Methods for Evaluating
Neurotoxicity," In Neurotoxicology, Abou-Donia, Ed., CRC Press, Boca
Raton, FL, pp. 509 - 525.

Allen, J.R., Barsotti, D.A., Van Miller, J.P., Abrahamson, L.J., and
Lalich, J.J., 1977, "Morphological changes in Monkeys Consuming a DIet
Containing Low Levels of 2,3,7,8-Tetrachlorodibenzo-p-Dioxin," Food and
Cosmetic Toxicology, Vol. 15, pp. 401 - 410.

Allred, P.M. and Strange, J.R., 1977, "The Effects of 2,4,5-
Trichlorophenoxyacetic Acid and 2,3,7,8-Tetrachlorodibenzo-p-Dioxin on
Developing CHicken Embryos," Archives of Environmental Contamination and
Toxicology, Vol. 5, pp. 483 - 489.

Beatty, P.W., Vaughn, W.K., Neal, R.A., 1978, "Effect of Alteration of
Rat Hepatic Mixed-Function Oxidase (MFO) Activity on the Toxicity of
2,3,7,8-Tetrachlorodibenzo-p-Dioxin (TCDD)," Toxicology and Applied
Pharmacology, Vol. 45, pp. 513 - 519.

Birnbaum, L.S., 1991, "Developmental Toxicity of TCDD and Related
Compounds: Species Sensitivity and Differences," In Biological Basis
for Risk Assessment of Dioxins and Related Compounds, Gallo, M.A.,
Scheuplein, R.J., and van der Heijden, C.A.,, Eds, Banbury Report 35,
Cold Spring Harbor Laboratory, Cold Spring Harbor, N.Y., pp. 51 - 68.

Brunstrom, B., Darnerud, P.O., 1983, "Toxicity and Distribution. in Chick
Embryos of 3,3',4,4'-Tetrachlorobiphenyl injected into the eggs,"
Toxicology, Vol. 27, pp. 103 - 110.

Brunstrom, B. and Lund, J., 1988, "Differences Between Chick and Turkey Embryos in Sensitivity to 3,3',4,4'-Tetrachlorobiphenyl and in Concentration Affinity of the Hepatic Receptor for 2,3,7,8-Tetrachlorodibenzo-p-Dioxin," Comparative Biochemistry and Physiology , Vol. 91C, pp. 507 - 512.

Brunstrom, B., 1989, "Toxicity of Coplanar Polychlorinated Biphenyls in Avian Embryos," Chemosphere, Vol. 19, pp. 765 - 768.

Cheung, M.O., Gilbert, E.F., and Peterson, R.E., 1981, "Cardiovascular Teratogenicity of 2,3,7,8-Tetrachlorodibenzo-p-Dioxin in the Chick Embryo," Toxicology and Applied Pharmacology, Vol. 61, pp. 197   204.

Colburn, T., 1991, "Epidemiology of Great Lakes Bald Eagles", Journal of Toxicology and Environmental Health, Vol. 33, Number 4, pp 395 - 453.

Colburn, T., vom Saal, F.S., Soto, A.M., 1993, "Developmental Effects of Endocrine-Disrupting Chemicals in Wildlife and Humans," Environmental Health Perspectives, Vol. 101, pp. 378 - 384.

Couture, L.A., Harris, M.A., and Birnbaum, L.S., 1990, "A Critical Review of the Developmental Toxicity and Teratogenicity of 2,3,7,8-Tetrachlorodibenzo-p-Dioxin: Recent Advances Toward Understanding the Mechanism," Toxicology, Vol. 42, pp. 619 - 627.

Denison, M.S., Okey, A.b., Hamilton, J.W., Bloom, S.E., and Wilkinson, C.F., 1986, "Ah Receptor for 2,3,7,8-Tetrachlorodibenzo-p-Dioxin: Ontogeny in Chick Embryo Liver," Journal of Biochemical Toxicology, Vol. 1, pp. 39 - 49.

Food and Drug Administration (FDA), 1993, Toxicological Principles for the Safety Assessment of Direct FOod Additives and Color Additives Used in Food (FDA Redbook II), USFDA, Center for Food Safety and Applied Nutrition DRAFT

Frankos, V.H., 1985, "FDA Perspectives on the Use of Teratology Data for Human Risk Assessment," Fundamental and Applied Toxicology, Vol. 5, pp. 615   622.

Gilbertson, M., 1988, "Epidemics in Birds and Mammals Caused by Chemicals in the Great Lakes," In Toxic Contaminants and Ecosystem Health: A Great Lakes Focus, Evans, M.S., Editor, John Wiley and Sons, New York, pp. 133 - 152.

Greig, J.B., Jones, G., Butler, W.H., and Barnes, J.M., 1973, "Toxic Effects of 2,3,7,8-Tetrachlorodibenzo-p-Dioxin," Food and Cosmetic Toxicology, Vol. 11, pp. 585 - 595.

Hassoun, E., d'Argy, R., Dencker, L., Lundin, L.-G., Borwell, P., 1984, "Teratogenicity of 2,3,7,8-tetrachlorodibenzofuran in BVD recombinant inbred strains," Toxicology Letters Vol. 23, pp. 37 - 42.

Henck, J.M., New, M.A., Kociba, R.J., Rao, K.S., 1981, "2,3,7,8-Tetrachlorodibenzo-p-Dioxin: Acute Oral Toxicity in Hamsters," Toxicology and Applied Pharmacology, Vol. 59, pp. 405 - 407.

Henshel, D.S., 1993a, "LD50 and Teratogenicity Studies of the Effects of TCDD on Chicken Embryos," Society for Environmental Toxicology and Chemistry Abstracts , Vol. 14, pp. 280.

Henshel, D.S., 1993b, "Dysmyelination in 2,3,7,8-Tetrachlorodibenzo-p-Dioxin Exposed Chicken Embryos," The Toxicologist, Vol. 13, p. 172.

Henshel, D.S., Hehn, B.M., Vo, M.T., Steeves, J.D., 1993c, "A Short-Term Test for Dioxin Teratogenicity Using Chicken Embryos," Environmental Toxicology and Risk Assessment: 2nd Volume, ASTM STP 1216, J.W. Gorsuch, F.J. Dwyer, C.G. Ingersoll, T.W. La Point, Eds., American Society for Testing and Materials, Philadelphia, pp. 159 - 174.

Hill, E.F. and Hoffman, D.J., 1984, "Avian Models for Toxicity Testing," Journal of the American College of Toxicology, Vol 3, pp. 357-376.

Hoffman, D.J., Rice, C.P., Kubiak, T.J., 1996, "PCBs and Dioxins in Birds," Interpreting Environmental Contaminants in Animal Tissues, W.N. Beyer, G.H. Heinz and A.W. Redmon, Eds., Lewis Publishers, CRC Press, Boca Raton, FL, Chapter 7, pp 167 - 209.

Hood, R.D., 1990, "Animals Models of Effects of Prenatal Insults," In Hood, R.D. (Ed.), Developmental Toxicology: Risk Assessment and the Future, sponsored by the Reproductive and Developmental Toxicology Branch, Human Health Assessment Group, Office of Health and Environmental Assessment, Office of Research and Development, US Environmental Protection Agency, Washington, D.C.

Inveresk Research International (IRI), 1990a, "Reproductive Toxicity," Regulatory Guidelines Number 4.

Inveresk Research International (IRI), 1990b, "Rodent Carcinogenicity and Chronic Toxicity," Regulatory Guidelines Number 1.

Klaassen, C.D. and Eaton, D.L., 1991, "Principles of Toxicology," In Casarett and Doull's Toxicology: The Basic Science of Poisons, Amdur, M.O., Doull, J., and Klaassen, C.D., Eds, McGraw-Hill, New York, pp. 12 - 49.

Martin, S., Duncan, D., Thiel, D., Peterson, R., and Lemke, M., 1989, "Evaluation of the Effects of Dioxin-Contaminated Sludges on Eastern Bluebirds and Tree Swallows," Report prepared for Nekoosa Papers, Inc, Port Edwards, WI, as quoted in Peterson, R., Health Assessment for 2,3,7,8-Tetrachlorodibenzo-p-Dioxin (TCDD) and Related Compounds: Chapter 5. Reproductive and Developmental Toxicity, Workshop Review Draft, August 1992, Environmental Protection Agency, EPA/600/AP-92/001e.

Mineau, P., Fox, G.F.A., Norstrom, R.J., Weseloh, D.V., Hallett, D.J., and Ellenton, J.A., 1984, "Using the Herring Gull to Monitor Levels and Effects of Organochlorine Contamination in the Canadian Great Lakes," In Toxic Contaminants in the Great Lakes   Advances in Environmental Sciences and Technology, Nriagu J.O. and Simmons, M.S., Eds., John Wiley and Sons, New York, pp. 425 - 452.

Moore, J.A., McConnell, E.E., Dalgard, D.W., Harris, M.W., 1979, "Comparative Toxicity of Three Halogenated Dibenzofurans in Guinea Pigs, Mice and Rhesus Monkeys," Annals of the New York Academy of Science, Vol. 320, pp. 151 - 163.

Nikolaidis, E., Brunstrom, B., and Dencker, L., 1988, "Effects of the TCDD Congeners 3,3',4,4'-Tetrachlorobiphenyl and 3,3',4,4'-Tetrachloroazoxybenzene on Lymphoid Development in the Bursa of Fabricus of the Chick Embryo," Toxicology and Applied Pharmacology, Vol. 92, pp. 315 - 323.

Nikolaidis, E., Brunstrom, B., and Dencker, L., 1988a, "Effects of TCDD and its Congeners 3,3,',4,4'-Tetrachloroazoxybenzene and 3,3',4,4'-Tetrachlorobiphenyl on Lymphoid Development in the Thymus of Avian Embryos," Pharmacology and Toxicology, Vol. 63, pp. 333 - 336.

Nosek, J.A., Craven, S.R., Peterson, R.E., Sullivan, J.R., Hill, G., 1989, "Dioxin Toxicity in Adult Hen and Hatchling Ring-Necked Pheasants," Socity for Environmental Toxicology and Chemistry Abstracts, Vol 10, p. 224.

Petreas, M.X., Goldman, L.R., Hayward, D.G., Chang, R.R., Flattery, J.J., Wiesmuller, T., Stephens, R.D., Fry, D.M., Rappe, C., 1991, "Biotransfer and Bioaccumulation of PCDD/PCDFs From Soil: Controlled Exposure Studies of Chickens," Chemosphere, Vol, 23, pp. 1731 - 1741.

Poland, A., and Glover, E., 1980, "2,3,7,8-Tetrachlorodibenzo-p-dioxin: Segregation of Toxicity with the Ah Locus," Molecular Pharmacology, Vol. 17, pp. 86 - 94.

Rifkind, A.B., Sassa, S., Reyes, J., Muschick, H., 1985, "Polychlorinated Aromatic Hydrocarbon Lethality, Mixed Function Oxidase Induction, and Uroporphyinogen Decarboxylase Inhibition in the Chick Embryo: Dissociation of Dose-Response Relationships," Toxicology and Applied Pharmacology, Vol. 78, pp. 268 - 279.

Sanger, V.L., Scott, L., Hamdy, A., Gale, C., and Pounden, W.D., 1958, "Alimentary Toxemia in Chickens," Journal of the American Veterinary Medicine Association, Vol. 132, pp. 172 - 176.

Schmittle, S.C., Edwards, H.M., and Morris, D., 1958, "A disorder probably due to a toxic feed -- Preliminary report," Journal of the American Veterinary Medicine Association, Vol. 132, pp. 216 - 219.

Schwetz, B.A., Norris, J.M., Sparschu, G.L., Rowe, V.K., Gehring, P.J., Emerson, J.L., and Gerbig, C.G., 1973, "Toxicology of Chlorinated Dibenzo-p-Dioxins," Environmental Health Perspectives, Vol. 5, pp. 87 - 99.

Summer, C.L., 1992, "An Avian Ecosystem Health Indicator: The Reproductive Effects Induced by Feeding Great Lakes Fish to White Leghorn Laying Hens," M.S. Thesis, Michigan State University.

Vos, J.G., Moore, J.A., Zinkl, J.G., 1973, "Effect of 2,3,7,8-Tetrachlorodibenzo-p-Dioxin on the Immune System of Laboratory Animals," Environmental Health Perspectives, Vol. 5, pp. 149 - 162.

Walker, M.K., Spitsbergen, J.M., Olson, J.R., and Peterson, R.E., 1991, "2,3,7,8-Tetrachlorodibenzo-p-Dioxin Toxicity During Early Life Stage Development of Lake Trout (Salvelinus namaycush)," Canadian Journal of Fish. and Aquatic Science, Vol. 48, pp. 875 - 883.

Yamashita, F., and Hayashi, M, 1985, "Fetal PCB Syndrome: Clinical Features, Intrauterine Growth Retardation and Possible Alteration in Calcium Metabolism," Environmental Health Perspectives, Vol. 59, pp. 41 - 45.

Diane S. Henshel[1,3], J. William Martin[1], Dave Best[2], Kimberley M. Cheng[3], John E. Elliott[3,4], Diana Rosenstein[5], James Sikarskie[5]

EVALUATING GROSS BRAIN ASYMMETRY: A POTENTIAL BIOMARKER FOR 2,3,7,8-TETRACHLORODIBENZO-p-DIOXIN-RELATED NEUROTOXICITY

REFERENCE: Henshel, D. S., Martin, J. W., Best, D., Cheng, K. M., Elliott, J. E., Rosenstein, D., and Sikarskie, J., **"Evaluating Gross Brain Asymmetry: A Potential Biomarker for 2,3,7,8-Tetrachlorodibenzo-p-Dioxin-Related Neurotoxicity,"** *Environmental Toxicology and Risk Assessment: Biomarkers and Risk Assessment—Fifth Volume, ASTM STP 1306,* David A. Bengtson and Diane S. Henshel, Eds., American Society for Testing and Materials, 1996.

ABSTRACT: Recent evidence indicates that avian embryonic exposure to polychlorinated dibenzodioxins (PCDDs) and related compounds is associated with the development of a gross brain asymmetry which can be quantified.   Three methods can be used to quantify the asymmetry, including external measurements of the intact brain, measurements of brain cross-sections and measurements of computer tomography (CT) - generated images of brain sections. All three methods produce reliable results. The whole brain measurements do not require specialized equipment, and are the most flexible. However, the possibility for unintentional bias is greatest for this technique. The CT scan technology is non-invasive, but requires access to specialized equipment and may be expensive. The cross-sectional measurements, which are similar to the CT scan measurements, require careful processing prior to measurement.

KEYWORDS: TCDD, PCBs, asymmetry, teratogen, bird, nervous system

According to ASTM Subcommittee E47.09 on Biomarkers, biomarkers are "biological measures (within organisms) of exposure to, effects of, or susceptibility to environmental stress [determined] using molecular,

[1] Indiana University, School of Public and Environmental Affairs, Bloomington, IN

[2] U.S. Fish and Wildlife Service, East Lansing Field Office, East Lansing, MI.

[3] University of British Columbia, Department of Animal Science, Vancouver, B.C., Canada

[4] Pacific Wildlife Research Centre, Canadian Wildlife Service, Delta, B.C., Canada.

[5] Veterinary Clinical Center, Michigan State University, East Lansing, MI

genetic, biochemical, histological, or physiological techniques." There are a number of biomarkers which may be used as indicators of potential carcinogenic effects (e.g. DNA adducts) or of generalized cellular adverse effects (e.g. measures of reduced glutathione or of lipid peroxidation as indicators of oxidative stress or the histological evaluation of tissue edema as an indicator of tissue damage[McCarthy and Shugart, 1990; Huggett et al, 1992]). The observation of specific patterns and types of teratogenic abnormalities induced after exposure to certain chemicals or stressors (e.g disruption of myelin after exposure to thallium) may also be considered a biomarker of effect (Abou-Donia, 1992). There are few specific biomarkers, however, which may be used as indicators of developmental nervous system toxicity.

Recent evidence indicates that the development of a gross brain asymmetry may be a specific indicator for developmental neurological changes induced by exposure to 2,3,7,8-tetrachlorodibenzo-p-dioxin (TCDD) and related chemicals (Henshel et al, 1993, 1994, 1996; Henshel and Martin, 1995). Experimental observations on avian nestlings (great blue heron, double-crested cormorants, bald eagle)exposed in ovo in the wild to TCDD-like compounds paired with studies of chicken embryos injected with known doses of TCDD from the start of incubation indicate that there is a consistent correlation between exposure to TCDD and TCDD-like compounds and the development of grossly asymmetric brains. The brain asymmetry is primarily seen as an increase in several measures of the birds' left forebrain region (cerebral hemisphere) compared to the right forebrain region.

The main parameters which are consistently affected include a medio-lateral width at approximately the level of the pineal and an oblique measure ("angle") which is measured from the same medial point just rostral to the pineal and ending on the lateral aspect of the forebrain where the lateral edge of the forebrain just starts to parallel the midline (Figure 1). A third parameter which is generally affected is the dorso-ventral depth of the brain at approximately the point where the thalamic/hypothalamic region joins the ventral forebrain region. This is generally measured at the level of the pre-optic area since the brain has easily identifiable landmarks at that point. Rostro-caudal "height" of the forebrain is inconsistently asymmetric, depending on the species. In addition, the tectum also is enlarged on the left side of the brain. Tectal height (or length) is most readily measured from the lateral aspect of the brain.

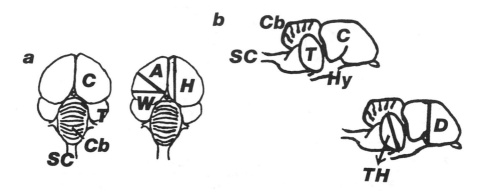

Figure 1. Depiction of the avian brain from a dorsal and lateral perspective illustrating the major brain regions and the measurements made on the whole brains. Brain regions: C cerebrum (telencephalic hemispheres), Cb cerebellum, Hy hypothalamus, SC spinal cord, T tectum. Brain measurements: A angle, D depth, H height, TH tectal height, W width.

Three methods have been used to document these changes, including measurements of the whole, uncut brain, computer tomographic (CT) scans of the brain in cross-section, and cut cross-sections of the brain. The first and simplest method is to measure the uncut, fixed[6] brain using a finely graded ruler appropriate to the size of the brain. An engineering ruler with 0.5 mm markings is acceptable for many medium-sized (e.g. chicken hatchling and great blue heron)or large (e.g. bald eagle) avian brains. Rulers must be held parallel to the medio-lateral plane of the brains. For accurate measurement it is important to ensure that the brain is essentially parallel to the supporting surface. This may be accomplished by positioning the brain on little pieces of cork or pipette tips. To make measurements, the ruler is then placed parallel to the brain at a level as close to the surface of the brain as possible. When the measurements are made, one eye must be centered over the midline of the brain. The other eye then determines the measurement. If the eyes are not centered over the brain in this way, one can skew the measurements depending on how far the ruler is away from the surface of the brain, how large a brain is being measured, and how far away from the midline is each eye. To ensure consistency, the measurements are made twice, and recorded separately. This forces the measurer to move his/her head and reposition the head between measurements. If the two measurements do not agree, then the measurement needs to be made three more times (total n=5) and the resultant measurements averaged. This happens infrequently once the measurer becomes more experienced.

Width and angle measurements may be made from the ventral as well as the dorsal aspect of the brain. As seen in Figure 3, the correlation between the ventral and dorsal difference measurements on the same brain is excellent. The asymmetry is easiest to visualize on the ventral surface of the brain as well. The angle difference is seen as a flattening of the arc on the lateral edge of the forebrain (illustrated in Figure 2). The tectal width measurement may also be most easily made from the ventral surface of the brain, depending on the brain morphology.

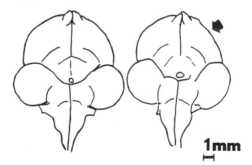

Figure 2. Tracing of the ventral surface of a control (left) and a TCDD-exposed chicken brain (right) illustrating the flattened arc (arrow) which is measured by the angle measurement.

---

[6] Brains may be fixed in any appropriate fixative. Neutral buffered formalin (10%) or 4% paraformaldehyde made up in buffered saline (pH 7 - 7.5) are two such appropriate fixatives. If the brain will be processed for histopathology, whichever fixative is appropriate for the stains to be used will probably be appropriate for both the CT scans (if the animal is dead) and the gross external measurements.

Two methods may be used for fixation, cardiac or carotid perfusion of saline followed by fixative, or immersion fixing. If the brain is to be immersion fixed, it must be placed gently in the fixative, and not pushed into a small space where the soft tissue of the brain could be easily distorted by pressure prior to and during fixation.

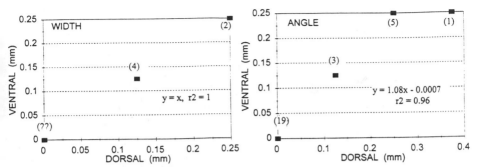

Figure 3. Graphs illustrating the high degree of correlation between the dorsal and ventral width and angle measurements made as gross external measurements on cormorant hatchling brains from Lake Ontario (high PCBs, generally asymmetric), Lost Mountain Lake, Saskatchewan (low PCBs, symmetric; see Henshel et al, 1996) and the Strait of Georgia, British Columbia (varying). Birds from all colonies are pooled in the graph. The numbers in parentheses above each point indicate the sample size for that point.

The second method entails evaluation of sequential computer tomographic (CT) scans of the brain in cross section (Henshel et al, in preparation). The CT scans may be made of anesthetized intact animals or of the brain while still in the skull of an isolated head (see Figure 4). Theoretically the CT scans could also be made of the whole dissected brain. Given that ice crystal formation may only damage tissue at the light microscopic level, it is possible that CT scans of frozen brains remaining in the braincase could be used to evaluate the symmetry of previously frozen archived specimens. The caveat here would be that the brains must have been frozen once only and never thawed, and that the brains must be kept frozen during the scanning procedure. Again theoretically, the brains, heads or entire body might be freeze-dried and maintain internal structure sufficiently to be evaluated using computer tomography. The brain is aligned properly within the chamber, and multiple imaged cross-sections of the brain are then made. CT scans must be done using appropriate facilities, and must be carried out with the aid of a radiologist or computer tomographic technician. Scans are printed on X-ray film which can then be evaluated manually (with a fine ruler, a linen tester, or a microscope graticule) or, ideally, with the aid of computerized imaging software. The films can be printed and the prints may also be measured. CT scans can also be evaluated using the hardware and imaging software with which the scans were made. This, however, requires that the evaluator have access to this hardware for extended periods of time, a situation which may not be feasible for most investigators. Interestingly, of the CT scans which have been measured (on bald eagles only) the most consistent measurements which demonstrate the visually observable asymmetry are the depth measurements (dorso-ventral depth in the brain) and the measurements of the tectum, both length and width (as measured in the CT scan). The tectum is likely to only be visualized in one, or maybe two, imaged cross-sections (Figure 4). To increase the number of measurements made on each imaged section (for statistical comparisons), the depth measurements may be made at two places within each section. The first depth measurement starts dorsally mid-wulst (the medial "ridge" on the dorso-medial aspect of the avian forebrain, seen as a "bump" on the dorso-medial surface of a CT scanned or histological cross-section) and ends at the most medial point of the ventral indentation of the forebrain (Figure 4B). Note that this depth measure is angled away from the midline and does not run parallel to the midline. The second depth measurement starts at the lateral point two-thirds of the width of the demi-brain (that side of the brain) in that image (see Figure 4B) and is made parallel to the dorso-ventral midline. Both depth measurements appear to consistently reflect asymmetry throughout the image planes of the forebrain.

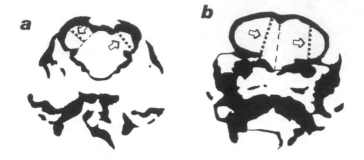

Figure 4. Tracings of two CT scan images made of the asymmetric brain of a 6 month old bald eagle from Michigan (near Lake Huron) manifesting a gross abnormality (crossed bill; Eagle 2 in Figure 5). CT scans were made of the whole head in cross-section. The brain is the white area outlined in the center of the upper half of each image. The measurements are indicated by the dashed lines. 4a illustrates the tectal measurements (tectal width [dashed line on the left side, arrow] and tectal length [dashed line on the right side, arrow]). 4b illustrates the two forebrain depth measurements (forebrain depth [dashed line on the left side, arrow], and forebrain depth at 2/3 width [dashed line on the right side, arrow]) that most consistently manifest the brain asymmetry. Bone is blackened in.

Surprisingly, the medio-lateral width measurement is not consistently useful as a measure of gross brain asymmetry throughout the forebrain (Figure 5, Image 9), although it does seem to more con- sistently illustrate the asymmetry in the more rostral part of the forebrain (Figure 5, Image 12).

One would expect the width measure of the appropriate image (the virtual cross section through the brain at a given point) to be equivalent to the width measurement made on the whole brain (the gross external width measurement). This does not seem to be the case, as illustrated in Figure 6A. Whereas the depth measurements (depth and depth at 2/3 width) were both consistent between the gross external measurements and the measurements made from the CT scans, the width measurements were not consistent in all brains. Both sets of measurements were double-checked when this discrepancy was noted, and both sets of measurements held true. It is possible that the discrepancy may be due to the fact that each CT scanned image is an average of 3 mm (rostro-caudally) of each brain, whereas the gross external width measurement is made in one medio-lateral plane, just rostral to the pineal.

The third method for evaluation of gross brain asymmetry is to make the measurements on histological cross-sections. In essence, these measurements are very similar to the CT scan measurements because one is again making serial cross-sections through the brain and measuring each cross-section. The thickness of the cross-sections to be cut will depend on the size of the brain as well as whether the cross-sections will be used for other purposes (such as the histological or immunohistochemical evaluation of cellular or tissue abnormalities). Measurements may be made using the graticule of the microscope, image analysis software, measuring photographs of each section, or drawing each section with the aid of a drawing tube or an image projector and measuring the drawing.

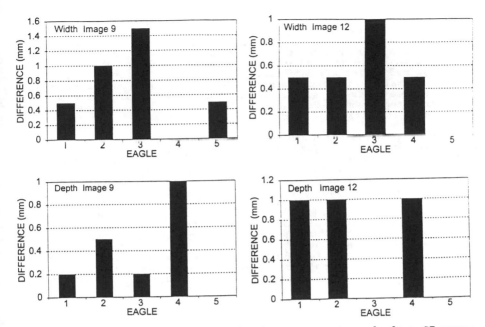

Figure 5. Histograms of width and depth measurements made from CT scans of five eagles from Michigan and Wisconsin, four of which manifested developmental abnormalities (Eagles 2,4: severe crossed-bills; Eagle 1: mild crossed-bill; Eagle 3: deformed claws). Eagle 5 was the relatively uncontaminated control eagle who had been raised in captivity for several years. Image 9 is relatively caudal compared to Image 12.

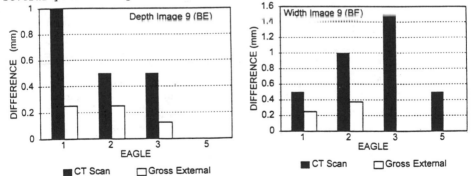

Figure 6. Histograms comparing the width and depth measurements made at equivalent points in the brain using the gross external method and by measuring CT scans. Gross external width measurements were made at the medio-lateral plane just rostral to the pineal as viewed from the dorsal aspect of the brain. External depth measurements were made from the dorsal-most part of the brain to the junction of the hypothalamus and the forebrain (the pre-optic area). Depth measurements were made from the CT scans (Image 9 of 13) as illustrated in Figure 4b. Width measurements were made at the widest point in the forebrain in Image 9. Measurements were made from the same set of bald eagle brains. Eagles are numbered as above. Eagle 4 was not used as it is still alive.

This last method, however, introduces the possibility of additional
error in the accuracy of the drawing. It can be very difficult to draw
the lines precisely on the edge of the projected section, especially for
an inexperienced investigator. Yet a slip of the wrist or the pencil
while tracing the projected image which produces a line which appears
visually insignificantly different from the projected image could
potentially affect the measurement. The measurements made are similar
to those made on the CT scans. Again, the depth measurement seems to be
more consistent (show less asymmetry in the controls) than the width
measurement (Lipsitz et al, 1996).

    The strengths and drawbacks of each measurement method are
summarized in Table 1. The choice of measurement may well depend on the
circumstances. Given access to computer tomographic facilities, the CT
scans are an excellent non-invasive method which may be used to evaluate
live specimens which can be released back to the wild. However, the
cost ($200 per scan) may be prohibitive, depending on the budget for the
project. If the animal is to be euthanized, the choice of method may
well depend on whether the investigator has the time or the means to
carry out the histological evaluation. As this is, at this time,
specialized work, it cannot be carried out by routine histopathological
requests to a contract laboratory. However, the measurements are not
difficult for a trained technician and could theoretically be added to
the histopathological analysis for an added cost(presumably). Depending
on the laboratory, slides are processed for $10 - 30 per specimen, so
costs would be below that of CT scans, but above that for gross external
measurements. If the processing is being done within the laboratory and

Table 1. Comparison of the methods for analyzing brain asymmetry.

	Gross External	CT Scan	Cross-Sections
Potential Resolution	Depends on ruler/divider	Depends on how measured – excellent if using computer imaging	Using microscope graticule – better than for gross external. Equal to CT scans if use computer imaging
Ease of Measurement	Very easy with training.	Need a technician/ radiologist to produce CT scans –relatively easy to measure scans	Need training to make slides. Time consuming to prepare slides. Relatively easy to measure once slides are made.
Potential for Bias	Relatively higher due to 3D aspect of brains	Relatively low – 2D images	Relatively low – 2D images
Availability of Equipment	High	Low – speciallized equipment, need to contract out	Moderate – many laboratories have the capabilities
Costs	Low	High	Moderate
Other Comments	May be done as an "add-in" to necropsy	Non-invasive – can use live specimens	May be done as an "add-in" to histopathology

not contracted out, the costs will be significantly less. Depending on the equipment available, costs will include those for slides, processing and staining chemicals, and the cost of the person doing the processing (student, post-doctoral fellow, principle investigator, technician). Regardless, given a fixed brain, it is probably a good idea to measure the whole brain as that is the only way to evaluate the difference in the angle measurement. The angle measurement, which is relatively readily visualized from the ventral surface of the whole brain, is not measureable or visualizable once the brain has been sectioned histologically. Costs for the gross external brain measurements are very low, including the cost of an engineering ruler ($3 - 8) and the measurer's time. A lighted table top magnifier ($30 - 75) may also facilitate making the measurements.

DISCUSSION

Gross brain asymmetry is a relatively new technique which is being used to evaluate a gross brain dysmorphism which appears to develop in avian brains in response to TCDD and related compounds (Henshel et al, 1993, 1995). Because it is such a new technique, the best methods for making the measurements are still being developed. As discussed in this paper, the most appropriate method to use may depend on the circumstances. The method used most often, and on the largest datasets to date, is the gross external method. This method is easily added onto the necropsy protocol, and is thus relatively easy to add into large cooperative studies. The CT scan method, however, holds a lot of promise for the future. Deformed birds are sometimes caught or found, and the damage needs to be documented. It is not always desirable, however, to kill the bird just to document a potential contaminant-induced deformity. In these cases, the CT scan may be used to document effects non-invasively. Due to the cost and relative inaccessibility of the computer tomography equipment, only one study has been done using the CT scans. Clearly, more studies need to be carried out using this measurement method in order to continue to validate its usefulness in measuring gross brain asymmetry. Similarly, only one major study has used the histological cross-section method to analyze brain asymmetry (Lipschitz et al, 1996). As with the CT scan method, more studies still need to be carried out to determine how best to characterize asymmetry in cross sections of brain.

REFERENCES

Abou-Donia, M.B., Ed., 1992, Neurotoxicology, CRC Press, Inc., Boca Raton.

Henshel, D.S., Cheng, K.M., Norstrom, R., Whitehead, P., and Steeves, J.D., 1993, Morphometric and histological changes in brains of Great Blue heron hatchlings exposed to PCDDs: Preliminary Analyses. In Lewis, M et. al., Eds, ASTM STP #1179: Environmental Toxicology and Risk Assessment. American Society for Testing and Materials (ASTM), Philadelphia, pp. 262-280.

Henshel, D.S. and Martin, J.W., 1995, Brain asymmetry as a potential biomarker for developmental TCDD intoxication: a dose-response study, Seventh International Congress of Toxicology, Seattle, WA, July 2 - 6, 1995, and submitted to Biomarkers.

Henshel, D.S., Martin, J.W., DeWitt, J., Norstrom R., Elliott, J.E., and Cheng, K.M., 1996, Brain asymmetry in Double-Crested Cormorants exposed in ovo to PCBs and related compounds. Submitted to J. Great Lakes

Research.

Henshel, D.S., Martin, J.W., Norstrom, R., Whitehead, P. and Cheng,
K.M., 1995, Morphometric abnormalities in brains of Great Blue Heron
hatchlings exposed to PCDDs. Environmental Health Perspectives, Vol. 103
Suppl. 4:61-66.

Henshel, D.S., Martin, J.W., and Rapp, K., 1994, Brain asymmetry
measured in birds after in ovo exposure to TCDD related compounds.
Society for Environmental Toxicology and Chemistry, 15th Annual Meeting,
Denver, CO, October 30- November 3, 1994.

Henshel, D.S., Martin, J.W., Nelson, C., Rosenfield, D., Sikarski, J.,
Bolander, R., Bowerman, W., Best, D., Using computer tomography to
detect gross brain asymmetry induced by exposure to environmental
pollutants, in preparation.

Huggett, R.J., Kimerle, R.A., Mehrle, P.M., Jr., Bergman, H.L.,Eds.,
1992, Biomarkers Biochemical, Physiological, and Histological Markers of
Anthropogenic Stress., Lewis Publishers, Boca Raton.

Lipsitz, L., Powell, D., Bursian, S., Tanaka, D. Jr., 1996, Assessment
of cerebral hemispheric symmetry in hatchling chickens exposed in ovo to
polychlorinated biphenyl congeners. Archives of Environmental
Contamination and Toxicology. In press.

McCarthy, J.F. and Shugart, L.R., Eds, 1990, Biomarkers of Environmental
Contamination, Lewis Publishers, Boca Raton.

Janis T. Eells [1], Michele M. Salzman [2], Michael F. Lewandowski [3] and Timothy G. Murray [4]

DEVELOPMENT AND CHARACTERIZATION OF A NONPRIMATE ANIMAL MODEL OF METHANOL-INDUCED NEUROTOXICITY

REFERENCE: Eells, J.T., Salzman, M.M., Lewandowski, M.F., and Murray, T.G., "**Development and Characterization of a Nonprimate Animal Model of Methanol-Induced Neurotoxicity**," *Environmental Toxicology and Risk Assessment: Biomarkers and Risk Assessment—Fifth Volume, ASTM STP 1306*, David A. Bengtson and Diane S. Henshel, Eds., American Society for Testing and Materials, 1996.

ABSTRACT: Humans and nonhuman primates are uniquely sensitive to the toxic effects of methanol. The toxic syndrome in these species is characterized by formic acidemia, metabolic acidosis and blindness or serious visual impairment. Nonprimate species are normally resistant to the accumulation of formate and associated metabolic and visual toxicity. We have developed a nonprimate model of methanol toxicity using rats in which formate oxidation has been selectively inhibited. Methanol-intoxicated rats developed formic acidemia, metabolic acidosis and visual toxicity analogous to the human methanol poisoning syndrome. Visual dysfunction was manifested as reductions in the flash evoked cortical potential and electroretinogram which occurred coincident with blood formate accumulation. Histopathologic studies revealed mitochondrial disruption and vacuolation in the retinal pigment epithelium, photoreceptor inner segments and optic nerve. The establishment of this nonprimate animal model of methanol intoxication will facilitate research into the mechanistic aspects of methanol toxicity as well as the development and testing of treatments for human methanol poisoning. (Supported by The American Petroleum Institute and NIH grants RO1-ES06648 and P30-EYO1931).

KEYWORDS: methanol, formic acid, retina, visual toxicity, electroretinogram

Methanol is an important public health and environmental concern because of its selective neurotoxic actions on the retina and optic nerve in acute intoxication and because of its potential as a developmental neurotoxin following chronic exposure. Blindness or

[1] Associate Professor, Dept. of Pharmacology and Toxicology, Medical College of Wisconsin, Milwaukee, WI 53226

[2] Research Technologist, Dept. of Pharmacology and Toxicology, Medical College of Wisconsin, Milwaukee, WI 53226

[3] Assistant Adjunct Professor of Ophthalmology, Department of Ophthalmology Medical College of Wisconsin , Milwaukee, WI 53226

[4] Assistant Professor, Bascom Palmer Eye Institute, University of Miami School of Medicine, Miami, FL 33136

serious visual impairment is a well-known effect of acute human methanol poisoning. In addition, some studies have suggested that chronic low level exposures to methanol may also disrupt visual function (Frederick *et al.*, 1984; Andrews *et al.*, 1987, Kavet and Nauss, 1990, Lee *et al.*,1994b). Although methanol has been recognized as a human neurotoxin for more than a century, the mechanisms responsible for the toxic actions of this agent on retinal and optic nerve function are not understood (Tephly and McMartin, 1984; Eells, 1992).

Our understanding of the pathogenesis of methanol poisoning has been limited by the lack of animal models which mimic the human poisoning syndrome. Humans and non-human primates are uniquely sensitive to methanol poisoning. The toxic syndrome in these species is characterized by formic acidemia, metabolic acidosis and ocular toxicity. In humans, the acute effects of methanol toxicity appear after an asymptomatic latent period of about 24 hours and consists of formic acidemia, uncompensated metabolic acidosis, visual toxicity, coma and in extreme cases death. Visual disturbances generally develop between 18 and 48 hours after methanol ingestion and range from mild photophobia and misty or blurred vision to markedly reduced visual acuity and complete blindness (Buller and Wood, 1904; Benton and Calhoun, 1952; Roe, 1955).

In all mammalian species studied, methanol is metabolized in the liver by sequential oxidative steps to form formaldehyde, formic acid and CO_2 (Fig. 1) (Tephly, 1991; Eells, 1992). Although this metabolic sequence is identical for all species studied there are profound differences in the rate of formate oxidation in different species which determine the sensitivity to methanol (Palese and Tephly 1975; McMartin *et al.*, 1977 a, b; Eells *et al.*, 1981, 1983).

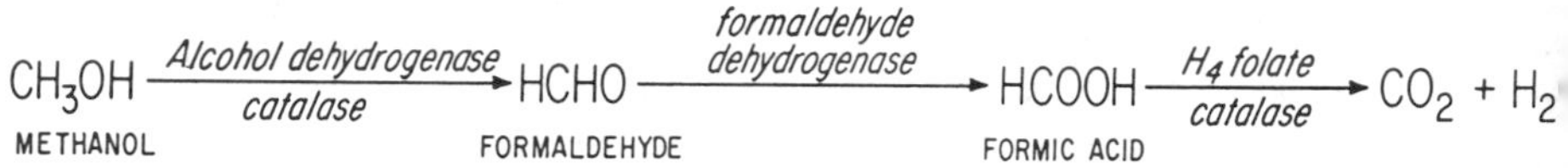

$$CH_3OH \xrightarrow[\text{catalase}]{\text{Alcohol dehydrogenase}} HCHO \xrightarrow[\text{dehydrogenase}]{\text{formaldehyde}} HCOOH \xrightarrow[\text{catalase}]{H_4 \text{ folate}} CO_2 + H_2$$

METHANOL   FORMALDEHYDE   FORMIC ACID

FIG. 1: Biochemical reactions in the oxidation of methanol to carbon dioxide in mammals

Formic acid is the toxic metabolite responsible for the metabolic acidosis observed in methanol poisoning in humans (McMartin *et al.*, 1980; Jacobsen and McMartin, 1986) and nonhuman primates (McMartin *et al.*, 1975, 1977; Eells *et al.*, 1983) as well as for the ocular toxicity produced in nonhuman primates (Martin-Amat *et al.*, 1977, 1978). Formic acid is also believed to be the toxic metabolite responsible for the ocular toxicity seen in methanol poisoned humans (Sharpe *et al.*, 1982). Nonprimate species do not accumulate formic acid following methanol administration and exhibit only central nervous system depression following methanol administration.

Formic acid accumulates in species susceptible to methanol poisoning and does not accumulate in species resistant to the toxicity due to differences in formic acid metabolism (Tephly, 1991; Eells, 1992). Formic acid is oxidized to carbon dioxide through a tetrahydrofolate-dependent pathway which functions more efficiently in rats than in humans and nonhuman primates (Eells *et al.*, 1981, 1983; Black *et al.*, 1985; Johlin *et al.*, 1987). Both dietary and chemically mediated depletion of endogenous folate cofactors in rats have been shown to increase formate accumulation following methanol administration (Makar and Tephly, 1976; Eells 1991; Lee *et al.*, 1994a, b) and to result in the development of metabolic acidosis and ocular toxicity similar to that observed in human intoxication (Eells, 1991: Murray *et al.*, 1991; and Lee *et al.*, 1994a, b).

We report on the development and characterization of a methanol-sensitive rodent model that manifests the formic acidemia, metabolic acidosis and retinal and optic nerve toxicity typical of human methanol poisoning. In this rodent model, formate oxidation has been selectively inhibited by treatment with nitrous oxide (Eells *et al.*, 1981; Eells, 1991; Murray *et al.*, 1991). Subanesthetic concentrations of nitrous oxide inactivate the enzyme methionine synthase (Deacon *et al.*, 1980) reducing the production of tetrahydrofolate, the cosubstrate for formate oxidation thus allowing formate to accumulate to toxic concentrations following methanol administration (Eells *et al.*, 1981). Methanol-intoxicated rats developed formic acidemia, metabolic acidosis and visual toxicity within 36 hours of methanol administration analogous to the human methanol poisoning syndrome. Visual dysfunction was measured as reductions in the flash evoked cortical potential and electroretinogram which occurred coincident with blood formate accumulation. Alterations in the electroretinogram occurred at formate concentrations lower than those associated with other visual changes and provide functional evidence of formate-induced retinal toxicity (Eells, 1991). Histopathologic studies revealed mitochondrial disruption and vacuolation in the retinal pigment epithelium, photoreceptor inner segments and optic nerve (Murray *et al.*, 1991). Similar electroretinographic and retinal and optic nerve histopathologic changes have recently been reported by our laboratory in a fatal human case of methanol poisoning, thus further validating this model. (Eells *et al.*, 1991; Murray *et al.*, 1996). We believe that this rodent model of methanol toxicity will be valuable in elucidating the mechanisms responsible for the selective neurotoxic actions of formic acid.

EXPERIMENTAL METHOD

Materials: Methanol (HPLC grade) obtained from Sigma Chemical Co. (St. Louis, MO) was diluted in sterile saline and administered as a 20% w/v solution. Sodium pentobarbital was purchased from Steris Laboratories (Phoenix, AZ) and tiletamine HCl / zolazepam HCl [1:1] (Telazol) was obtained from A.H. Robbins Co. (Richmond, VA). Phenylephrine HCl, 2.5% (Neosynephrine) was acquired from Winthrop Pharmaceuticals (New York, NY). All other chemicals were reagent grade or better.

Animals: Male Sprague-Dawley (formate metabolism studies) or Long Evans (all other studies) rats (Harlan Sprague-Dawley, Madison, WI) which weighed 250-300 g were used throughout these experiments. Formate metabolism studies were conducted in Sprague-Dawley rats and methanol intoxication and visual function studies were conducted in Long Evans rats since visual function measurements have been shown to be more reproducible in animals with pigmented retinas (Creel *et al.*, 1970). No differences in methanol or formate oxidation rates were apparent in the two strains of rats. All animals were supplied food and water *ad libitum* and maintained on a 12-hour light/dark schedule in a temperature and humidity controlled environment. Animals were handled in accordance with the Declaration of Helsinki and/or with the Guide for the Care and Use of Laboratory Animals as adopted and promulgated by the National Institutes of Health.

Formate Metabolism studies: Rats were placed in glass metabolic chambers and exposed to a mixture of N_2O/O_2 (1:1; flow rate 2 liters/min) for 4 hours prior to the administration of sodium ^{14}C-formate (500 mg/kg, 40,000 dpm/mg). Control groups were allowed to breathe room air. Expired $^{14}CO_2$ was collected at timed intervals and analyzed as described by McMartin *et al.*, (1975).

Methanol-intoxication protocol: Rats were placed in a Plexiglas chamber (22 x 55 x 22 cm) and exposed to a mixture of N_2O/O_2 (1:1; flow rate 2 liters/min) for 4 hours prior to the administration of methanol or saline. N_2O/O_2 exposure was continued throughout the course of the experiment. Methanol (20% w/v methanol in saline) was administered by intraperitoneal injection at a dose of 4g/kg followed by supplemental doses of 2g/kg at 12 hour intervals. This dosage regimen was designed to maintain blood formate concentrations between 8-15 mM for 30-40 hours in the methanol-treated animals. Similar concentrations of blood formate over these time periods have been shown to produce ocular toxicity experimentally in monkeys and are associated with visual toxicity in human methanol intoxication (Martin-Amat et al., 1977; Jacobson and McMartin, 1986). Controls for these experiments included groups of rats treated with saline and exposed to nitrous oxide (N2O-control); rats treated with methanol, but not exposed to nitrous oxide (methanol-control); and untreated rats (untreated-control). Blood samples for blood gas determinations and formate analysis and electrophysiological measurements of FEP and ERG were obtained prior to N_2O exposure, after 4 hours of N_2O exposure and at predetermined intervals following methanol administration for 60 hours. Rats were periodically removed from the exposure chamber for behavioral observations (6-8 hour intervals), electrophysiological measurements (12-24 hour intervals) and to obtain blood samples (12 hour intervals). Behavioral observations included non-quantitative assessments of exploratory behavior, righting reflex and withdrawal-response to paw pressure. Blood samples for formate analysis and blood gas measurements were obtained from the tail or orbital sinus (under Telazol anesthesia, 10 mg/kg) after the electrophysiological recording sessions.

Surgical procedures and flash-evoked cortical potential measurements: For measurement of flash-evoked cortical potentials (FEP), rats were anesthetized with sodium pentobarbital (50 mg/kg, ip) and indwelling electrodes were stereotaxically implanted over the visual cortices (Eells and Wilkison, 1989). All electrodes were attached to an Amphenol connector and the entire assembly was secured to the skull with dental acrylic. Recording sessions were initiated following a one week recovery period. Pupils were dilated by ocular administration of neosynephrine 2.5% and mydriacyl 1%. Rats were placed in a shielded cage with mirrored panels on the sides and the floor. The animals were dark adapted for 20 min and the averaged FEP was measured in response to 50 flashes (3.2×10^3 lux), 10 μsec in duration presented at 0.2 Hz. (Eells and Wilkison, 1989). The amplitude of the P20-N30 complex of the FEP was measured in microvolts from the peak of the first positive wave (P20 wave) to the peak of the first negative wave (N30 wave) and the latency was measured as the interval between the stimulus onset and the peak of the N30 wave. Two baseline recordings of FEP were obtained in each rat. Treatment effects were calculated as percentage of the control (mean of baseline measurements) amplitude or latency of P20-N30 complex of the FEP and averaged across animals (Eells and Wilkison, 1989).

Electroretinogram measurements: Electroretinograms (ERGs) were recorded from lightly anesthetized rats (pentobarbital, 10 mg/kg) using circular silver wire electrodes (Murray et al., 1991). Tetracaine 0.5% was used as a topical anesthetic followed by pupillary dilation with neosynephrine 2.5% and mydriacyl 1%. Two baseline recordings were obtained from each rat and experimental ERGs were recorded at 24, 48 and 60 hours after methanol administration. Animals were dark adapted for 30 min and the averaged ERG was recorded using a Nicolet system (CA1000 Flash DC200) in response to 4 flashes (3.2×10^3 lux), 10 msec in duration presented at 0.03 Hz. ERG amplitudes were measured in microvolts from the baseline to the peak for the negative a-wave (a-wave amplitude) and from the peak of the a-wave to the peak of the positive b-wave (b-wave amplitude). Implicit times were measured as the interval between the stimulus onset and the peak of the corresponding a- or b-wave of the ERG. Treatment effects were calculated as percentage of the control (mean of baseline measurements) a- or b-wave amplitude and averaged across animals (Eells, 1991).

Histopathologic Analysis: Animals were anesthetized with sodium pentobarbital (60 mg/kg) and perfused (intracardiac) with phosphate-buffered 2.5% glutaraldehyde/2.5% formaldehyde, pH 7.4. Eyes were enucleated and immersed in the above fixative for 72 hours. The anterior segment and vitreous were removed, then full thickness pieces of eye wall were dissected from the posterior pole, including the optic nerve. Tissues were postfixed in phosphate-buffered 2% OsO_4, dehydrated in a graded ethanol series and embedded in epoxy resin. Thick sections (1 μ) for light microscopy were stained with toluidine blue; thin sections for electron microscopy were stained with uranyl acetate and lead citrate.

Analytical Procedures: Blood gases and blood pH were measured on orbital sinus blood samples using a blood gas analyzer (Radiometer, ABL2). Bicarbonate values were calculated from pH and pCO_2 values using the Henderson-Hasselbach equation. Formate concentrations were determined on orbital sinus or tail blood samples (McMartin et al., 1975) using the fluorometric assay of Makar and Tephly (1982). Endogenous concentrations of hepatic folate cofactors were determined by using high pressure liquid chromatography for the separation of folate monoglutamate forms with specific quantitation of folate cofactors by microbiological analysis of the eluted fractions as described by McMartin et al., (1981).

Statistical analysis: Statistical comparison of group means were made by using a group Student's t test if only one comparison was made between two groups. In all cases in which several comparisons were required, one-way analysis of variance with repeated measures was performed. This was followed by a Dunnett's test procedure for multiple comparisons with a control. In all cases, the minimum level of significance was taken as $p < 0.05$.

RESULTS

Reduction of hepatic tetrahydrofolate concentrations and inhibition of formate oxidation by nitrous oxide treatment. Formate is oxidized to CO_2 *in vivo* in mammals primarily by a tetrahydrofolate-dependent pathway (Fig. 2). Formate enters this pathway by combining with tetrahydrofolate to form 10-formyl-tetrahydrofolate in a reaction catalyzed by formyl-tetrahydrofolate synthase. 10-formyl-tetrahydrofolate may then be further oxidized to CO_2 and tetrahydrofolate by formyl-tetrahydrofolate dehydrogenase (Kutzbach and Stokestad 1968). The concentration of tetrahydrofolate is a major determinant of the rate of formate oxidation (Eells et al., 1981, 1982). A key enzymatic reaction responsible for the generation of tetrahydrofolate is catalyzed by the enzyme methionine synthase (Huennekens et al., 1976). Exposure of rats to the anesthetic gas, nitrous oxide, produces an irreversible inhibition of methionine synthase activity (Banks et al., 1968; Deacon et al., 1980) and a significant reduction in the production of tetrahydrofolate (Eells et al., 1983). As shown in Fig.3, hepatic tetrahydrofolate concentrations are significantly reduced in rats following 4 hours of exposure to a mixture of N_2O/O_2 (1:1). Importantly, the concentrations of hepatic tetrahydrofolate in N_2O-exposed rats are comparable to those measured in the livers of cynomolgus monkeys and humans (Eells et al., 1981, 1982; Black et al., 1985, Johlin et al., 1987). The data in Fig. 3 also show that the rate of formate oxidation (500 mg/kg dose of formate) in N_2O-treated rats is reduced to 50% of the rate of formate oxidation measured in air breathing control rats and is comparable to the rate of formate oxidation determined at this same dose of formate in cynomolgus monkeys (Eells et al., 1983).

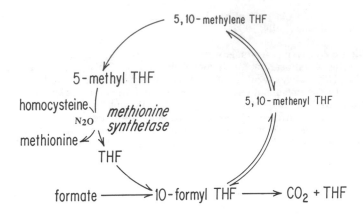

FIG. 2: Site of action of N2O in the metabolic pathway of folate-dependent formate oxidation

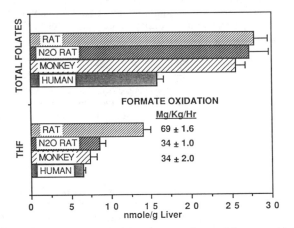

FIG. 3: Effect of N2O on hepatic tetrahydrofolate concentrations and formate oxidation. Data compiled from studies conducted by Eells *et al.*, (1981, 1982) and Johlin *et al.*, (1987).

Development of formic acidemia and metabolic acidosis in methanol-intoxicated rats: Methanol (4 g/kg plus 2 g/kg at 12- hour intervals) was administered to male Long Evans rats exposed to subanesthetic concentrations of nitrous oxide [N2O/O2 (1:1)]. Methanol-intoxicated rats developed formic acidemia, metabolic acidosis and visual toxicity analogous to the human methanol poisoning syndrome. Methanol administration produced an initial mild CNS depression which was followed by a latent period of 12-18 hours, during which the behavior of methanol intoxicated rats was indistinguishable from saline-treated control rats. Following this latent period, methanol-intoxicated rats became progressively more lethargic and unresponsive. Some animals became comatose and died between 48-60 hrs after the initial methanol dose. Sixty hours after methanol administration blood formate concentrations in surviving animals were 16.1 ± 0.7 mM ; blood bicarbonate values were 7.7 ± 1.2 mEq/l and blood pH had declined to 6.90 ± 0.06. (Table 1). Similar blood formate concentrations and blood bicarbonate and pH values have been reported in methanol-intoxicated monkeys (Martin-Amat et al., 1977) and in severe cases of human methanol poisoning (McMartin et al., 1980; Murray et al., 1996). Saline-treated rats exposed to N_2O/O_2 exhibited no differences in behavior from that observed in animals breathing room air. In addition, no alterations in blood formate concentrations, blood pH or blood bicarbonate concentrations were observed in these animals.

Metabolic Parameter	N_2O-treated Rats	Monkeys	Humans
Blood Formate (mM) [normal values]	16.1 ± 0.7 [0.5 ± 0.1]	11.4 ± 1.2 [0.5 ± 0.2]	19.3 ± 4.4 [0.6 ± 0.2]
Blood Bicarbonate (mM) [normal values]	7.7 ± 1.2 [25.6 ± 1.4]	6.5 ± 0.5 [21.0 ± 2.1]	3.2 ± 0.4 [22-28]
Blood pH [normal values]	6.90 ± 0.06 [7.34 ± 0.03]	7.22 ± 0.02 [7.41 ± 0.02]	6.93 ± 0.02 [7.40 ± 0.02]

TABLE 1: Formic Acidemia and Metabolic Acidosis in Methanol-Intoxicated Rodents, Primates and Humans Blood formate, blood bicarbonate and pH values were determined in methanol-intoxicated rats 60 hrs after the initial dose of methanol. The monkey data was compiled from studies by Martin-Amat et al., (1977) and the human data was compiled from studies conducted by McMartin et al., (1980) and Murray et al., (1996).

Development of Visual Dysfunction in Methanol-Intoxicated Rats:

Visual dysfunction following methanol intoxication was evaluated by measurement of flash-evoked cortical potentials (FEP) and electroretinograms (ERG). The FEP is a measure of the functional integrity of the primary visual pathway from the retina to the visual cortex and the ERG is a global measure of retinal function in response to illumination (Creel et al., 1970; Green, 1973; Dowling, 1987). The averaged FEP measured prior to methanol intoxication consisted of a primary (P20-N30) component (mean amplitude : 93 ± 12 μV; mean latency : 31.7 ± 0.5 msec) and additional more variable secondary components (Fig. 4). Microelectrode studies have shown that the P20-N30 component of the FEP is the result of retinogeniculostriate activity whereas the secondary components arise from central modulatory systems (Creel et al., 1970). The amplitude of the P20-N30 component of the FEP was progressively diminished (Fig. 4) with a corresponding increase in latency (Eells, 1991) in methanol-intoxicated rats. These findings are indicative of a disruption of neuronal conduction along the primary visual pathway from the retina to the visual cortex. Retinal function was evaluated by ERG analysis. The averaged ERG measured prior to methanol intoxication consisted of a negative a-wave (mean amplitude: 176 ± 30 μV; mean implicit time: 17.5 ± 1.0 msec) followed by a positive b-wave (mean amplitude: 508 ± 70 μV; mean implicit time: 48.5 ± 1.9 msec). The a-wave of the ERG reflects photoreceptor activation and the b-wave results from the depolarization of the Muller glial cells secondary to activity of the bipolar cells (Dowling, 1987). ERG analysis in methanol-intoxicated rats revealed an early deficit in b-wave amplitude followed by a temporally delayed lesser reduction in a-wave amplitude (Fig. 5). No significant alterations were observed in the implicit times of the a- or b-wave in methanol-intoxicated rats. Reductions in the b-wave of the ERG were observed as early as 12-24 hours after the initial dose of methanol at a time when formate concentrations were below concentrations associated with other visual changes (Eells, 1991, Murray et al., 1991). Forty-eight hours after the initial dose of methanol, b-wave amplitude was 25% of control values and at 60 hours the b-wave was less than 5% of control values. Significant reductions in a-wave amplitude (40% of control values) were apparent at 60 hours in methanol-intoxicated rats. Both FEP and ERG alterations occurred coincident with the accumulation of blood formate suggestive of a causal relationship between formate induced metabolic and visual disturbances. A highly significant negative correlation was demonstrated between blood formate concentration and each of these parameters of visual function (Eells, 1991; Eells *et al.*, 1996).

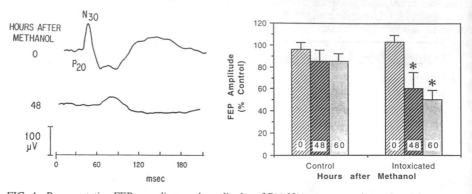

FIG. 4: Representative FEP recordings and amplitudes of P20-N30 component in methanol-intoxicated (methanol and N2O-treated) and control (saline and N2O-treated) rats. Data are expressed as percent of mean zero time control values of FEP amplitude. Shown are the mean values ± SE (n = 6). Significant decreases in amplitude from control measurements are denoted with an asterisk.

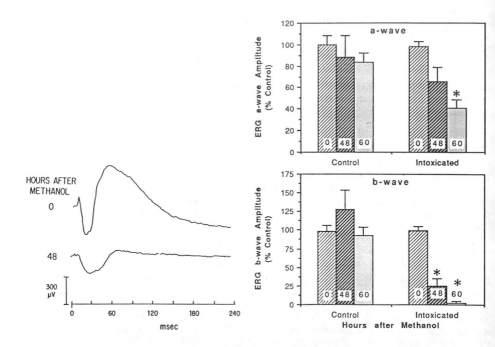

FIG. 5: Representative ERG recordings and amplitudes of a-waves and b-waves in methanol-intoxicated (methanol and N2O-treated) and control (saline and N2O-treated) rats. Data are expressed as percent of mean zero time control values of ERG *a*-wave or *b*-wave amplitude. Shown are the mean values ± SE (n = 4). Significant decreases in amplitude from control measurements are denoted with an asterisk.

Evidence of Retinal and Optic Nerve Damage in Methanol-Intoxicated Rats: In addition to electrophysiologic changes, structural alterations suggestive of direct toxicity to the retina and optic nerve were also observed in the methanol-treated rats. Histologic evaluation of the eyes 60 hours after methanol administration revealed optic nerve changes similar to those reported in methanol and formate intoxicated primates (Baumbach *et al*, 1977, Hayreh *et al.*, 1980) and also showed distinctive retinal changes at the level of the RPE and neurosensory retina. Light microscopic evaluation showed generalized retinal edema and vacuolation in the photoreceptors and retinal pigment epithelium (Fig. 6). Ultrastructural examination showed swelling and disruption of the mitochondria in the optic nerve, retinal pigment epithelium and photoreceptor inner segments (Fig. 7) (Murray *et al.*, 1991). These findings are consistent with a disruption in ionic homeostasis in the RPE and photoreceptors secondary to inhibition of mitochondrial function (Siesjo, 1992; Trump *et al.*, 1989). It is interesting to note that similar changes are observed in retinas from patients with mitochondrial diseases that affect the electron transport chain (McKechnie *et al.*, 1985; Runge *et al.*, 1986; McKelvie *et al.*, 1991) and in some forms of light induced retinal degeneration associated with inactivation of cytochrome oxidase (Rapp *et al.*, 1990; Pautler *et al.*, 1990).

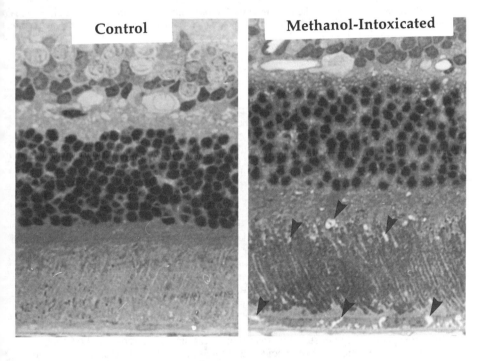

FIG. 6: Light micrographs of retina from an untreated control animal (left) and from a methanol-intoxicated (methanol and N2O-treated) (right). The retina from the methanol-intoxicated rat shows evidence of diffuse edema and vacuolation (arrows) at the junction of the inner and outer segments of the photoreceptor cells and in the retinal pigment epithelial cells (x 210).

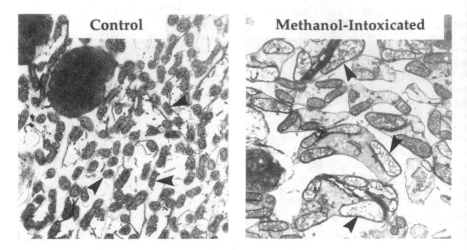

FIG. 7: Electron micrographs of the photoreceptor layers of untreated control (left) and methanol and N2O-treated experimental retinas (right). Photoreceptor mitochondria from control animals showed normal morphology with well defined cristae. In contrast, photoreceptor mitochondria from methanol intoxicated rats were swollen with expanded or disrupted cristae (x 10,000).

Controls for these experiments included groups of rats which were treated with saline and exposed to nitrous oxide (N2O-control); rats which were treated with methanol, but not exposed to nitrous oxide (methanol-control); and untreated rats. No alterations in visual function (ERG and FEP), metabolic parameters (blood formate concentrations, blood pH, bicarbonate, body temperature), or histology were observed in any of the control groups with the exception of subtle alterations in the mitochondria of the optic nerve observed in the methanol control group (Eells *et al.*, 1981, 1983; Eells, 1991; Murray *et al.*, 1991). These results suggest that the mitochondria of the optic nerve may be particularly sensitive to methanol poisoning.

DISCUSSION

Methanol has been recognized as a serious human neurotoxin for nearly a century and the clinical features of human methanol poisoning have been extensively documented. Despite numerous clinical reports on ocular findings, the pathogenesis of methanol poisoning has remained obscure. In addition, many questions remain regarding the nature and extent of retinal and optic nerve injury and the mechanism of action of methanol's toxic metabolite, formic acid. Attempts to produce experimental models of ocular toxicity have yielded results with little relevance to the poisoning of humans. The principal difficulty has been that in most commonly employed laboratory animals, the type of poisoning induced by methanol differs significantly from that observed in humans. In nonprimate species, large doses of methanol induce a state of narcosis and death, but without the manifestation of formic acidemia, metabolic acidosis and retinal and optic nerve damage similar to that reported in humans. The only exception has been work conducted in nonhuman primates in which methanol administration results in the production of a syndrome similar to that observed in human methanol intoxication. However, observations on retinal involvement from primate animal studies show some inconsistencies because of variations in methanol dosage, individual animal variation, and the limitations on numbers of animals which were studied imposed by cost and availability. We report on the development and characterization of a methanol-sensitive

·odent model which we have used to investigate the metabolic and visual system toxicity ıssociated with methanol intoxication. As in human and nonhuman primate poisonings, he response of rats to methanol in this model is characterized by a latent period followed ɔy accumulation of formate within the blood. The formate accumulation parallels the ɹevelopment of a metabolic acidosis with decreasing bicarbonate and blood pH, and can ead to death (Tephly and McMartin, 1984; Eells et al., 1981; Eells, 1991; Jacobson and ʼʌcMartin, 1986).

The alterations in visual function observed in our studies suggest that the retina is a ɔrimary site of formate toxicity. They also provide an important functional correlate of ·etlnal and/or optic nerve damage reported in human cases of methanol poisoning and in ıon-human primate studies (Benton and Calhoun, 1952; Sharpe et al., 1982; Hayreh et ıl., 1980). Disruptions in the P20-N30 component of the FEP have been associated with ɹirect retinal actions as well as effects on optic nerve function (Eells and Wilkison, 1989). ʼʌore specifically, the reductions of the a-wave and b-wave of the ERG observed in the methanol-intoxicated rats indicate that retinal function is directly disrupted by formate. The a-wave of the ERG reflects the hyperpolarization of the photoreceptors and the b-wave is generated by the depolarization of Muller glial cells and reflects synaptic activity at level of the bipolar cells (Dowling, 1987). The ERG is not affected by lesions in the optic nerve or retinal ganglion cells (Dowling, 1987). The alterations in the ERG observed in methanol-intoxicated rats in this study as well as those reported in humans (Eells et al., 1995; Murray et al., 1996) and non-human primates (Ingmannsson, 1983) are therefore indicative of a toxic action of formate on retinal function which is primarily manifested as a disruption of glial or bipolar cell function and to a lesser extent a disruption of photoreceptor function.

Similar, although not identical, alterations in retinal function have been reported by Lee and colleagues (Lee et al., 1994a, b) in methanol intoxicated folate-deficient rats . In these studies, rats were maintained on a folate-deficient diet for 18 weeks, resulting in a 90% reduction in total hepatic folate concentrations. Following methanol administration (3.5 g/kg, po), folate-deficient rats developed formic acidemia and visual toxicity. Visual ɹysfunction was manifested 48 hours after methanol administration as an increase in the latency of the P20-N30 component of the FEP and a reduction in the amplitude of the b-wave of the ERG. However, no alterations in the amplitude of the P20-N30 component of the FEP or the a-wave of the ERG were observed in these animals. Formic acid accumulation was comparable in both methanol-sensitive rodent models, therefore, the discrepancies in methanol-induced retinal toxicity observed in N_2O-treated tetrahydrofolate deficient and dietary folate depleted rats are most likely due to the differences in stimulation and recording parameters. Flash intensity was substantially greater in the studies by Lee and colleagues (4.5×10^7 lux compared to 3.2×10^3 lux in our studies) producing a more intense visual stimulation and eliminating more subtle responses observed at the lower stimulus intensities employed in our studies. In addition, the studies by Lee et al., (1994a, b) did not examine the effects of methanol-intoxication on visual function beyond 48 hours. Significant reductions in a-wave amplitude were apparent only after 48 hours in our studies. Electroretinographic studies are currently being conducted in our laboratory to define the time-course and stimulus-response relationships in methanol-intoxicated rats over an extended range of stimulus intensities.

In addition to electrophysiologic changes, structural alterations suggestive of direct toxicity to the retina were also observed in the methanol-treated rats. The most pronounced alteration was a severe vacuolation at the base of the photoreceptor outer segments, just distal to the outer limiting membrane formed by the junctional complexes between photoreceptors and Muller glia. Also prominent was dilation of the extracellular space at the bases of the pigment epithelium. Diffuse retinal edema which was seen here has been observed by ophthalmoscopic evaluation in methanol intoxicated humans and nonhuman primates (Benton and Calhoun, 1952; Potts, 1955). Baumbach et al., (1977) documented mitochondrial swelling and disruption in the optic nerve of methanol-intoxicated primates. In agreement with these findings, the optic nerve in this rodent model also appears to be sensitive to formate exposure. In this study, mitochondrial changes were also seen in other tissues, notably photoreceptors and RPE.

An important obstacle in understanding the pathogenesis of methanol poisoning has been the lack of animal models which mimic the human poisoning syndrome. Methanol poisoning occurs in humans and non-human primates; the two species that uniquely accumulate formic acid after methanol exposure (Eells, 1992; Tephly and McMartin, 1984). Formate accumulation coincides with the classic presentation of methanol toxicity. The initial delay in symptoms followed by an uncompensated metabolic acidosis, visual disturbances ranging from visual blurring to blindness, and central nervous system alterations occasionally leading to coma and even death may all be directly attributable to formate (Eells, 1992; Tephly and McMartin, 1984; Sharpe et al, 1982). We have developed a rodent model of methanol toxicity by selective inhibition of formate oxidation in this species (Eells et al., 1981, 1982; Murray et al., 1991; Eells, 1991). Methanol-intoxicated rats developed formic acidemia, metabolic acidosis and visual toxicity characterized by reductions in the visual evoked potential and electroretinogram. Histopathology of these animals revealed abnormalities at the level of the photoreceptors and retinal pigment epithelium in addition to optic nerve changes. Our laboratory has also obtained electroretinographic and morphologic evidence of similar retinal toxicity in a fatal case of human methanol poisoning (Eells et al., 1991; Murray et al., 1996) thus further substantiating the clinical and toxicological relevance of this nonprimate model of methanol poisoning.

Formate has been hypothesized to produce retinal and optic nerve toxicity by disrupting mitochondrial energy production (Martin-Amat et al., 1977, 1978; Sharpe et al., 1982). In vitro studies have shown that formate inhibits the activity of cytochrome oxidase, a vital component of the mitochondrial electron transport chain involved in ATP synthesis (Nicholls, 1975, 1976; Eells et al., 1995). Formic acid binds to cytochrome aa3 and inhibits cytochrome oxidase activity with inhibition constant values between 5 and 30 mM (Nicholls, 1975, 1976). Concentrations of formate present in the retina and vitreous humor of these methanol-intoxicated rats are within this range as are the concentrations of formate measured in the blood, vitreous humor and CSF of methanol poisoned humans and monkeys (McMartin et al., 1980; Sejersted et al., 1983; Martin-Amat et al., 1977). Selective inhibition of mitochondrial function in the retina and optic nerve is consistent with both the functional and morphological findings in methanol intoxication. However, further investigations are needed to confirm or refute this hypothesis and to delineate the mechanisms through which formate induces ocular toxicity. The development of this non-primate animal model of methanol toxicity will greatly facilitate research into the mechanistic aspects of methanol toxicity and may prove valuable in developing and testing treatments for human methanol poisoning.

REFERENCES

Andrews, L.S., Clary, J.J., Terrill, J.B., and Bolte, H.F., 1987, "Subchronic inhalation toxicity of methanol," Journal of Toxicology and Environmental Health ,Vol. 20, pp.117-124.

Banks, R.G.S., Henderson, R.J. and Pratt, J.M., 1968, "Reactions of gases in solution. Part III. Some reactions of nitrous oxide with transition-metal complexes," Journal of the Chemical Society, (A): pp. 2886-2898.

Baumbach, G.L., Cancilla, P.A., Martin-Amat, G., Tephly, T.R., McMartin, K.E., Makar, A.B., Hayreh, M.S. and Hayreh, S.S., 1977, "Methyl alcohol poisoning. IV. Alterations of the morphological findings of the retina and optic nerve," Arch. Ophthalmology, Vol. 95, pp. 1859-1865.

Benton, C.D. and Calhoun, F.P., 1952, "The ocular effects of methyl alcohol poisoning. Report of a catastrophe involving three hundred and twenty persons," Trans. Am. Acad. Ophthalmology, Vol. 56, pp. 875-883.

Black, K.A., Eells, J.T., Noker, P.E., Hawtrey, C.A. and Tephly, T.R., 1985, "Role of hepatic tetrahydrofolate in the species difference in methanol toxicity," Proc. Natl. Acad. Sci. USA, Vol. 82, pp. 3854-3858.

Buller, F. and Wood, C.A., 1904, "Poisoning by wood alcohol. Cases of death and blindness from Columbian spirits and other methylated preparations,"J. Am. Med. Association, Vol. 43, pp. 1058-1062, 1117-1123, 1213-1221, 1289-1296.

Creel, D.J., Dustman, R.E. and Beck, E.C., 1970, "Differences in visually evoked responses in albino versus hooded rats," Experimental Neurology, Vol. 29, pp. 298.

Deacon, R., Lumb, M., Perry, J., Chanarin, B., Minty, M.J. and Nunn, J., 1980, "Inactivation of methionine synthase by nitrous oxide," Eur. J. Biochem., Vol. 104, pp. 419.

Dowling, J.E., 1987, "The electroretinogram and glial responses,"In The Retina: An Approachable Part of the Brain by J. E. Dowling, pp 164-186, Belknapp Press of Harvard University Press, Cambridge.

Eells, J.T., 1991, "Methanol-induced visual toxicity in the rat," J. Pharmacol. Exp. Ther., Vol. 257, pp. 56-63.

Eells, J.T., 1992, "Methanol," In Browning's Toxicity and Metabolism of Industrial Solvents, Vol IV: Alcohols and Esters, ed R.G. Thurman and F.C. Kaufmann, pp. 3-15. Elsevier Biomedical Press, Amsterdam.

Eells, J.T., Black, K.A., Makar, A.B., Tedford, C.E. and Tephly, T.R., 1982, "The regulation of one-carbon oxidation in the rat by nitrous oxide and methionine," Arch. Biochem. Biophys., Vol. 219, pp. 316-326.

Eells, J.T., Black, K.A., Tedford, C.E. and Tephly, T.R., 1983, "Methanol toxicity in the monkey: effects of nitrous oxide and methionine," J. Pharmacol. Exp. Ther., Vol. 227, pp. 349-353.

Eells, J.T., Lewandowski, M.F., and Murray, T.G., 1996, "Formate-induced retinal dysfunction in methanol-intoxicated rats," Toxicology and Applied Pharmacology, (in press).

Eells, J.T., Makar, A.B., Noker, P.E. and Tephly, T.R., 1981, "Methanol poisoning and formate oxidation in nitrous oxide treated rats," J. Pharmacol. Exp. Ther., Vol. 217, pp. 57-61.

Eells, J.T., Murray, T.G., Lewandowski, M.F., Stueven, H.A. and Burke, J.M., 1991, "Methanol poisoning: clinical and morphologic evidence of direct retinal dysfunction. Invest. Ophthalmol. Vis. Sci. Vol. 32, p. 689.

Eells, J.T., Salzman, M.M.and Trusk T..C., 1995, " Inhibition of retinal mitochondrial function in methanol intoxication," The Toxicologist, Vol 15, p. 21.

Eells, J.T. and Wilkison, D.W., 1989, "Effects of Intraocular mescaline and LSD on visual-evoked responses in the rat," Pharm. Biochem. Behav., Vol. 32, pp. 191-196.

Frederick, L.J., Schulte, P.A. and Apol, A., 1984, "Investigation and control of occupational hazards associated with the use of spirit duplicators,"Am. Ind. Hyg. Assoc. Journal, Vol. 45, pp. 51-55.

Green, D., 1973, "Scotopic and photopic components of the rat electroretinogram," Journal of Physiol. (Lond)., Vol. 228, pp. 781.

Hayreh, M.M., Hayreh, S. S., Baumbach, G.L., Cancilla, P., Martin-Amat, G., and Tephly, T.R., 1980, "Ocular toxicity of methanol: an experimental study," In Neurotoxicity of the Visual System, ed. by W. Merigan and B. Weiss, pp. 35-53, Raven Press, New York.

Huennekens, F.M., Digirolama, P.M., Fujii, K., Jacobsen, D.W. and Vitols, K.S., 1976, "B-12 dependent methionine synthetase as a potential target for cancer chemotherapy," Advances in Enzyme Regulation, Vol. 14, pp. 187-205.

Ingemansson, S.O., 1983, "Studies on the effect of 4-methylpyrazole on retinal activity in the methanol poisoned monkey by recording the electroretinogram," Acta Ophthalmol. Suppl. (Copenh), Vol. 158, pp. 5-24.

Jacobsen, D. and McMartin, K.E., 1986, "Methanol and ethylene glycol poisonings: mechanism of toxicity, clinical course diagnosis and treatment," Medical Toxicology, Vol. 1, pp. 309-334.

Johlin, F.C., Fortman, C.S. Nghiem, D. D. and Tephly, T.R., 1987, "Studies on the role of folic acid and folate-dependent enzymes in human methanol poisoning," Molec. Pharm., Vol. 31, pp. 557-661.

Kavet, R. and Nauss, K.,.1990, "The toxicity of methanol vapors," Crit. Rev. Tox., Vol. 21, No. 1, pp. 21-50.

Kutzbach, C. and Stokstad, E.L.R., 1968, "Partial purification of a 10-formyl tetrahydrofolate: NADP oxidoreductase from mammalian liver," Biochem. Biophy. Res. Commun., Vol. 30, pp. 111.

Lee, E.W., Garner, C.D. and Terzo, T.S., 1994 a, "Animal model for the study of methanol toxicity: Comparison of folate-reduced rat responses with published monkey data," Journal of Toxicology and Environmental Health, Vol. 41, pp. 71-82.

Lee, E.W., Garner, C.D. and Terzo, T.S., 1994 b, "A rat model manifesting methanol-induced visual dysfunction suitable for both acute and long-term exposure studies," Toxicology and Applied Pharmacology, Vol. 128, pp. 199-206.

Makar, A.B. and Tephly, T.R., 1976, "Methaol poisoning in the folate-deficient rat," Nature, Vol. 261, pp. 715-716.

Makar, A. B. and Tephly, T. R., 1982, "Improved estimation of formate in body fluids and tissues," Clin. Chem., Vol. 28, pp. 385.

Martin-Amat, G., McMartin, K.E., Hayreh, S.S., Hayreh M.S. and Tephly, T.R., 1978, "Methanol poisoning: Ocular toxicity produced by formate," Toxicol. Appl. Pharmacol., Vol. 45, pp. 201-208.

Martin-Amat, G., Tephly, T.R., McMartin, K.E., Makar, A.B., Hayreh, M.S.,Hayreh, S.S., Baumbach, G. and Cancilla, P., 1977, "Methyl alcohol poisoning. II. Development of a model for ocular toxicity in methyl alcohol poisoning using the Rhesus monkey," Arch. Ophthalmol., Vol. 95, pp. 1847-1850.

McKechnie, N. M., King, M. and Lee, W. R., 1985, "Retinal pathology in the Kearns-Sayre syndrome," Br. J. Ophthalmol., Vol. 69, pp. 63.

McKelvie, P.A., Morley, J.B., Byrne, E. and Marzuki, S. 1991, "Mitochondrial encephalomyopathies: a correlation between neuropathological findings and defects in mitochondrial DNA," J. Neurol. Sci., Vol. 102, pp. 51-60.

McMartin, K.E., Ambre, J.J. and Tephly, T.R., 1980, "Methanol poisoning in human subjects: Role of formic acid accumulation in the metabolic acidosis," Am. J. Med., Vol. 68, pp. 414-418.

McMartin, K.E., Makar, A.B., Martin-Amat, G., Palese, M. and Tephly, T.R., 1975, "Methanol poisoning. I. The role of formic acid in the development of metabolic acidosis in the monkey and the reversal by 4-methylpyrazole," Biochem. Med., Vol. 13, pp. 319-333.

McMartin, K.E., Martin-Amat, G. Makar, A.B. and Tephly, T.R., 1977, "Methanol poisoning. V. Role of formate metabolism in the monkey," J. Pharmacol. Exp. Ther., Vol. 201, pp. 564-572.

McMartin, K.E., Virayotha, V. and Tephly, T.R., 1981, "High-pressure liquid chromatography separation and determination of rat liver folates," Arch. Biochem. Biophys., Vol. 209, pp. 127-136.

Murray, T.G., Burke, J.M., Lewandowski, M.F., Steuven, H.A. and Eells, J.T., 1996, "Clinical and morphologic evidence for retinal dysfunction in methanol poisoning," Retina, (in review).

Murray, T. G., Burton, T. C., Rajani, C., Lewandowski, M. F., Burke, J. M. and Eells, J. T., 1991, "Methanol poisoning: a rodent model with structural and functional evidence for retinal involvement," Arch. Ophthalmol., Vol. 109, pp. 1012-1016.

Nicholls, P., 1975, "Formate as an inhibitor of cytochrome c oxidase," Biochem. Biophys. Res. Comm., Vol. 67, pp. 610-616.

Nicholls, P., 1976, "The effects of formate on cytochrome aa3 and on electron transport in the intact respiratory chain," Biochim. Biophys. Acta , Vol. 430, pp. 13-29.

Palese, M. and Tephly, T.R ,1975, "Metabolism of formate in the rat, J. Toxicol. Environ. Health, Vol. 1, pp. 13-24.

Pautler, E.L., Morita, M. and Beezley, D., 1990, "Hemoprotein(s) mediate blue light damage in the retinal pigment epithelium," Photochem. and Photobiol., Vol. 51, No. 5, pp. 599-605.

Potts, A.M., 1955, "The visual toxicity of methanol. VI. The clinical aspects of experimental methanol poisoning treated with base," Am. J. Ophthalmol., Vol. 39, pp. 86-92.

Rapp, L.M., Tolman, B.L. and Dhindsa, H.S., 1990, "Separate mechanisms for retinal damage by ultraviolet-A and mid-visible light," Invest. Ophthalmol. Vis. Sci., Vol. 31, No. 6, pp. 1186-1190.

Roe, O., 1955, "The metabolism and toxicity of methanol," Pharmacol. Rev., Vol. 7, pp. 399-412.

Runge, P., Calver, D., Marshall, J. and Taylor, D., 1986, "Histopathology of mitochondrial cytopathy and the Laurence-Moon -Biedl syndrome," Br. J. Ophthalmol., Vol. 70, pp. 782-796.

Sejersted, O.M., Jacobsen, D., Ovrebo, S. and Jansen, H., 1983, "Formate concentrations in plasma from patients poisoned with methanol," Acta Med. Scand., Vol. 213, pp. 105-110.

Sharpe, J., Hostovsky, M., Bilbao, J. and Rewcastle, N.B., 1982, "Methanol optic neuropathy: A histopathological study," Neurology, Vol. 32, pp. 1093-1100.

Siesjo, B., 1992, "Pathophysiology and treatment of focal cerebral ischemia. Part I: Pathophysiology," J. Neurosurg., Vol. 77, pp. 169-184.

Tephly, T., 1991, "The toxicity of methanol," Life Sci., Vol. 48, pp. 1031-1041.

Tephly, T.R. and McMartin, K.E., 1984, "Methanol Metabolism and Toxicity," In Aspartame: Physiology and Biochemistry, ed by L.D. Stegink and L.J. Filer, pp. 111-140, Marcel, Dekker, New York.

Trump, B.F., Berezesky I.K., Smithe, M.W., Phelps, P.C. and Elliget, K.A., 1989, "The relationship between cellular ion deregulation and acute and chronic toxicity," Toxicol. Appl. Pharmacol., Vol. 97, pp. 6-22.

Aquatic and Sediment Toxicology, Behavior, and Risk Assessment

Suzanne M. Lussier,[1] Denise Champlin,[1] Anne Kuhn[1], and James F. Heltshe[2]

MYSID (*MYSIDOPSIS BAHIA*) LIFE-CYCLE TEST: DESIGN COMPARISONS AND ASSESSMENT

REFERENCE: Lussier, S. M., Champlin, D., Kuhn, A., and Heltshe, J. F., "Mysid (*Mysidopsis bahia*) Life-Cycle Test: Design Comparisons and Assessments," *Environmental Toxicology and Risk Assessment: Biomarkers and Risk Assessment—Fifth Volume, ASTM STP 1306,* David A. Bengtson and Diane S. Henshel, Eds., American Society for Testing and Materials, 1996.

ABSTRACT: This study examines ASTM Standard E1191-90, "Standard Guide for Conducting Life-cycle Toxicity Tests with Saltwater Mysids", 1990, using *Mysidopsis bahia*, by comparing several test designs to assess growth, reproduction, and survival. The primary objective was to determine the most labor efficient and statistically powerful test design for the measurement of statistically detectable effects on biologically sensitive endpoints. Five different test designs were evaluated varying compartment size, number of organisms per compartment, and sex ratio. Results showed that while paired organisms in the ASTM design had the highest rate of reproduction among designs tested, no individual design had greater statistical power to detect differences in reproductive effects. Reproduction was not statistically different between organisms paired in the ASTM design and those with randomized sex ratios using larger test compartments. These treatments had numerically higher reproductive success and lower within tank replicate variance than treatments using small compartments where organisms were randomized, or had a specific sex ratio. In this study, survival and growth were not statistically different among designs tested. Within tank replicate variability can be reduced by using many exposure compartments with pairs, or few compartments with many organisms in each. While this improves variance within replicate chambers, it does not strengthen the power of detection among treatments in the test. An increase in the number of true replicates (exposure chambers) to eight will have the effect of reducing the percent detectable difference by a factor of two. The results indicate that, of the five test designs compared, test design two, with randomized sex ratios using larger test compartments, employed the same number of test organisms in fewer compartments, produced good survival and growth, yielded reproduction comparable with the ASTM method, and required less animal handling and monitoring time. We recommend adoption of this test design with the incorporation of an increase in the number of true replicates to eight.

KEYWORDS: mysid, *Mysidopsis bahia*, life-cycle test, toxicity test methods

[1] U.S. Environmental Protection Agency, ORD/NHEERL, Atlantic Ecology Division, 27 Tarzwell Drive, Narragansett, RI 02882 (EPA Contribution No. 1645)
[2] University of Rhode Island, Kingston, RI 02881

The mysid life-cycle test was first developed with *Mysidopsis bahia* by Nimmo et al. (1977). Since then the method has been revised by several investigators (Breteler et al. 1982, McKenney et al.1982, Lussier et al. 1985, Cripe et al. 1981). It is the most widely used chronic test with a marine organism, having been tested with over 40 substances in more than 60 studies. In 1987, "The Standard Guide for Conducting Life-Cycle Toxicity Tests with Saltwater Mysids" was initially published as ASTM Standard E1191-87, after five years of discussions and data analyses by the ASTM workgroup (Subcommittee E47.01). This method, revised in 1990 (ASTM E1191-90), has been used for the development of Water Quality Criteria (Federal Register 1980, 1985), registration of pesticides, and hazard evaluations of many substances or conditions. On review of some of these data, it was determined that, due to the inherent variability of the reproduction endpoint, differences from the control sometimes could not be detected even though reproduction was completely absent in other treatments. This problem of reproductive variability had been demonstrated in an earlier field verification study conducted for Black Rock Harbor, Connecticut, (Gentile et al. 1985) when large differences in reproduction did not show statistical significance until the experimental design was changed. The new design increased pairs of test animals from six to thirty, and replicates from two to eight per treatment, thereby reducing the replicate to replicate variability, and increasing overall statistical power. An analysis of nine most recently conducted mysid life-cycle tests at U.S. EPA, Atlantic Ecology Division, Narragansett, R.I., using the ASTM method (which uses two replicate aquaria and eight mysid pairs per replicate), revealed that the range of detectable differences from control was from 22 to 208%, with a mean of 104%.

Based on these data, it was determined that the ASTM method should be reexamined to determine whether the test design could be modified to reduce the reproductive variability and improve the power of detection. The present study consists of a life-cycle test to compare five different test designs (one per treatment), developed based on previous unpublished data which contributed to the development of the ASTM method. Data were compared to evaluate the effects of test design under control conditions, on survival, growth, and reproduction in mysid life-cycle exposures.

METHODS

Culture and Exposure Systems

Mysidopsis bahia were obtained from laboratory cultures maintained in filtered (15μ) Narragansett Bay seawater in a flow-through (100 mL/ min) system (Lussier et al. 1991). Seawater was maintained at $25 \pm 1°$ C, $30 \pm 2\%$. salinity, and a pH of 7.8-8.2, in 76-L glass aquaria with undergravel filters and a dolomite substrate with gentle aeration. Taxonomic identification of cultured animals was reverified by Wayne Price and Richard Heard at the Mysid Taxonomy Workshop in 1989. *M. bahia* has recently been renamed *Americamysis bahia* (Price *et al.* 1994) in the designation of a new genus, *Americamysis,* to separate the several *Mysidopsis* species which were often confused. *Artemia* sp. nauplii (24 h posthatch) were provided as food at about 7×10^4 nauplii per day to each aquarium, with the amount adjusted according to mysid density to provide ad libitum food to prevent cannibalism.

In the exposure system, each treatment utilized two replicate glass chambers (15.5cm x 47cm x 15.5cm), which received water from a mini-diluter system modified from Benoit et al. (1982). A siphon-flush mechanism (Sosnowski et al. 1979) was used to produce a 40ml/min flow rate per replicate chamber; approximately 14 volume additions per day. Test chambers are defined as the "smallest physical units between which there are no water connections. Screens and cups may be used to create two or more compartments within each chamber" (ASTM E1191-90). Three exposure compartment designs were tested: (1) large netted compartments; fabricated from 14 cm diameter glass petri dishes each with a 320μ Nitex* screen collar fastened with clear silastic sealant; (2) small netted compartments; fabricated identically only using 9 cm diameter glass petri dishes; and (3) small glass compartments, 6.5 cm diameter of glass jars with two opposing 3cm diameter holes covered with 320μ Nitex screen.

Test Designs

Five different test designs, using exposure compartments, were compared to evaluate the possible effects on survival, growth (measured as dry weight), and reproduction in life-cycle exposures (Figure 1). All treatments employed two replicate exposure chambers. The effects of compartment size, sex ratio, animal density, and handling were compared using filtered Narragansett Bay seawater. The design used in ASTM E1191-90, served as the standard test design to which other four designs were compared. The test using all designs (treatments) was initiated using newly hatched (12-24 h) *M. bahia* juveniles that were fed *Artemia* sp. nauplii ad libitum. Test organisms as close to the same age as possible were used, as required by ASTM, to minimize variation in growth and reproduction.

Treatment 1 (ASTM method): Days 0-14, 15 animals were held in each of two large (14 cm diameter) netted compartments per duplicate chamber (N = 30). On day 14 (at sexual maturity), animals were paired by sex, and redistributed into each of eight small glass (6.5 cm diameter) compartments per duplicate chamber (N = 16), for the remainder of the test (days 15-28). Extra males not used for pairing were held in separate netted compartments within the exposure chambers. To ensure fertility of females, these males were used to replace paired males that died during the reproductive phase of the test, but were not counted in quantification of survival. Dead females were not replaced.

Treatment 2: Days 0-14, 10 animals were held in each of three large (14 cm diameter) netted compartments per duplicate chamber (N = 30). On day 14, animals were not redistributed, but left in the same configuration, regardless of sex ratio, for the remainder of the test.

---

*Mention of commercial products does not constitute endorsement by the U.S. Environmental Protection Agency.

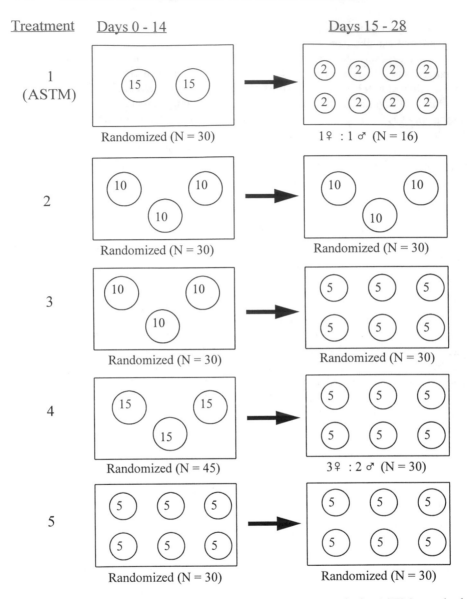

FIG. 1-- Five test treatments were compared; treatment 1 is the ASTM standard method. The number of animals (n) in each exposure compartment is shown before and after redistribution on day 14. N equals total animals in each replicate of the treatment. Only one of two replicates per treatment is shown.

Treatment 3: Days 0-14, 10 animals were held in each of three large (14 cm diameter) netted compartments per duplicate chamber (N = 30). On day 14, animals were randomly redistributed, five animals to each of six small (9 cm diameter) netted compartments per replicate chamber, for the remainder of the test.

Treatment 4: Days 0-14, 15 animals were held in each of three large (14 cm diameter) netted compartments per duplicate chamber (N = 45). On day 14, (at sexual maturity), animals were examined, sorted by sex, and redistributed, five animals to each of six small (9 cm diameter) netted compartments with a 3 female: 2 male sex ratio (N = 30) for the remainder of the test.

Treatment 5: Days 0-14, 5 animals were held in each of six small (9 cm diameter) netted compartments per duplicate chamber (N = 30). On day 14, animals were not redistributed, but left in the same configuration for the remainder of the test (N = 30).

Biological Measurements

All exposure compartments were monitored daily throughout the entire test. Dead adults and young mysids (after day 14) were counted and removed. Feeding was adjusted according to the number of live adults. Survival was quantified during the entire test but, because it was nearly 100% in all treatments during the first phase of the test, was statistically compared among treatments only for the reproductive phase (days 15 to 28).

Growth was measured as dry weight as required in the ASTM method (E1191-90). Males and females were removed from each exposure compartment at the end of the test, rinsed with deionized water, placed on tared pans according to sex, dried at 60° C for at least 72 hours, and weighed to obtain a mean dry weight separately for male and female mysids.

Reproduction in the life-cycle toxicity test is usually measured as the number of young produced per available female reproductive day (AFRD) which adjusts for differences in young produced caused by toxicant related mortality of females. In this test, no toxic substances were used, the number of females varied among the designs, and some were not distributed according to sex ratio. Therefore, we measured the cumulative number of young produced per number of females at the start of the reproductive period (day 15) through the end of the test (day 28), resulting in a mean productivity per female.

Statistical Measurements

Statistical differences (P = 0.05) among treatments were detected by analysis of variance (Snedecor and Cochran 1980) and Fisher's protected least significant difference test (1960). Coefficients of variation and detectable differences were calculated for each treatment using within and between replicate variability.

RESULTS

Results from analyses of the five test treatments are presented for the biologically important endpoints of survival, growth, and reproduction.

Survival

The pattern of survival was similar among treatments (Figure 2). Female survival during the reproductive period (83 to 97%) was better than male survival, (64 to 79%), a trend we have observed previously. Total percent survival (for both sexes) in all treatments ranged from 74 to 88% and was within the acceptable limit of >70% established by ASTM. Analysis of variance showed no significant differences in survival of females, males, or both sexes among treatments.

Growth

Dry weights of males, females, and all mysids at the end of the test ranged from 0.9 to 1.5μg (Figure 3). The ASTM mysid life-cycle test has no established criteria for acceptable dry weight. No significant differences were observed among the treatments.

Reproduction

The mean number of young per female during the reproductive period (day 15-28) ranged from 3.76 to 11.38 among the five test designs (Table 1). Figure 4 shows the pattern of reproduction for each of the test designs. Analysis of variance showed a significant difference in reproduction among the five test designs (P<0.05). Females from treatment 1 (the ASTM method) averaged 11.38 young each, which was significantly greater than the number of young released by females in treatments 3, 4, and 5. The mean number of young released in treatment 2 (8.75 young/female) did not differ from any other treatment. Some females in each of treatments 1 and 2 released a second brood during the reproductive period.

TABLE 1-- Mean and coefficient of variation (CV) on the number of young released per female mysid from day 15 to 28 of a life-cycle test

Treatment	Young / Female	CV%
1	11.38	59
2	8.75	58
3	3.77	58
4	3.95	64
5	5.79	52

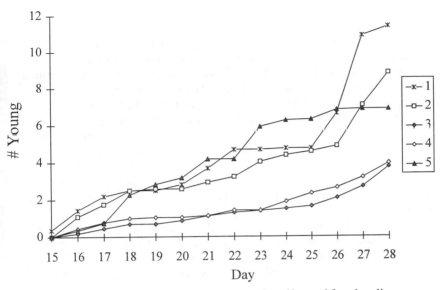

FIG. 4--Cumulative number of young produced by total females alive at start of reproductive period (Day 15) in each treatment.

Power of Detection

In a life-cycle test, after a significant difference among treatments is determined, it is necessary to identify which treatment concentrations of a toxic substance have caused an adverse biological effect. Statistical tests for significant differences between each treatment and the control, or reference treatment, are then conducted. The lower the variability, the more powerful the test, and the smaller the difference from control that can be detected. Tests designs with a greater power of detection will be better predictors of chemical effects. The detectable percent difference of a statistical test is that percent difference between two treatment means that can be detected "P" percent of the time. This "P" percent being the power of the statistical test. The desired power can either be fixed to compute effect size or vice versa. The results of these five treatment configurations show that while treatment 1 (ASTM) had the highest reproduction, the between replicate variability was also very high (Table 1). The five treatments had similar coefficients of variance for reproduction implying that each test design has approximately the same percent detectable difference between duplicates.

Coefficients of variance were also calculated within duplicate tanks in each treatment. Varability within treatments can be reduced by the configuration of exposure chambers and organisms as demonstrated in the five test designs used in this study. Coefficients of variance were lower in test designs 1 and 2 (67% and 61%, respectively), compared with designs 3, 4, and 5 (79%, 78%, and 128%, respectively). This reduction in within duplicate variance was not observed between duplicates, and so the power of detection remained unaffected.

DISCUSSION

The test designs devised for this study examined a number of factors that may control reproductive success, inherent variability of reproduction, ease of testing, and therefore the power to predict effects in the *M. bahia* life-cycle test. In our reevaluation of the ASTM (E1191-90) test design, we reviewed our unpublished test information which had contributed to the development of the original test method. Experimental designs were chosen for this study to integrate and test some of those same design factors with the goal of providing data required to modify the ASTM method. For example, results from previous research showed that survival and reproduction were significantly improved when fewer animals (6 vs 12) were employed per exposure compartment (unpublished data). Those results were corroborated in this study with increased reproduction in test designs 1 and 2 (Figure 1), which offered the greatest compartment surface area per animal (33.2 cm^2 and 30.7 cm^2, respectively). All other designs offered only 25.4 cm^2 per animal. Some females in treatments 1 and 2 also released a second brood during the reproductive period, indicating a faster development rate. Previous studies also showed a significant improvement in survival and reproduction when animals were exposed in larger compartments (14 vs 9 cm diameter) regardless of density. In this study, test design 2 with the larger netted compartments had numerically double the reproduction of test designs 3, 4, and 5, with small compartments, but did not differ significantly from design 1. Previous results (unpublished) showed no improvement in survival or reproduction when sex ratios within exposure compartments were varied. Likewise in this study, test designs 3 and 4 (random vs 3F:2M) showed no differences. We theorized that the additional handling involved in redistribution of animals into a particular sex ratio might adversely effect survival. However, no difference in survival was detected among the designs tested (Figure 2).

A statistical factor that may be related to design options, minimum significant difference, was also reviewed. Upon examination of previous tests which were conducted at our laboratory in accordance with the ASTM method, we found that the detectable difference in reproduction from control ranged from 22 to 208%, with a mean of 104%. This is a result of the high variability between duplicate chambers in the treatments. Because the tests were conducted over a period of several years, there may have been other factors which contributed to this variability, such as culture conditions, seasonal seawater changes, etc. The present study removed those variables, affording the opportunity to compare test designs under the same controlled laboratory conditions, without exposure to a toxic material. The between duplicate variability in this study was similar for all treatments, i.e., coefficients of variation 52 to 64% (Table 1).

Lower variability for survival and growth measurements usually enable differences among treatments to be detected statistically. However reproduction, often the most sensitive indicator of effects, has an innately high variability which often impedes statistical detection of differences among treatments. It is for this reason that the reproductive parameter was emphasized in this study, to explore ways to enhance female productivity and reduce sources of variance due to test design. Because of the variability associated with the reproductive endpoint, one comparative test is only an indicator, not a predictor, of the ability to detect differences in reproduction. While a repeat of this test

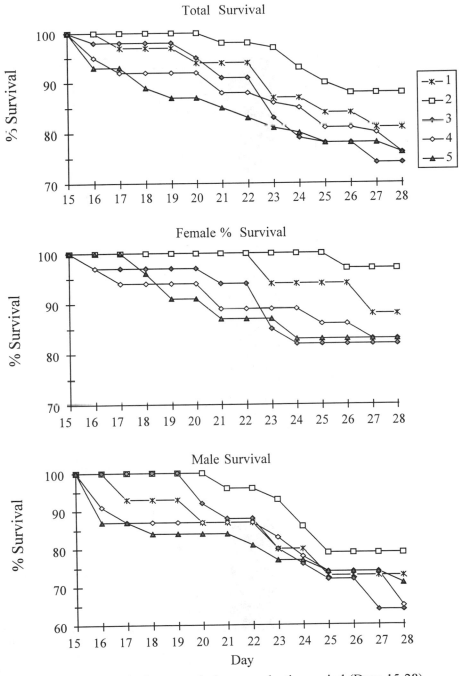

FIG. 2--Survival pattern during reproductive period (Days 15-28)

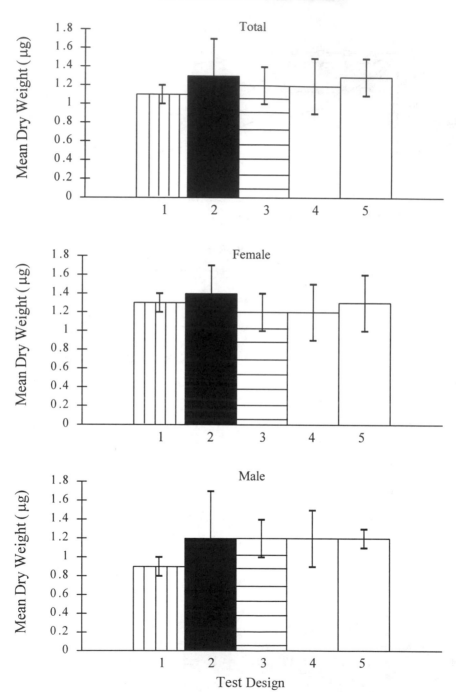

FIG. 3--Growth (as dry weight) results from five test designs.

could give somewhat different results, there was no significant difference in detectability of reproductive effects among the five test designs with only duplicate chambers. Therefore, the use of only two replicates is a more important constraint on the power of the test than the experimental design used for reproductive assessment. Even though the variability within replicate tanks was reduced in treatments 1 and 2 compared with treatments 3, 4, and 5; the reduction reflected variance among exposure chambers sharing the same exposure water and had no effect on the detectable difference for the test. True replicates (n), which by definition have no water connection, are used in the calculation of the power of detection of the test (ASTM E1191-90). Increasing the number of **true** replicates to eight is calculated to have the effect of reducing the percent detectable difference by a factor of two. All Minimum Significant Differences (MSD) are functions of coefficients of variance and sample sizes. The sample size enters the calculation in the form $(2/n)^{1/2}$ for equal number of replicates per treatment. Clearly, as we increase n from two to eight, this reduces the MSD by a factor of two. The MSD is halved for $n=8$ versus $n=2$. For reproduction data, the MSD for $n=2$ (two replicates) was 166%, if n is increased to 8 replicates, the MSD is 83%. This expected increase in sensitivity is similar to that empirically determined in the Black Rock Harbor experiments with eight true replicates, noted earlier (Gentile et al. 1985).

Practical and economic aspects are also important determinants of a test design. The number of animals required, time involved checking and handling test organisms, maintenance of the test system, etc., all add cost. To better compare these attributes, they are listed in Table 2. The important note is, there are pros and cons to each design, and one must be chosen that produces statistical resolution, balanced with ease of conducting the test.

TABLE 2--Comparison of test design attributes

Treatment	Number of Mysids	Handling Time	Number of Chambers	Mean Young/ Female	Mean % Survival	Mean Dry Weight (μg)
1	60	High (pairing)	20	11.38	81	1.1
2	60	Low	6	8.75	88	1.3
3	60	Medium	18	3.77	74	1.2
4	90	High (sex ratio)	18	3.95	76	1.2
5	60	Low	12	5.79	76	1.3

Test design 2 used a reasonable number of test organisms and compartments, and produced good survival and growth. Reproduction was not significantly different from the ASTM method, and with pairing eliminated, less animal handling was required during the test. Due to the high inherent variability in reproduction, the ability to detect differences among test treatments can be improved only by increasing the number of true replicates. It is for these reasons we recommend adoption of test design 2, with the incorporation of an increase in the number of true replicate chambers to eight. We believe that the time saved by eliminating the pairing requirement will compensate for the increased number of replicates, and a better power of detection will reduce the necessity for repeating tests.

ACKNOWLEDGEMENTS

We greatly appreciate the efforts of Sherry Poucher for her assistance in the interpretation of the data, and to David Hansen who provided the impetus for this study and critical examination of the results.

REFERENCES

American Society for Testing and Materials, 1990, "Guide for Conducting Life-cycle Toxicity Tests with Saltwater Mysids," E1191-90 Annual Book of ASTM Methods, ASTM, Philadelphia, pp. 735-751.

Benoit, D.A., Mattson, V.R., and Olson, D.L., 1982, "A Continuous-flow Mini-diluter System for Toxicity Testing," Water Research, Vol 18, pp. 457-464.

Breteler, R.J., Williams, J.W., and Buhl, R.L., 1982, "Measurement of Chronic Toxicity Using the Opossum Shrimp Mysidopsis bahia," Hydrobiologia, Vol 93, pp. 189-194.

Cripe, G.M., Nimmo, D.R., and Hamaker, T.L., 1981, "Effect of Two Organophosphate Pesticides on Swimming Stamina of the Mysid Mysidopsis bahia," Biological Monitoring of Marine Pollutants, Academic Press, N.Y., N.Y., Vernberg F.J., Thurberg, F., Calabrese, A., and Vernberg, W., eds., pp. 21-36.

Federal Register, November 28, 1980, Vol 45, pp. 79318-79279.

Federal Register, July 29, 1985, Vol 50, pp. 30784-40796.

Fisher, R.A., 1960, The Design of Experiments, 7th ed., Oliver & Boyd, Edinburgh.

Gentile, J.H., Scott, K.J., Lussier, S., and Redmond, M., 1985, "Application of Laboratory Population Responses for Evaluating the Effects of Dredged Material," US EPA Technical Report D-85-8, pp. 39-46.

Lussier, S.M., Gentile, J.H., and Walker, J., 1985, "Acute and Chronic Effects of Heavy Metals and Cyanide on *Mysidopsis bahia* (Crustacea: Mysidacea)," Aquatic Toxicology, Vol 7, pp. 25-35.

Lussier, S.M., Kuhn, A., Chammas, M.J., and Sewall, J., 1991, "Life History and Toxicological Comparisons of Temperate and Subtropical Mysids," American Fisheries Society Symposium, Vol 9, pp. 169-181.

McKenney, C.L., 1982, "Interlaboratory Comparison of Chronic Toxicity Testing Using the Estuarine Mysid (*Mysidopsis bahia*): A Final Report," (ERL, GB, 182, unpublished), U.S. Environmental Protection Agency, Environmental Research Laboratory, Gulf Breeze, FL, 35 pp.

Nimmo, D.R., Bahner, L.H., Rigby, R.A., Sheppard, J.M., and Wilson, A.J., Jr., 1977, "*Mysidopsis bahia*: An Estuarine Species Suitable for Life-Cycle Toxicity Tests to Determine the Effects of a Pollutant," Aquatic Toxicology and Hazard Evaluation, First Annual Symposium, ASTM STP 634, Mayer, F.L., and Hamelink, J.L., eds., ASTM, pp. 109-116.

Price, W.W., Heard, R.W., and Stuck, L., 1994. "Observations on the Genus *Mysidopsis* Sars, 1864 with the Designation of a New Genus, *Americamysis*, and the Descriptions of *Americamysis alleni* and *A. Stucki* (Peracarida:Mysidacea: Mysidae), from the Gulf of Mexico," Proceedings of the Biological Society of Washington, Vol 107(4), pp. 680-698.

Snedecor, G.W. and W.G. Cochran, 1980, Statistical Methods, 7th ed., Iowa State University Press, Ames, Iowa, 507 pp.

Sosnowski, S.L., Germond, D.L., and Gentile, J.H., 1979 "The Effect of Nutrition on the Response of Field Populations of the Calanoid Copepod *Acartia Tonsa* to Copper," Water Research, Vol 13, pp. 449-452.

Julia S. Lytle[1] and Thomas F. Lytle[1]

RESPONSES OF THE ESTUARINE PLANT *SCIRPUS OLNEYI* TO TWO HERBICIDES, ATRAZINE AND METOLACHLOR

REFERENCE: Lytle, J. S. and Lytle, T. F., "Responses of the Estuarine Plant *Scirpus Olneyi* to Two Herbicides, Atrazine and Metolachlor," *Environmental Toxicology and Risk Assessment: Biomarkers and Risk Assessment—Fifth Volume, ASTM STP 1306*, David A. Bengtson and Diane S. Henshel, Eds., American Society for Testing and Materials, 1996.

ABSTRACT: The phytotoxicity of atrazine and metolachlor was tested using rhizome cultures of *Scirpus olneyi*, a major salt marsh emergent macrophyte that has wide distribution around Gulf estuaries. A variety of types of exposure media and methods of toxicant addition were employed. Test systems included: (1) rhizomes placed in biochambers with atrazine-spiked "clean" estuarine sediment; (2) rhizomes placed in biochambers containing composited estuarine sediment with grain sizes ranging from sands to clays; (3) young shoots placed in biochambers prepared as in (2); and; (4) young shoots placed in biochambers in seawater diluted to varying salinities. Metolachlor was the test pesticide in systems 2-4. Plant responses measured included peroxidase activity (POD), peroxidation products, chlorophyll, and growth. All responses to atrazine-spiked sediments were clearly related to the dose, whereas responses to metolachlor showed high variability with increasing salinity and low variability with varying grain size. At 12‰, salinity effects completely masked the metolachlor effects (as measured by growth) at all test levels, indicating that growth as an ecological endpoint used to evaluate a chemical stressor is ineffective under certain salinity regimes.

KEYWORDS: emergent macrophytes, pesticides, estuarine variables, biomarkers

Estuarine marsh plants play an extremely important role in estuaries. They are the nursery grounds for many important fish and avian species, and they act as powerful buffers against storm erosion. Though they are very vulnerable to agricultural runoff, little scientific data exist regarding their pesticide sensitivities. To assess effects of pesticides on plants within an estuary, it is critical to understand how estuarine variables such as fluctuating salinity and variable sediment regimes affect pesticide toxicities.

[1]Head, Environmental Chemistry and Head, Analytical Chemistry, respectively, Gulf Coast Research Laboratory, 703 E. Beach, Ocean Springs, MS 39564

Standardized test protocols have not been developed to evaluate chemicals for the protection of emergent estuarine macrophytes for various reasons. The culturing of young plants for toxicity testing of emergent estuarine species is problematic in that seeds are difficult to secure, techniques for breaking seed dormancy are not well documented, seed germinations are often long and sporadic, and seedling growth can be excessively slow. The objectives of the studies reported are several-fold: to develop a technique for propagating large numbers of young emergent estuarine macrophytes, to carry out phytotoxicity tests on the cultured species with two extensively used agricultural herbicides, to measure and compare plant responses to herbicide toxicity under varying salinity and sediment grain size regimes, and to evaluate biochemical assays for suitability of use under field conditions.

PROCEDURES

Plant Propagation

Scirpus olneyi, *Juncus roemerianus*, and *Spartina alterniflora* (emergent macrophytes) are major marsh plants along the Mississippi coast. *J. roemerianus* seeds are exceedingly small and difficult to physically separate from the spikelets, and when successful in germination, seedling growth is slow. *S. alterniflora* can be germinated from seed, if seeds are collected near peak maturity and properly stored using an after-ripening process (Woodhouse et al. 1974).   No known cultivation techniques are available for *S. olneyi*, commonly known as three square sedge. All three marsh plants spread naturally through rhizome emergence. To test feasibility of cultivating young plants from rhizomes, rhizomes from each of the three species were collected throughout 1993 and placed in shallow trays of water under greenhouse conditions (air circulated and temperature ranging from 23° to 28°C depending on season) until vegetative shoots emerged. *S. olneyi* was the only species which was easily cultivated from rhizomes, and rhizomes clipped in either spring or summer produced a large number of healthy plants. In May, 1994 small select stands of *S. olneyi* were removed from a pristine area in Davis Bayou, MS, and rhizomes were carefully washed and clipped at each node and placed in trays of water in the greenhouse until young shoots were 3-5 cm in height. Though this technique is successful in producing large numbers of young shoots having identical genetic material, it is labor intensive. Removal of *S. olneyi* stands causes no lasting detrimental effects since recolonization occurs within the growing season. Studies utilized either rhizomes or young plants grown from rhizomes.

Herbicide Preparation

Atrazine (2-chloro-4-ethylamino-6-isopropylamine-*s*-triazine, 97.1% pure, from Ciba-Geigy Corp., Greensboro, NC) was used without carrier and metolachlor, 2-chloro-N-(2-ethyl-6-methylphenyl)-N-(2-methoxy-1-methylethyl)acetamide, was a commercial liquid preparation of Pennant® (Ciba-Geigy, 85.1% active ingredient). In Test 1, three dose levels of atrazine were prepared as follows. Three aliquots weighed to yield approximately 1, 10 and 100 ppm (when added to sediment) were dissolved in 95% ethanol. Dissolved atrazine aliquots were transferred to 10 g fine quartz sand which had been precleaned by heating at 400°C for 24 hours. Atrazine/sand aliquots were slurried

TABLE 1--Exposure bioassay conditions.

		Test		
	1	2	3	4
Pesticide	Atrazine	Metolachlor	Metolachlor	Metolachlor
Level	1,10,100 ppm	0.1,1,10 ppm	0.01,0.1,1 ppm	0.01,0.1,1 ppm
Duration	24 days	28 days	16 days	16 days
Medium	Estuarine sediment	5 mixtures sands & clays	3 mixtures sands & clays	Seawater with Hoagland solution
Method of Toxicant Addition	Coated quartz sand mixed in sediment	Distilled water atop sediment	Hoagland solution atop sediment	In medium
Renewal	None	None	7 days	7 days
Culture	Rhizomes	Rhizomes	Rhizome plants	Rhizome plants
Measured Responses	Growth* Peroxidases Peroxidation Chlorophyll	Growth* Chlorophyll	Growth* Peroxidases Chlorophyll	Growth* Peroxidases Chlorophyll

*total biomass, shoot biomass, shoot length (mean & total), root length

and air dried under the fume hood for 8 hours to remove all ethanol. The sand coatings in Table 1 are nominal values that were not further verified. Before spiking with atrazine, wet sediments were thoroughly homogenized and divided into four-3 kg portions. Atrazine/sand and sand only (control) aliquots were added to 3 kg sediment portions and thoroughly homogenized. In Tests 2, 3 and 4, a concentrated solution of metolachlor was prepared and diluted with well water and sufficient nutrients to yield a 10% Hoagland solution (Hoagland and Arnon 1950).

Test Systems

All tests were carried out in a controlled temperature greenhouse during the months of May through September. Natural light was used throughout the testing. Air temperatures were monitored daily using a max/min thermometer. Temperatures ranged between 23°C and 28°C, which is a typical diurnal range of temperatures for this locale. Conditions for each test are described in Table 1. Sediments used in formulation of grain size tests were collected from two locations within Weeks Bay, AL, one dominated by clay (65.3% clay, 22.2% silt, and 12.5% sand) and the other by sand (39.6% coarse,

55.0% medium, 2.5% fine, 1.2% very fine sands, and 1.7% silt and clay). The clay-rich sediments were used for the atrazine-spiked tests. Wet sediments were refrigerated at 7°C prior to preparation of test media, and were stored less than 7 days before use. Both sediments were washed to remove salts before use in Test 3. Water pumped from a deep well was used for dilutions of seawater and for preparation of test solutions. Seawater was collected 3 miles offshore from Pensacola, Fl. Before use of well water and seawater, chemical analysis were performed for trace metals, pesticides and water quality (Strickland and Parsons 1968). Chemical characteristics (mean value reported) of well water were: hardness, 1.8 mg/L as $CaCO_3$; alkalinity, 210 mg/L as $CaCO_3$, pII, 7.8, total suspended solids, <1 mg/L; total organic carbon (TOC), 0.3 mg/L; unionized NH_3, 0.006 mg-N/L. Chemical characteristics of seawater were as follows: suspended solids, 125 mg/L; TOC, 7.8 mg/L; unionized NH_3, 0.003 mg-N/L. At laboratory detection limits for atrazine and metolachlor, 0.1 µg/L and 3.0 µg/L, respectively, neither were detected. Weeks Bay sediments used as sediment media were considered reference sediments.

Tests were run in the chronological order 1 to 4. Elements of test procedures constant in all systems were as follows. All treatment replicates were randomized within blocks and placed as blocks in an area of the greenhouse away from windows. Each treatment level contained five replicate biochambers, each of which contained 12 plants (n=60). Water levels were kept constant by daily addition of well water after initial herbicide application. Sediments were collected 2 days prior to preparation as a test medium and held wet at 7°C. Sediment pH was measured after homogenization prior to atrazine-spiking in Test 1 and after homogenization of sediment preparation of various grain size mixtures in Tests 2 and 3, and at the end of each study. No adjustments were made since the pH was within the optimum growing range of 6.0 to 7.5. Concentrations of herbicides in water solution were confirmed by gas chromatography. Sediments were collected before and after tests and frozen immediately for archiving. A brief description of each test system follows.

Test 1--Rhizomes/atrazine-spiked sediments.   Sixty rhizome sections (one node per section) per treatment/control were counted and carefully examined to assure all were healthy and approximately equal in size. Each treatment level and control contained 5 replicate biochambers, and were prepared by placing 600 mL of appropriate atrazine-spiked or control clay-rich sediments into each container. Sediment composition is reported under Test Systems. Blocks were randomized in a given area of the greenhouse. At the end of the test, shoot height was recorded for each plant. Plants were carefully removed, washed and wet weights recorded. Tissue from growing tips were clipped and kept separated by individual biochambers for triplicate analyses of peroxidase activity (POD), chlorophylls, and peroxidation products. Primary root length on each plant was measured and recorded.

Test 2--Rhizomes/metolachlor/grain sizes.   For further toxicity testing, metolachlor, in a water-borne route of testing, was tested using a commercial formulation to more closely mimic field application conditions. Test 2 required 1200 rhizomes. Five grain size fractions, each containing 5 replicates, were tested with 3 treatment levels of metolachlor, 0.1, 1, and 10 ppm and a control. Each treatment and control block, therefore, contained 5 blocks of variable sediment sizes. Sediment grain size fractions were prepared by utilizing 100% sand, 100% clay and 75:25% sand:clay, 50:50% sand:clay, 25:75% sand:clay. Six hundred mL of appropriate wet sediment were placed into each biochamber. Three hundred rhizomes were utilized within each treatment block. Appropriate concentrations of metolachlor were diluted with well water and 200 mL placed atop the sediments in each biochamber, and well water only was placed atop control sediments. Duration of Test 2 was 24 days. Procedure for plant measurements, separations and analyses followed that of Test 1.

Test 3--Young rhizome plants/metolachlor/grain size. Because sediments were not washed to remove salts prior to preparation of grain size fractions, and because no rhizome emergence occurred at the highest test level in Test 2, the test was repeated making the following changes in test design. Young rhizome plants having 3-5 cm growth tips arising from rhizome nodes were used instead of rhizomes not yet having vegetative shoots (as in Tests 1 and 2). Hoagland solution was added to the metolachlor/well water test solution. Only 3 grain size fractions were used in testing, 100% sand, 50:50% sand:clay, and 100% clay, allowing the test to be run with fewer rhizomes. Test concentrations were lowered by a factor of 10 to include 0.01, 0.1, and 1 ppm. A renewal of metolachlor test solution was made on day 7 to better maintain herbicide concentrations which permitted shortening the test duration to 16 days. Procedure for plant measurements, separations and analyses followed that of Test 1.

Test 4--Young rhizome plants/metolachlor/salinity. To examine the effect of salinity on plant responses to metolachlor, each treatment level and control utilized four salinity regimes, 0, 4, 8, and 12‰. Each regime contained five replicates, each replicate with 12 young rhizome plants. Metolachlor was prepared in seawater diluted with well water and Hoagland solution. Test concentrations included 0.01, 0.1, and 1 ppm. Four hundred mL of test solution were placed into each biochamber after which 12 rhizome plants were placed into the test solution. A renewal of test solution was made on day 7. Test duration was 16 days. Procedure for plant measurements, separations and analyses followed that of Test 1.

Biochemical Assays

Estimation of lipid peroxidation--To estimate lipid peroxidation, 1 g leaf tissue was homogenized in chilled 0.15 M KCl. One mL of the homogenate was incubated at 37°C for 2 h after which 1 mL of 10% w/v trichloroacetic acid was added. After thorough mixing, the reaction mixture was centrifuged at 2000 rpm for 10 min. One mL of supernatant liquid was added to one mL of 0.67% w/v 2-thiobarbituric acid (Sigma Chemical Co., St. Louis, MO), placed in a boiling water bath for 10 min, cooled and diluted with 1 mL of distilled water. Spectrophotometric readings at 535 nm were converted to μmoles malonaldehyde/g by the method of Utley et al. (1967).

Peroxidase enzyme activity--POD activity was measured using a modified version of the assay by Maehly and Chance (1954). A 1 g leaf sample was ground in 0.5 M CaCl$_2$. To 200 μL of the extract was added 1.4 mL of a solution containing 22.7 mg phenol (as substrate) and 0.70 mg 4-amino-antipyrine and 1.5 mL of 0.3% (w/v) H$_2$O$_2$ in a pH 6 buffer of 2-[N-Morpholino]ethanesulfonic acid. The rate of increase of absorbance was measured at 30 s intervals at 510 nm with a Perkin-Elmer UV/Vis Lambda 3B Spectrophotometer (Perkin-Elmer Co., Norwalk, CT) and converted to POD activity units by comparison with authentic horseradish peroxidase undergoing an identical bioassay.

Chlorophylls--Plant shoots were weighed (approximately 0.3 g) and ground using an all-glass tissue homogenizer. Chlorophylls were extracted using 20 mL of 90% aqueous spectrophotometric grade acetone over a 24 h period in the dark at 7°C; the mixture was centrifuged at 1200 rpm for 10 min and the supernatant brought up to exactly 20 mL. Absorbances were measured at 750, 663, 645, and 630 nm using a Perkin-Elmer UV/Vis Lambda 3B Spectrophotometer (Perkin-Elmer Co., Norwalk, CT). Chlorophylls a and b were quantified using SCOR/UNESCO equations (Strickland and Parsons 1968). Concentrations were converted to mg/g wet weight of leaf material.

Statistical Interpretation

For each of the responses, means and standard errors were computed for each treatment. One-way analysis of variance (ANOVA) was then applied to these data to establish statistically significant differences (Manugistics, Inc. 1994). When a difference did exist among a set of means, a least significant difference multiple range test was applied with a 95% confidence level ($p < 0.05$) to identify subsets within the set of means that were statistically indistinguishable. Toxicity was assessed as a statistically significant decrease relative to appropriate controls, in chlorophylls and all growth parameters, or a statistically significant increase in peroxidase activity or peroxidation products.

RESULTS

Test 1 _Scirpus_ rhizomes/atrazine

In Test 1, a 1 ppm atrazine-spiked sediment significantly inhibited photosynthesis leading to chlorophyll degradation and diminished levels of chlorophylls a and b and significantly increased POD, decreased total biomass and root length were noted at 10 ppm. As shown in Fig. 1, POD activity increased with each increasing exposure concentration relative to controls, and a significant toxic response was produced at 1 ppm. Peroxidation products increased significantly with each higher exposure concentration (Fig. 2). A significant decrease in both chlorophyll a and b resulted at the 1 ppm exposure level (Fig. 3). Since atrazine can inhibit photosynthesis (Moreland, 1980), one would expect biomass production to decrease with decrease in photosynthetic activity. This trend was demonstrated by a significant reduction in root length and by a significant decrease in total biomass at 10 ppm as shown in Fig. 4.

Test 2 _Scirpus_ rhizomes/grain size/metolachlor

Fig. 5 shows POD response to metolachlor exposure under test conditions using 5 different grain size sediment regimes. Results are not reported for the highest exposure level due to complete inhibition of shoot emergence in all grain size regimes. POD activity increased significantly at the 1 ppm test level in all sediment grain size regimes and at all test levels in sediments with high sand components. POD activity, however, as a function of grain size, was not significantly different between control, 1 and 10 ppm in the high clay regime but was significantly different in the high sand regime between control, 1 and

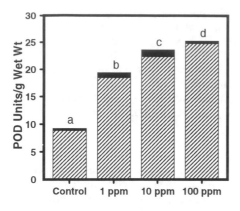

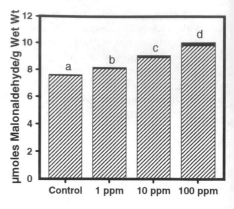

FIG. 1--Peroxidase activity units in *S. olneyi* exposed to atrazine (Test 1). Means and standard error (solid bar) are shown in units equivalent to horseradish peroxidase units. Letters indicate all bars significantly different (p<0.05).

FIG. 2--Peroxidation products in *S. olneyi* exposed to atrazine (Test 1). Means and standard error (solid bar) are in units of malonaldehyde with letters over bars in each group indicating all significantly different (p<0.05).

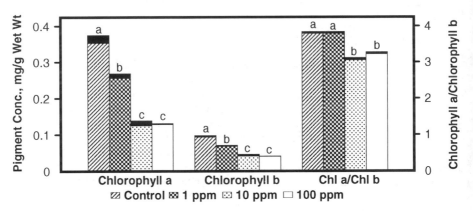

FIG. 3--Chlorophyll a and b in *S. olneyi* following exposure to atrazine (Test 1). Means and standard error (solid bar) are shown for three groups of data, with shared letters over bars signifying no significant difference (p<0.05).

10 ppm. Chlorophylls and various growth response measurements resulted in similar trends but showed no significant differences between concentration test levels. These confounding results, in conjunction with inhibition of shoot emergence at the highest test level, prompted us to repeat this experiment with important modifications. Variables other than grain size and concentration levels of metolachlor in Test 2 (salts in sediments, more nutrients in clay fractions than sands) were eliminated in Test 3. Note changes in Test 3 design as described under Test systems.

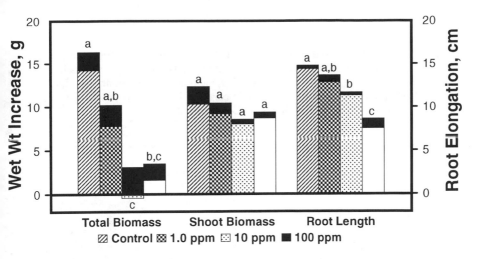

FIG. 4--Growth responses of *S. olneyi* following exposure to atrazine (Test 1). Three growth responses are depicted as means and standard error (solid bar) for change in total biomass, total shoot biomass, and mean root length. Shared letters in the three groups denote no significant difference (p<0.05).

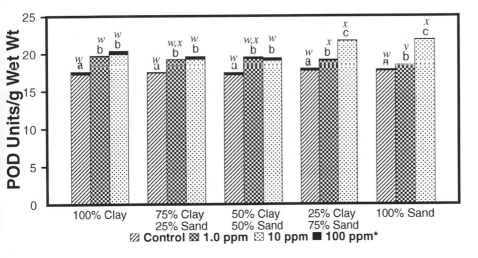

FIG. 5--Peroxidase activity units in *S. olneyi* grown in sediments of 5 grain sizes following exposure to metolachlor (Test 2). Means and standard error (solid bar) are shown for results of each sediment type. Bars sharing letters a-c indicate no significant differences (p<0.05) within group of same value of environmental parameter; shared letters w-y indicate no significant differences within group of identical exposure level (bars with same shading).

Test 3 Young *Scirpus* rhizome plants/metolachlor/grain size

In Test 3, *Scirpus* exposed to 0.1 ppm metolachlor under different sediment regimes significantly inhibited photosynthesis with resulting diminishment of chlorophylls a and b (not shown) and significantly increased POD activity; at 1 ppm metolachlor significantly decreased total shoot length and mean root length (not shown) in at least one grain size sediment regime. Fig. 6 shows POD response to metolachlor

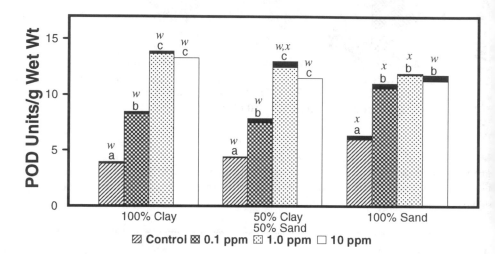

FIG. 6--Peroxidase activity in *S. olneyi* grown in sediments of 3 grain sizes following exposure to metolachlor (Test 3). See Fig. 5 notes.

exposure under test conditions using 3 different grain size regimes. POD activity significantly increased with increasing concentrations of metolachlor (control, 0.1, 1, 10 ppm) in both clay regimes, but only from control to 0.1 ppm in 100% sand. In examining differences between grain size regimes, POD responses were indistinguishable at all test levels in both of the clay regimes, i.e., grain size variability did not affect POD response when tested in clays. However, POD responses in the sand regime were distinguishable from other grain size regimes at 0.1 and 1 ppm exposure levels. At the highest test level (10 ppm), differences in mean shoot length (Fig. 7) are indistinguishable among all sediment regimes.

Test 4 Young *Scirpus* rhizome plants/metolachlor/salinity

In Test 4, *S. olneyi* exposed to 0.1 ppm metolachlor contained significantly less chlorophylls a and b (not shown), significantly elevated POD, and significantly decreased total shoot length and root length (not shown) in one or more salinity regimes. POD activity in *Scirpus* shoots resulting from metolachlor exposure in varying salinity regimes is shown in Fig. 8. Results are shown to illustrate the confounding nature of salinity effects on POD activity in *Scirpus*. A trend of increasing POD activity with increasing exposure concentration to metolachlor is observed when tested under freshwater

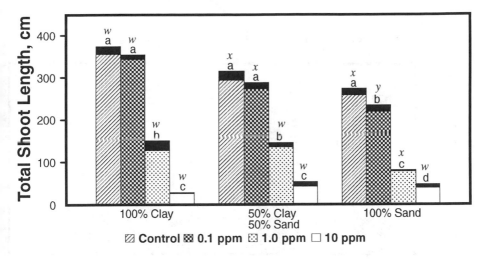

FIG. 7--Total shoot length of *S. olneyi* exposed to metolachlor in 3 grain size regimes (Test 3). See Fig. 5 notes.

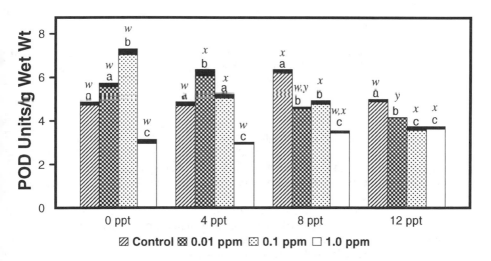

FIG. 8--POD activity in *S. olneyi* following exposure to metolachlor in 4 salinity regimes (Test 4). See Fig. 5 notes.

conditions though POD activity was inhibited at highest concentrations. However, POD activity shows a possible inhibition of the POD enzyme system that occurs at a lower test level as salinity increases i.e., inhibition at 1 ppm at 0‰, 0.1 ppm at 4‰ and 0.01 ppm at 8‰ and 12‰. Similarly, shoot lengths decreased with increasing metolachlor concentrations under freshwater and low salinity regimes (Fig. 9). With increasing salinities, however, growth responses are dampened with increasing exposure levels until

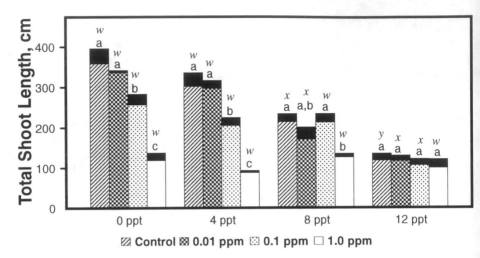

FIG. 9--Total shoot length of *S. olneyi* exposed to metolachlor in 4 salinity regimes (Test 4). See Fig. 5 notes.

at highest salinity, there are no differences in shoot length between any concentration test level. Though not shown, root lengths and shoot weights showed a similar response.

DISCUSSION

Atrazine is a herbicide which inhibits electron transport through photosystem II (Moreland 1980; Boger and Sandmann 1990). The inhibition of photosynthesis in turn also affects processes that are indirectly dependent on photosynthesis which may lead to substantial disruptions of overall metabolism, affecting RNA, enzyme, and protein synthesis (Huber 1993).

Various investigators (Correll and Wu 1982; Cunningham et al. 1984; Kemp et al. 1985) have reported atrazine growth inhibition in the aquatic macrophytes *Potamogeton perfoliatus* and *P. pectinatus* at concentrations ranging from 30-907 µg/L of atrazine, a concentration range similar to that found to elicit a suite of responses in *S. olneyi*. However, the TOC (2.32%) and the fine-grain clay sediment used in our test medium possibly make atrazine less bioavailable to the plant since atrazine is lipophilic and would adsorb to organics. Concentration levels used in this test, though higher than one would expect to find in estuarine sediments, up to 1.5 ppm (Huber 1993), were used to assure toxic concentrations. Testing should be repeated using a lower range of atrazine concentrations to fine tune biomarker responses to assess lowest observed effect concentration (LOEC) under similar sediment toxicity testing.

Metolachlor is classified as a chloroacetamide preemergent herbicide that inhibits protein and lipid (Jaworski 1975) synthesis but does not inhibit photosynthesis.

Metolachlor is stable even at pH of 1 making it unlikely to be decomposed readily. It has been reported to be stable in loamy soil for 64 days. As a nonionic herbicide, it also adsorbs to organic matter and clay in soils at pH above 4, thus ground water contamination as a result of metolachlor leaching is highly unlikely (Gerber et al. 1974). Like atrazine, adsorption of metolachlor can reduce bioavailability, hence toxicity to plants. Walsh et al. (1991a) reported a LOEC for survival of 0.5 mg/kg metolachlor in natural and synthetic sediments with *Echinochloa crusgalli crusgalli* and 2.5 mg/kg in synthetic and 7.5 mg/kg in natural sediments with *S. alterniflora*. *E. crusgalli crusgalli* was tested using freshwater and *S. alterniflora*, using 4‰ diluted seawater that contained the herbicide. These concentrations are slightly higher than those reported with *S. olneyi* in our studies. However, toxicity was reported as a significant change in measured plant responses as compared to controls in our studies rather than survival, and length of exposure in our studies was 16 days vs 4 weeks.

POD is a non-specific measurement of plant stress. Plant peroxidases are ubiquitous in the plant kingdom and catalyze the oxidation of a large number of, as well as diverse classes of, endogenous and exogenous substrates (Higashi 1988). Peroxidases have a variety of functions in plant tissue, some of which include oxidation of exogenous compounds that enter the plant cell, regulation of dormancy and bud break and regulation of plant development (Del Grosso et al. 1987; Higashi 1988; Wang et al. 1991). Stress induced changes in peroxidase activity have been reported for plants that have been injured by fungi (Johnson and Cunningham 1972; Kawashima and Uritana 1963), ozone-induced necrosis (Patton and Garraway 1986) and air pollutants (Markkola et al. 1990). Byl and Klaine (1991) investigated the use of POD as an indicator of sublethal stress in *Hydrilla verticillata*, a rooted aquatic vascular plant, and concluded that POD was a good indicator of chemical stress due to exposure to sublethal concentrations of copper and sulfometuron methyl, a sulfonylurea herbicide. In our studies POD activation was an effective and sensitive measurement of an induced stress response by *S. olneyi* with exposure to atrazine and metolachlor under freshwater or low salinity test conditions. However, POD would not be effective as a biomarker if used under a wide range of salinity regimes.

In plants, increased production of oxygen free radicals and the accumulation of lipid peroxidation products have been associated with a variety of types of environmental stress (Barclay and McKersie 1994). It has been suggested that pesticides are oxidized in plants by plant peroxidases (Lamoureux and Frear 1979; Stiborova and Anzenbacher 1991). The most commonly used method to monitor oxidation of lipids is the thiobarbituric acid (TBA) assay. This method measures the relative degree of lipid oxidation since TBA reacts with many lipid peroxidation products (Tamura and Shibamoto 1991). Use of this assay in Test 1 was effective. However, even though this measurement was significant with each increasing exposure concentration and variability (standard error) was very small, the absolute differences in the response were also very small. Further testing under a broader range of conditions is needed before assessment for use as a biomarker under field conditions.

Chlorophyll responses as a biomarker were very effective in assessing toxicity of atrazine, but yielded confounding results in assessing toxicity to metolachlor. As a biomarker, chlorophylls are most effective when the mode of action of the herbicide directly affects photosynthesis, particularly when measuring acute responses following a short exposure duration.

Surprisingly, when tested under low salinity or freshwater regimes, growth responses were as effective in assessing toxicity of atrazine and metolachlor to *S. olneyi* as were the biochemical responses. However, because nutrients can become available to plants under certain field conditions such as effluents released from chemical and sewage treatment plants (Walsh et al. 1991b), and because exposure to very low concentrations of certain pesticides can act to stimulate growth (Lytle and Lytle, manuscript in preparation), growth responses cannot always be used to assess exposure to very low concentrations of pesticides.

Acknowledgments--We acknowledge the help provided by J. D. Caldwell in culturing plants and maintaining greenhouse conditions; we thank E. Otvos for providing grain size analysis and to Lea Sharp and Hong Cui for laboratory technical assistance. This work was supported by U.S. Environmental Protection Agency grant No. CR820666-01-3.

REFERENCES

Barclay, K. D., and McKersie, B. D., 1994, "Peroxidation Reactions in Plant Membranes: Effects of Free Fatty Acids," Lipids, Vol. 29, No. 12, pp. 877-882

Boger, P., and Sandmann, G., 1990, In Chemistry of Plant Protection, Vol. 6, W.S. Bowers, W. Ebing, D. Martin, and R. Wegler, Eds., Springer-Verlag, Berlin, p. 173

Byl, T. D., and Klaine, S. J., 1991, "Peroxidase Activity as an Indicator of Sublethal Stress in the Aquatic Plant *Hydrilla verticillata* (Royle)," Plants for Toxicity Assessment: Second Volume, ASTM STP 1115, J.W. Gorsuch, W.R. Lower, W. Wang, and M.A. Lewis, Eds., American Society for Testing and Materials, Philadelphia, pp. 101-106

Correll, D. L., and Wu, T. L., 1982, "Atrazine Toxicity to Submersed Vascular Plants in Simulated Estuarine Microcosms," Aquatic Botany, Vol, 14, pp. 151-158

Cunningham, J. J., Kemp, W. M., Lewis, M. R., and Stevenson, J. C., 1984, "Temporal Responses of the Macrophytes, *Potamogeton perfoliatus* L.,and its associated Autotrophic Community to Atrazine Exposure in Estuarine Microcosms," Estuaries, Vol. 7, pp. 519-530

Del Grosso, E., Grazia, S., and Maraldi, A. C., 1987, "Peroxidase Activity in *Phaseolus vulgaris* Seedling Tissues and Callus Cultures: A Comparison of Genotypes and Developmental Stages," Environmental and Experimental Botany, Vol. 27, No. 4, pp. 387-394

Gerber, H. R., Muller, G, and Ebner, L., 1974, "CGA-24705. A New Grasskiller Herbicide," Proceedings of 12th British Weed Control Conference, Vol 3, pp. 787-794

Higashi, K., 1988, "Metabolic Activation of Environmental Chemicals by Microsomal Enzymes of Higher Plants," Mutation Research, Vol. 197, pp. 273-288

Huber, W., 1993, "Ecotoxicological Relevance of Atrazine in Aquatic Systems," Environmental Toxicology and Chemistry, Vol. 12, pp. 1865-1881

Jaworski, E.G., 1975, In Herbicides: Chemistry, Degradation and Mode of Action, P. C. Kearney and D. D. Kaufman, Eds., Dekker, New York, pp. 349-376

Johnson, L. B., and Cunningham, B. A., 1972, "Peroxidase Activity in Healthy and Leaf-rust Infected Wheat Leaves," Phytochemistry, Vol. 11, pp. 547-551

Kawashima N., and Uritana, I., 1963, "Occurrence of Peroxidases in Sweet Potato Infected by the Black Rot Fungus," Agricultural and Biological Chemistry, Vol. 27, pp. 409-417

Kemp, W. M., Boynton, W. R., Cunningham, J. J., Stevenson, J. C., Jones, T. W., and Means, J. C., 1985, "Effects of Atrazine and Linuron on Photosynthesis and Growth of the Macrophytes, *Potamogeton perfoliatus* L. and *Myriophyllum spicatum* L., in an Estuarine Environment," Marine Environmental Research, Vol. 16, pp. 255-280

Lamoureux, G. L., and Frear, D. S., 1979, "Pesticide Metabolism in Higher Plants: In Vitro Enzyme Studies," In Drug Metabolism, D. V. Parke and R. L. Smith, Eds., Taylor and Francis, London, pp. 191-217

Maehly, A. C., and Chance, B., 1954, In Methods of Biochemical Analysis, Vol. 1, D. Glick, Ed., Interscience, New York, p. 357

Manugistics, Inc., 1994, Statgraphics Plus 1994 Version 7.1, 2115 East Jefferson St., Rockville, MD

Markkola, A. M., Ohtonen, R., and Tarvainen, R., 1990, "Peroxidase Activity as an Indicator of Pollution Stress in the Fine Roots of *Pinus sylvestris*," Water, Air, and Soil Pollution, Vol. 52, pp. 149-156

Moreland, D. E., 1980, "Mechanisms of Action of Herbicides," Annual Review of Plant Physiology, Vol. 31, pp. 597-638

Patton, R. L., and Garraway, M. O., 1986, "Ozone-induced Necrosis and Increased Peroxidase Activity in Hybrid Poplar (*Populus* sp.) Leaves," Environmental and Experimental Botany, Vol. 25, No. 2, pp. 137-141

Stiborova, M. And Anzenbacher, P., 1991, "What are the Principal Enzymes Oxidizing the Xenobiotics in Plants: Cytochromes P-450 or Peroxidases? (A Hypothesis)," General Physiology and Biophysics, Vol. 10, pp. 209-216

Strickland, J. D. H., and Parsons, T. R., 1968, A Practical Handbook of Seawater Analysis, Fisheries Research Board of Canada, Ottawa, pp. 185-192

Tamura, H., and Shibamoto, T., 1991, "Antioxidative Activity Measurement in Lipid Peroxidation Systems with Malonaldehyde and 4-Hydroxy Nonenal," Journal of American Oil Chemists Society, Vol. 68, No. 12, pp. 941-943

Utley, H. G., Bernheim, F., and Hochstein, P., 1967, "Effect of Sulfhydryl Reagents on Peroxidation in Microsomes," Archives of Biochemistry and Biophysics, Vol. 118, pp. 29-32

Walsh, G. E., Weber, D. E., Simon, T. L., Brashers, L. K., and Moore, J. C., 1991a, "Use of Marsh Plants for Toxicity Testing of Water and Sediment," Plants for Toxicity Assessment: Second Volume, ASTM STP 1115, J. W. Gorsuch, W. R. Lower, W. Wang and M. A. Lewis, Eds., American Society for Testing and Materials, Philadelphia, pp. 341-354

Walsh, G. E., Weber, D. E., Simon, T. L., and Brashers, L. K., 1991b. "Toxicity Tests of Effluents with Marsh Plants in Water and Sediment," Environmental Toxicology and Chemistry, Vol. 10, pp. 517-525

Wang, S. Y., Jiao, H. J., and Faust, M., 1991, "Changes in the Activities of Catalase, Peroxidase, and Polyphenol Oxidase in Apple Buds During Bud Break Induced in Thidiazuron," Journal of Plant Growth Regulation, Vol. 10, pp. 33-39

Woodhouse, W. W. Jr., Seneca, E. D., and Broome, S. W., 1974, "Propagation of *Spartina alterniflora* for Substrate Stabilization and Salt Marsh Development," Technical Memorandum No. 46, U.S. Army, Corps of Engineers, Coastal Engineering Research Center, Fort Belvoir, VA. pp. 50-59

Meg R. Pinza[1], Nancy P. Kohn,[1] Stacy L. Ohlrogge,[1] Camari J. Ferguson,[1] and Jack Q. Word[1]

REDUCING THE EFFECTS OF TOTAL AMMONIA IN 10-DAY SEDIMENT TOXICITY TESTS WITH THE AMPHIPOD, *RHEPOXYNIUS ABRONIUS*

REFERENCE: Pinza, M. R., Kohn, N. P., Ohlrogge, S. L., Ferguson, C. J., and Word, J. Q., "Reducing the Effects of Total Ammonia in 10-Day Sediment Toxicity Tests with the Amphipod, *Rhepoxynius abronius*," *Environmental Toxicology and Risk Assessment: Biomarkers and Risk Assessment—Fifth Volume, ASTM STP 1306,* David A. Bengtson and Diane S. Henshel, Eds., American Society for Testing and Materials, 1996.

ABSTRACT: Sediment toxicity tests are used to measure the effects of contaminants in sediment and are important management tools for agencies that regulate dredging and dredged material disposal, wastewater discharges, and other activities that might affect the aquatic environment. The interpretation of the results of routine toxicity tests can, however, be confounded by naturally occurring factors, such as ammonia, sulfides, sediment grain size, and salinity. Ammonia has been suspected for many years to be a sediment toxicant. It is only recently that the sensitivity of routine test organisms to ammonia has been quantified, and even more recently that dose-responses have been related to ammonia concentrations that occur in standard sediment toxicity tests. The first objective of this study was to compare the effects of ammonia in sediment toxicity tests under two pore water ammonia reduction procedures. The first procedure reduced total pore water ammonia from test sediments by replacing overlying water two times in a 24-h period. The second procedure used natural bacterial processes to reduce pore water ammonia. The second objective was to evaluate the current no-effect concentrations (originally based on 96-h water-only toxicity tests) using the overlying-water-exchange procedure. The final objective was to determine whether ammonia concentrations would increase to toxic levels in sediments that had naturally reached no-effect concentrations, but that were then physically disturbed. The marine amphipod, *Rhepoxynius abronius,* was exposed to sediments with low (≈ 30 mg/L), moderate (≈ 100 mg/L), and high (≈ 200 mg/L) initial concentrations of pore water total ammonia in five separate 10-day toxicity tests. One test followed standard protocols (ASTM E 1367-90). Two tests were initiated after pore water ammonia concentrations were reduced by overlying water exchange to ≤ 30 mg/L and ≤ 20 mg/L. Two tests were initiated after pore water total ammonia decreased by natural reduction to <10 mg/L; half of the test chambers from the final test were disturbed by shaking before test organisms were placed in the test containers. Toxicity of sediments with higher initial concentrations of pore water ammonia decreased significantly when ammonia was reduced to ≤ 30 mg/L. Reaching 30 mg/L required up to 12 days with the reduction procedure (24 exchanges of overlying water) or up to 47 days under the natural-reduction procedure. There was no difference in toxicity between the naturally reduced and the disturbed samples.

KEYWORDS: pore water ammonia, toxicity, *R. abronius*, reduction, bioavailability

[1]Research scientist, research scientist, intern student, intern student, and group leader, respectively, for the Marine Ecological Processes Group, Battelle/Marine Sciences Laboratory, 1529 West Sequim Bay Road, Sequim, WA 98382.

INTRODUCTION

Sediment toxicity tests using sensitive indicator species such as the marine amphipod, *Rhepoxynius abronius*, provide a rapid and direct measure of the effects resulting from sediment contaminants. The results of these tests are used as a management tool by agencies that regulate dredging and dredged material disposal, sewage and wastewater discharges, and other activities that might affect the aquatic environment, and they are used to make decisions affecting sediment remediation and disposal. One problem with toxicity tests is that naturally occurring factors, such as grain size, salinity, and ammonia, may confound test interpretation by increasing the laboratory toxicity of sediments that might otherwise be considered nontoxic. This paper examines the effects of total ammonia measured in the pore water of sediments that are used in 10-day tests with *R. abronius*. Current guidance states that if ammonia is not a chemical of concern at the disposal site, ammonia levels should be reduced to a point where there are no species-specific effects before benthic organisms are tested (EPA-USACE 1994).

Although ammonia has been suspected for years to be a sediment toxicant, only recently has the sensitivity of various species of test organisms to ammonia been quantified. Ammonia is present in aquatic systems as total ammonia, which includes both NH_3 and NH_4^+. The most toxic form to most aquatic organisms is believed to be unionized ammonia, NH_3 (EPA 1989); however, this conclusion has been questioned (Spotte 1992). The percentage of NH_3's contribution to total ammonia is generally small (<10%), is not directly measurable, and is determined based upon a relationship with pH, salinity, and temperature of a given test system. The factors that increase the percentage of NH_3 in aquatic systems are higher pH values, higher temperatures, and lower salinities, which may result in an increase in the toxicity of a specific concentration of total ammonia (Bower and Bidwell 1978; Creswell 1993). In the following tests, both salinity and temperature were controlled within very small ranges (±2‰ or 2°C), whereas pH varied based upon the individual sediment or water characteristics (8.0±0.4 units). Therefore, for these tests, the predicted variation in the amount of NH_3 or unionized ammonia relative to the total measured ammonia is ≤5.3 % (Trussel 1972).

Previous experiments conducted at Battelle/Marine Sciences Laboratory (MSL) have shown that high concentrations of total ammonia are often encountered in core samples collected for dredged material evaluations. Total ammonia may be present at levels of toxicological importance in marine sediments, especially at depths that are below the surface sediments. This is particularly true of new work dredging projects that evaluate sediments that have been buried since pre- and interglacial periods, when man had virtually no environmental impact (Pinza et al. 1995). Total ammonia may be an issue when cores are collected from depths that are below the influence of benthic microflora and microfauna. In the uppermost layers of marine and freshwater sediments, ammonia is converted to nitrite and nitrate through bacterial processes (Barnes 1957; Riley and Chester 1971). When field samples are retrieved from depths below the influence of nitrifying bacteria, ammonia may be present at concentrations that influence toxicity test results. As an example, the MSL has collected core samples on both the east and west coast with core lengths ranging from 5 ft to greater than 20 ft. The pore water ammonia concentrations in these cores ranged from approximately 50 mg/L to greater than 200 mg/L of total ammonia.

The currently accepted no-effect concentration (based on 96-h water-only tests) for *R. abronius* is ≤30 mg/L of total ammonia (EPA 1994). As a result of the short exposure period upon which the no-effects level is based, the ≤30 mg/L of total ammonia value may be inappropriate for the 10-day sediment exposures. Although water-only exposures could be extended to 10-day periods to accommodate this issue, these tests would probably fail because the sediment-dwelling amphipod would not derive sufficient nourishment nor behave normally in the absence of sediment. Additional issues that need to be considered when accounting for ammonia toxicity include 1) the potential for removal of the water-soluble fractions of the contaminants of concern during the ammonia purging procedure, 2) the additional cost of performing the ammonia removal techniques during routine sediment evaluations, and 3) the adequacy of test conditions to represent the scenario under evaluation (i.e., in situ conditions or conditions that occur after the sediment has been collected and processed for testing).

The issue of the bioavailability of pore water total ammonia is relevant to toxicity testing of manipulated sediments. To address the bioavailability of pore water ammonia, two experiments were performed: a natural ammonia-reduction test and a disturbance test. The former was designed to represent marine surface sediments that were available to interact with organic materials, ammonia, and the bacterially controlled nitrogen cycle. The latter was designed to represent the same sediments, which were then disrupted to determine whether ammonia might again be released from the sediment by vigorous shaking. The results from these two tests were used to answer the following question: If ammonia is sequestered in sediments that have not been manipulated, does it become bioavailable after disturbance and affect test organism survival?

The experiments conducted during this study were designed to accomplish the following:

- Determine the time required to reduce concentrations of ammonia using two methods: 1) reduce ammonia from the system using two exchanges of overlying water per day (EPA 1994); and 2) allow ammonia to decrease naturally over time under static conditions.
- Compare the current no-effect concentration of pore water ammonia in 96-h water-only tests with pore water ammonia concentrations from 10-day sediment tests.
- Examine the bioavailability of ammonia under conditions where ammonia has naturally decreased to levels below the current no-effect concentration followed by disturbance of these same sediments.
- Compare sediment pore water total ammonia concentrations in 10-day sediment tests with a 96-h water-only dose-response curve.

METHODS

The marine amphipod, *R. abronius*, was exposed to three test sediments selected to represent low, medium, and high levels of pore water ammonia (Sediments 1, 2, and 3, respectively). A "native" control sediment (Sediment 4) and reference toxicant, cadmium chloride, were also tested to verify the health and response of the test organisms (EPA/USACE 1991). To address the objectives, the following 10-day sediment toxicity tests were conducted:

- Experiment 1--standard test with no ammonia-reduction protocols.
- Experiment 2--pore water ammonia concentrations reduced to ≤ 30 mg/L by two exchanges of overlying water per day.
- Experiment 3--pore water ammonia concentrations reduced to ≤ 20 mg/L by two exchanges of overlying water per day.
- Experiment 4--pore water ammonia concentrations reduced to ≤ 20 mg/L by natural bacterial activity.
- Experiment 5---pore water ammonia concentrations reduced to ≤ 20 mg/L by natural bacterial activity, followed by disturbance (shaking) of the sediment.

All of the 10-day tests followed ASTM E 1367-90 and were conducted under static conditions. Any modifications to ASTM E 1367-90 are described below.

R. abronius were collected by the MSL off West Beach, Whidbey Island, using the specially designed anchor dredge deployed from a 17-ft Boston Whaler. Sediment brought up with the dredge was sieved through a 2-mm mesh screen to remove large debris and predatory species. During sampling, the amphipods were kept in coolers partially filled with their native sediment and seawater until delivery to a holding tank at the MSL. The amphipods were kept in a large holding tank containing their native sediment with flowing 15°C seawater. Organisms were not fed during the holding period, which was less than 2 weeks before test initiation. Three different collections of wild-captured *R. abronius* populations were necessary to meet animal holding times for all of the tests. Collection 1 was for the standard 10-day test with no ammonia manipulation, Collection 2 was for the ammonia reduction tests to ≤30 mg/L and ≤20 mg/L, and Collection 3 was for the natural-reduction test and the disturbance test. In order to compare the results of the five different experiments using different populations of *R. abronius*, reference toxicant test with cadmium or ammonia was conducted as an indication of the relative health and sensitivity of each test population. Comparable sensitivity was assumed when the LC_{50} values were within our laboratory's normal control chart limits for that toxicant. The reference toxicant tests were conducted in the same manner as the 10-day solid-phase test. *R. abronius* were exposed to a seawater control plus four concentrations of cadmium chloride (0.38, 0.75, 1.5 and 3.0 mg/L as cadmium [Cd]). There were three replicates of each concentration.

The *R. abronius* test was conducted in 1-L glass jars placed in random positions on a water table maintained at 15°C. The test design included five replicates of each treatment plus two additional replicates for the measurement of pore water ammonia. Prior to test initiation, test sediment was added to the jars to a depth of 2 cm, and then 0.44-μm-filtered seawater was added to a volume of 750 mL. The jars were aerated and placed on the water table overnight to stabilize temperature to test conditions. After settling, initial water quality parameters were measured in each container.

The amphipods were gently sieved from the holding tank into clean seawater and counted into small transfer containers. The number of organisms was then confirmed by a second observer before the amphipods were transferred into the test container. Testing began by adding 20 *R. abronius* to each test container. *R. abronius* were observed daily during the test, and the number of organisms floating on the surface, swimming in the jar, or resting on the sediment surface was recorded on observation forms. Amphipods that were floating on the surface were gently pushed below the water surface with a pipette tip and observed as they either buried or did not rebury into the sediment.

Water temperature, salinity, pH, and dissolved oxygen (DO) were measured daily in one replicate of each sediment treatment, and in all containers at initiation and termination of the bioassay. Acceptable ranges for water quality parameters during the experiment were as follows:

DO	≥6.0 mg/L
pH	7.60 to 8.40
Salinity	30 ±2.0‰
Temperature	15.0°C ±2.0°C
Ammonia (pore water)	test-dependent, either ≤30 mg/L or ≤20 mg/L.

At the end of the test (Day 10), the contents of each jar were sieved through a 0.5-mm Nytex screen to collect the *R. abronius*. The number of live and dead organisms was counted, and organisms were examined under a dissecting microscope. The presence or absence of body parts recovered at the end of the test was also noted. If an individual organism did not respond to gentle probing, it was considered dead. At least 10% of the mortality counts were confirmed by a second observer.

Total ammonia in the overlying water and the pore water was measured using a Fisher Scientific Accumet 1003 meter and ammonia-ion-selective electrode. To measure pore water total ammonia in solid-phase tests, "surrogate" jars were filled with approximately 200 mL of wet sediment and 600 mL of seawater and then placed on the water table with the actual testing chambers. Test organisms were not added to the surrogate jars. Surrogate containers were used to measure the interstitial pore water ammonia of the sediment treatments prior to initiation of the organisms (Day O) and on the termination day (Day 10). Ammonia in the overlying water was measured on Days 0, 1, 3, 7, and 10. To extract pore water ammonia, the overlying water was siphoned from the test containers and the sediment was removed and placed in 500-mL Teflon containers. The pore water for measuring ammonia was obtained by low-speed centrifugation at 1750 rpm for 10 min, at a relative centrifugal force of approximately 1000 gravity.

The procedures for reducing pore water total ammonia concentrations to ≤30 mg/L or ≤20 mg/L followed interim guidelines established by a U.S. Environmental Protection Agency memorandum.[2] This memorandum suggested exchanging the overlying water in each test container twice a day until pore water ammonia concentrations were below the desired levels. To accomplish this, the overlying water was siphoned to approximately 1 cm above the sediment and replaced with filtered seawater that was maintained at 15°C. Once the desired pore water total ammonia concentrations were reached in all test containers, the test was initiated by placing 20 organisms into each container.

The procedure for the natural reduction of total ammonia over time involved placing test sediment into each test chamber, filling the chambers to the correct test volume with filtered seawater (no test organisms), placing the chambers on a water table, and maintaining them at test conditions. For both experiments, test containers were maintained at test conditions for 47 days; at that time the total pore water ammonia concentration was <10 mg/L in all test containers. The ammonia levels were periodically monitored to chart the reduction of ammonia over time. Once the desired ammonia levels were reached in all test containers, R. abronius were added to each test chamber, and the test was continued for 10 days. The natural reduction of ammonia over time followed by a disturbance test was carried out as described above, except that after pore water ammonia concentrations were reduced to <10 mg/L, each test chamber was vigorously shaken and allowed to settle for 24 h. The shaking was done to simulate maximum disturbance, such as a vigorous mixing by large infaunal organisms, or a dredging operation in which sediment is removed from one location and then disposed through the water column at another location. After the sediments had settled, test organisms were added to each container, and the test was continued for 10 days following ASTM E 1367-90.

It is important to note that all of the sediments were added to the test containers at the same time and that these containers were placed randomly on the water table and maintained at test conditions. There were different starting times for each experiment: each test was begun by the addition of test organisms when the appropriate, measured concentration of total pore water ammonia was attained in all containers for that particular experiment. For example, Experiment 2 was started only after all test containers were below the target value, ≤30 mg/L. This means that although they were variable, the pore water total ammonia concentrations were all ≤30 mg/L at test initiation.

The test sediments for these experiments were collected from several locations. Sediment 1 came from San Francisco Bay and represented the low ammonia sediment; Sediments 2 and 3 came from New York Harbor and were the medium and high ammonia sediments. Sediments 1 through 3 are representative of actual dredged materials from these waterways. Sediment 4 came from Whidbey Island, Washington, and was the native control sediment for R. abronius. This sediment is normally collected at the same time as the test organisms and has been demonstrated to provide excellent survival of R. abronius in tests conducted over the past decade at our laboratory.

Sediment grain size and total organic carbon (TOC), which is the amount of nonvolatile, partially volatile, volatile, and particulate organic carbon compounds in a sample, were measured for each sediment. Grain-size analysis was conducted by Soil Technology, Inc., of Bainbridge Island, Washington. Four grain-size fractions were

---

[2]Davies, T. T., Davis D. G., and Elmore J. P., unpublished memorandum to U.S. Environmental Protection Agency Regional Ocean Dumping Coordinators, Regional Wetlands Coordinators, and the U.S. Army Corps of Engineers, December 1993.

determined by a combination of sieve and pipette techniques (PSEP 1986). These methods are consistent with ASTM D217-85 and ASTM D422-72 (with the substitution of a No. 100 sieve for a No. 140 sieve). Analysis of TOC was performed by Global Geochemistry in Canoga Park, California. Each sediment treatment was dried and ball-milled to a fine powder. Before combustion, inorganic carbon in the sample was removed by acidification. The TOC in sediment was then determined by measuring the quantity of carbon dioxide released during combustion of the sample and reporting the release as percentage of dry weight (EPA 1986).

The percentage-survival results for each test sediment were compared across all five test designs using the Bonferroni/Dunn's multiple comparison method with an experimental-wise error rate of $\propto = 0.05$. This procedure makes all possible pairwise comparisons among a group of means. This method will detect as many differences in means as Fisher's Least Significant Difference approach but will detect more differences than the Tukey's Honestly Significant Difference method (Chew 1977).

RESULTS

Grain size, TOC, and initial total pore water ammonia concentrations for each sediment (measured prior to the start of the experiments) are presented in Table 1. The grain-size distribution indicates that Sediment 4 was predominantly sand, in contrast to the three test sediments, which were predominantly silty-clay.

TABLE 1--Summary of physical parameters.

Sediment Treatment	Grain-Size Distribution % Dry Weight				Total Organic Carbon (%)	Pore water Ammonia (mg/L)
	Gravel	Sand	Silt	Clay		
Sediment 1	8	14	45	33	0.85	29.4
Sediment 2	3	21	45	32	2.99	110
Sediment 3	2	9	54	36	2.71	200
Sediment 4	0	99	0	1	0.06	NM[a]

(a) Not measured; technician was unable to retrieve enough pore water to measure total ammonia. Previous experiments conducted at the MSL using this sediment indicated a mean total pore water ammonia concentration of 2 mg/L.

Both ammonia-reduction methods were effective for reducing total pore water ammonia concentrations. The method of two exchanges per day required between 2 and 12 days to reach ≤ 30 mg/L in the pore water, whereas the natural reduction test took between 16 and 40 days. As expected, the time needed for ammonia reduction was dependent on the amount of ammonia present in the sediments at the start of the test (Table 2; Figs. 1 and 2). At the time of these experiments, the current no-effect concentration of total ammonia (96-h water-only) for R. abronius was ≤ 30 mg/L. This value is shown in Figures 1 and 2 to provide a basis for comparison.

Survival of R. abronius exposed to each test sediment was compared using the standard 10-day test, the ammonia-reduction tests to ≤ 30 mg/L and ≤ 20 mg/L, and the natural ammonia-reduction test (Fig. 3). The most significant changes in R. abronius survival occurred with exposure to Sediments 2 and 3. The survival in Sediments 2 and 3

TABLE 2--The time (in days) to reduce the pore water ammonia concentration to
‹30 mg/L by a twice daily exchange of overlying water and by natural processes.

Sediment Treatment	Number of Days to reach ≤30 mg/L	
	Two Exchanges of Overlying Water/Day	Natural Reduction
Sediment 1	?	16
Sediment 2	9	34
Sediment 3	12	40
Sediment 4	0	0[a]

(a) The cause of the higher concentrations of total pore water ammonia between Days 20
and 40 is unknown.

for the standard 10-day test without reduction of pore water ammonia concentrations was
13% and 1%, respectively (Fig. 3). When total pore water ammonia was reduced to
≤30 mg/L prior to introduction of test organisms, the survival increased to 85% or greater
in both sediments, and when total pore water ammonia was reduced to ≤20 mg/L, survival
exceeded 90% for both sediments. This suggests that pore water ammonia concentrations
of >20 mg/L could have contributed to the effects observed for R. abronius exposed to
these sediments.

Sediments 1 and 4 did not show a statistically significant decrease in percentage of
survival in any of the tests. Survival of R. abronius exposed to Sediment 1 ranged from
65% to 70% throughout all experiments, suggesting that the toxicity of this sediment is
not attributable to ammonia. Survival of R. abronius exposed to Sediment 4 did not
change throughout all experiments, ranging from 95% to 98%. This sediment is the native
control sediment and is essentially free of contaminants, with typical total pore water
ammonia concentrations of ≤2 mg/L. During the course of these experiments, the total
pore water ammonia concentrations in the native control were <10 mg/L for the first 20
days. Between Days 20 and 40, the pore water ammonia concentration increased to >30
mg/L and gradually decreased to 2.7 mg/L by Day 47. The cause of the observed increase
in ammonia is unknown, but the increase demonstrates the need to measure pore water
ammonia concentrations during testing.

The survival of R. abronius did increase slightly, but not significantly in Sediments
1 through 3 when pore water ammonia concentrations were reduced to ≤20 mg/L.
Survival of R. abronius in Sediments 2 and 3 increased significantly in tests using two
exchanges of overlying water versus the standard test with no ammonia reduction. This
reduction in toxicity occurred in sediments with a relatively high silt and clay content
(78%-90%) and would be expected to have reduced survival because of the fine grain size
(DeWitt et al. 1988). Survival increased when the concentrations of pore water ammonia
or other covarying contaminants were reduced, regardless of grain size.

Survival of R. abronius in the natural reduction test was not significantly different
from that in tests in which ammonia was reduced to ≤20 mg/L using two exchanges of
overlying water per day. In the disturbance test, after a period of 47 days in which the
sediments were maintained under natural conditions, disturbance of the sediment by
shaking did not release ammonia at concentrations of toxicological importance during the
subsequent 10-day toxicity test (Table 3).

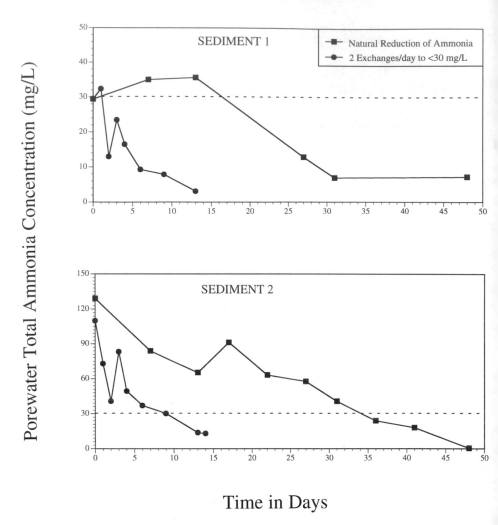

FIG. 1--Total pore water ammonia concentrations versus time during ammonia-reduction
phase for Sediments 1 and 2.

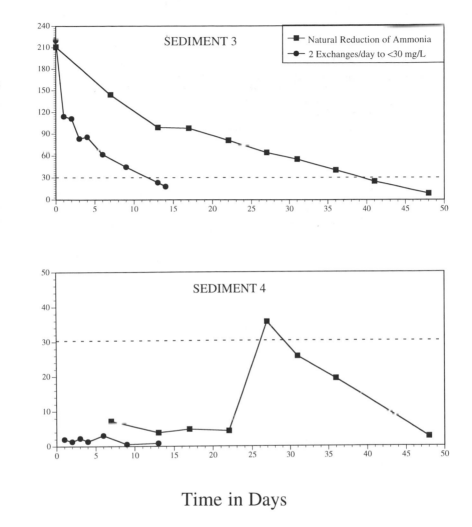

FIG. 2--Total pore water ammonia concentrations versus time during ammonia reduction
    phase for Sediments 3 and 4.

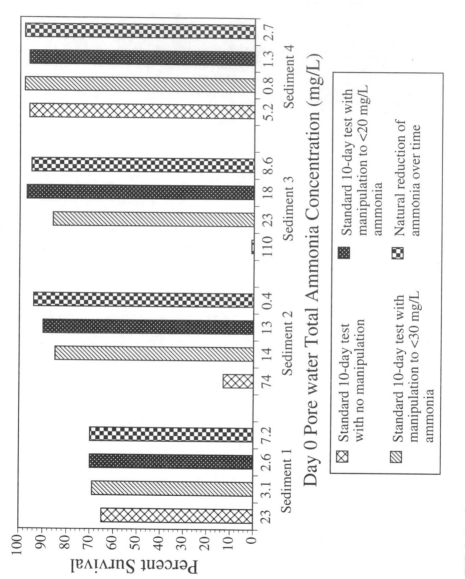

FIG. 3--*R. abronius* survival relative to total pore water ammonia concentrations in 10-day sediment toxicity tests.

TABLE 3--Results of the stability and disturbance tests.

Sediment Treatment	Initial Ammonia (mg/L)	Pore water Ammonia (mg/L)		Percent Survival
		Day 0	Day 10	
Natural Reduction Test				
Sediment 1	29.4	7.20	0.19	70
Sediment 2	110.0	0.36	0.51	94
Sediment 3	200.0	8.60	2.30	95
Sediment 4	NM[a]	2.70	NM	98
Disturbance Test				
Sediment 1	29.4	1.30	0.93	65
Sediment 2	110.0	0.89	0.71	94
Sediment 3	200.0	0.79	1.50	91
Sediment 4	NM	0.44	NM	97

(a)   Not measured; technician was unable to retrieve enough pore water to measure total ammonia. Previous experiments conducted at the MSL using this sediment indicated a mean total pore water ammonia concentration of 2 mg/L.

There was also no statistically significant difference in survival between the natural reduction and the disturbance test. After the sediments were disturbed, the pore water ammonia concentrations were slightly lower, whereas the overlying water concentrations were slightly higher than those in the nondisturbed-sediment tests. Ammonia concentrations did not return to the levels observed when the sediments were collected in the field, probably because the natural microbial populations that were established in the test containers were able to respond to the concentrations of total ammonia.

Table 4 presents a statistical comparison of the ammonia-reduction and disturbance experiments compared for each sediment treatment using the Bonferroni/Dunn method. The actual ammonia concentrations for each of the five ammonia-reduction tests are shown in Table 5. Concentrations in some of the test sediments were much lower than the target levels of ≤ 30 mg/L or ≤ 20 mg/L, because all of the test treatments were required to be below the specified concentrations prior to testing. For example, in Experiment 2, which employed overlying water exchange, it took the longest time to reduce ammonia concentration in Sediment 3 to ≤ 30 mg/L, and during the same time period, the concentrations in the other sediments were reduced to well below that level.

Three separate collections of R. abronius were used in these experiments. Reference toxicant tests were conducted with each new collection of amphipods to measure the health and relative sensitivity of each batch. The LC_{50}s for each of the three reference toxicant tests were 0.99 mgCd/L, 1.2 mgCd/L and 1.6 mgCd/L, respectively. The cadmium reference toxicant control chart from the MSL has a currently acceptable range of Cd sensitivity of 0.56 mgCd/L to 1.3 mgCd/L. The calculated LC_{50} for Collection 3 is above the control chart range and may indicate that the population of amphipods used for the stability and disturbance test was slightly less sensitive to Cd and possibly to other contaminants than typical test populations.

TABLE 4--Statistical summary of R. abronius survival in five experiments.

Sediment Treatment	Percent Survival[a]				
	Standard 10-day	≤30 mg/L	≤20 mg/L	Natural Reduction	Disturbance
Sediment 1	65	69	70	70	65
Sediment 2	13	85	90	94	94
Sediment 3	1	86	97	95	91
Sediment 4	96	98	96	98	97

(a) The underline indicates that the survival results were statistically different for this sediment compared with those of the same sediment tested under different conditions.

TABLE 5--Total pore water ammonia concentrations upon initiation of each experiment.

Sediment Treatment	Total pore water ammonia concentration in mg/L				
	Standard 10-day	≤30 mg/L	≤20 mg/L	Natural Reduction	Disturbance
Sediment 1	23	3.1	2.6	7.2	1.3
Sediment 2	74	14	13	0.36	0.89
Sediment 3	110	23	18	8.6	0.79
Sediment 4	5.2	0.84	1.3	2.7	0.44

One 96-h water-only dose-response test for ammonia was conducted at the same time as Experiment 1. The results from this experiment are shown on Figure 4 as points on a 96-h water-only dose-response curve generated from six separate ammonia 96-h tests (conducted independently of this study). The sensitivity of amphipods collected around the time of these experiments was comparable to the dose-response of ammonia established from the previous studies. This similar response enabled a comparison of survival data from four of the 10-day sediment tests to be plotted against the existing MSL dose-response curve for ammonia (Fig. 5). The results from this comparison showed that when the total pore water ammonia concentrations were >20 mg/L at test initiation for most of the test sediments, the survival observed in the 10-day tests was less than would be predicted from the 96-h water-only dose-response curve. Even when the total pore water ammonia concentration was reduced to ≤20 mg/L, survival of R. abronius exposed to Sediment 1 did not change significantly, as shown in the circled area in Figure 5. All of the points in this circle are for Sediment 1, and all the data points fall below the dose-response curve, showing that the reduction of ammonia did not change the toxicity of the sediment to R. abronius.

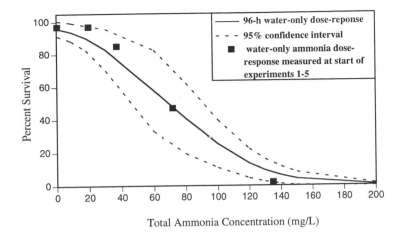

FIG. 4--Results of 96-h ammonia experiment conducted for these experiments compared with dose-response curve of *R. abronius* exposed to ammonia for 96 h.

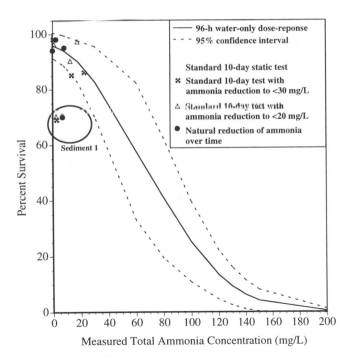

FIG. 5--Results of 10-day sediment toxicity tests compared with dose-response curve of *R. abronius* exposed to ammonia for 96 h.

DISCUSSION

It has been shown that ammonia-reduction procedures are effective and that they can reduce total pore water ammonia to below species-specific no-effects levels prior to testing; consequently, the interpretation of the results would not be driven by the amount of total ammonia present in the test sediments. This benefit may outweigh any additional expenses incurred to perform ammonia-reduction techniques. The experimental procedures that allow two exchanges of overlying water per day and those that make use of natural ammonia reduction were both effective at reducing the pore water ammonia concentrations and increasing test organism survival. *R. abronius* survival increased significantly for Sediments 2 and 3 using both reduction procedures, suggesting that ammonia was a major contributor to the toxicity of these sediments. The results of Experiment 4 also showed a slight improvement in amphipod survival over that in Experiment 2. The survival of *R. abronius* to Sediment 1 did not change significantly among the manipulation procedures, suggesting that ammonia was not the principal cause of toxicity in this sediment and that this toxicity was not diminished using either ammonia-reduction technique.

There are advantages and disadvantages to both ammonia-reduction methods. The advantage of overlying-water exchange is that it is much quicker than the natural-reduction method (14 to 28 days faster than the natural-reduction method). This would be desirable for sediments with stringent holding time requirements. The disadvantage is that there may be a potential of removing other contaminants from the test system during the flushing period. In contrast, the advantage to the natural ammonia-reduction method is that other potential contaminants are not physically removed. Future research needs to address whether the loss of contaminants by the overlying water exchange process is an issue. One disadvantage of the natural ammonia-reduction method is that the availability of contaminants may decrease while bacterial populations increase to levels that convert ammonia to nitrite and nitrate.

The 96-h water-only ammonia dose-response curve can be used as a screening tool for predicting whether pore water total ammonia will contribute to the toxicity of a particular test sediment. However, the toxicity of test sediment and total pore water ammonia over 10-day test periods is generally higher then would be predicted from the water-only, dose-response curve for the 96-h tests. There are several possible causes for the higher toxicity of total ammonia in the 10-day tests: the duration of testing is a factor, because the test organisms are exposed to ammonia over a longer period of time; sediment is not present in the 96-h water-only test to interact with total ammonia; and the test conditions, particularly pH, may tend to be slightly different between the two tests. However, in the experiments conducted at the MSL, the pH range is typically the same for both the 96-h water-only and the 10-day sediment test.

The implication of using the current no-effects concentration for ammonia is that it could be higher than that expected for a 10-day sediment toxicity test.

The conclusions from these experiments are as follows:

- Both the overlying-water-exchange and the natural-reduction method effectively reduced ammonia concentrations and increased *R. abronius* survival. The survival results using either method were comparable.

- The current no-effect concentration of ≤ 30 mg/L derived from 96-h water-only tests may be biased high for 10-day sediment tests, because it does not take into account the longer exposure period or physical and chemical interaction with the sediment. The reduction of total pore water ammonia to ≤ 20 mg/L seems to decrease the ammonia-related toxicity observed in Sediments 2 and 3 without compromising the responses (probably not related to ammonia) in Sediment 1.

- The pore water total ammonia concentrations did not become bioavailable during the disturbance test after periods of natural reduction.

- Standard 10-day sediment toxicity tests have established procedures for reducing pore water ammonia to below species-specific no-effect concentrations. These procedures should be used when total pore water ammonia concentrations are at or above levels that affect test species, so that regulators can make decisions about sediment remediation or disposal based on data that are not biased by pore water ammonia concentrations.

REFERENCES

Barnes, H., 1957, "Nutrient Elements," The Geological Society of America Memoir 67, Vol. 1, Ecology, National Sciences Academy, Washington, D.C., pp. 297-344.

Bower, C. E. and Bidwell, J. P., 1978, "Ionization of Ammonia in Seawater: Effects of Temperature, pH, and Salinity," Journal of Fish Research Board of Canada, Vol. 35, pp. 1012-1016.

Chew, V., 1977, Comparison Among Treatment Means in an Analysis of Variance, United States Department of Agriculture, Washington, D.C.

Creswell, R. L., 1993, Aquaculture Desk Reference, Van Nostrand Reinhold, New York.

DeWitt T. H., Ditsworth, G. R., and Swartz, R. C., 1988, "Effects of Natural Sediment Features on Survival of the Phoxcephalid Amphipod, *Rhepoxynius abronius*," Marine Environmental Research, Vol. 25, pp. 99-124.

(EPA) U.S. Environmental Protection Agency, 1986, Test Methods for Evaluating Solid Waste: Physical/Chemical Methods, EPA-955-001-00000, U.S. Environmental Protection Agency, Government Printing Office, Washington, D.C.

(EPA) U.S. Environmental Protection Agency, April 1989, Ambient Water Quality Criteria for Ammonia (Saltwater)-1989, EPA 440/5-88-004, Office of Water Regulations and Standards, Criteria and Standards Division, Washington, D.C.

(EPA) U.S. Environmental Protection Agency, June 1994, Methods for Assessing the Toxicity of Sediment-associated Contaminants with Estuarine and Marine Amphipods, EPA/600/R-94/025, Office of Research and Development, Washington, D.C.

(EPA-USACE) U.S. Environmental Protection Agency/U.S. Army Corps of Engineers, February 1991, Evaluation of Dredged Material Proposed for Ocean Disposal-Testing Manual, EPA-503/8-91/001, Office of Water, Washington, D.C.

(EPA-USACE) U. S. Environmental Protection Agency\U.S. Army Corps of Engineers, June 1994, Evaluation of Dredged Material Proposed for Discharge in Water on the U.S.-Testing Manual (Draft) Inland Testing Manual, EPA-823-B-94-002, Office of Water, Washington, D.C.

Pinza, M. R., Mayhew, H. L, and Word, J. Q., 1995, Evaluation of Older Bay Sediments from Richmond Harbor, California, Technical Report Prepared by Battelle/Marine Sciences Laboratory, Sequim, Washington.

(PSEP) Puget Sound Estuary Program, 1986, Recommended Protocols for Measuring Conventional Sediment Variables in Puget Sound, TC-3991-04, Tetra Tech, Inc., Bellevue Washington, pp. 23-27.

Riley, J. P. and Chester, R., 1971, "Micronutrient Elements," Introduction to Marine Chemistry, Chapter Seven, Academic Press, London and New York, pp. 152-181.

Spotte, S., 1992, Captive Seawater Fishes, Wiley Interscience Publication, New York.

Trussel, R. P., 1972, "Percent Un-Ionized Ammonia in Aqueous Ammonia Solutions at Different pH Levels and Temperatures," Journal of Fish Research Board of Canada, Vol. 29, pp. 1505-1507.

Dennis J. McCauley,[1] John E. Navarro,[1] and Trae A. Forgette[1]

A RAPID AND COST EFFECTIVE METHOD FOR FIELD/LABORATORY EXTRACTION OF
POREWATER FROM WHOLE LAKE SEDIMENT USING VACUUM EXTRACTION

REFERENCE: McCauley, D. J., Navarro, J. E., and Forgette, T. A., "A Rapid and Cost Effective
Method for Field/Laboratory Extraction of Porewater from Whole Lake Sediment Using
Vacuum Extraction," *Environmental Toxicology and Risk Assessment: Biomarkers and Risk
Assessment—Fifth Volume, ASTM STP 1306,* David A. Bengtson and Diane S. Henshel, Eds.,
American Society for Testing and Materials, 1996.

ABSTRACT: The use of an electric vacuum pump to extract porewater from
whole lake sediment was tested to determine if this method could be used
to collect a sample quickly and economically for determination of
sediment contamination. Multiple aquarium air stones (15 cm long) were
placed evenly throughout the sediment sample and attached to a vacuum
flask using aquarium tubing. An electric vacuum pump was used to create
a vacuum, which pulled sediment porewater from the sample into the
flask. In our investigation, sediment porewater was extracted at a rate
of 9.7 mL/min with minimal labor investment. Percent similarity of
duplicate chemical analyses ranged from 67 to 100% and percent
similarity of duplicate acute toxicity results was 96%. Increased
variability in both analytical and toxicological results was observed in
samples collected in close proximity and this variability increased as
sediment toxicity increased. Percent similarity of acute toxicity
results using porewater extracted by vacuum and centrifugation methods
were 84% for contaminated porewater and 100% for reference porewater.

KEYWORDS: porewater, sediment, toxicity, extraction

Because of the complicated physical nature of sediment, the
assessment of sediment toxicity is much more complicated than the
assessment of surface water or effluent toxicity. From a single matrix
(sediment) there are several sub-matrices used to determine sediment
toxicity, including testing of whole sediment, sediment elutriate and
sediment porewater using a wide variety of test organisms. Numerous
studies have compared different methodologies to determine their
effectiveness in determining sediment toxicity (Giesy et al. 1988, 1989,
1990; Hoke et al. 1990; Ross et al. 1992; Green et al. 1993; Harkey et
al. 1994). The use of resident benthic organism diversity as a stand
alone indicator or in conjunction with laboratory testing of sediment
toxicity has also been used (Malueg et al. 1984; Rosiu et al. 1989).

[1]Principal research scientist and environmental researchers,
respectively, Great Lakes Environmental Center, Inc., 739 Hastings,
Traverse City, Michigan 49686

The extraction of porewater from whole sediment is one of the more common procedures used to assess sediment quality (Hoke et al. 1990, 1993; Ankley et al. 1992; Ross et al. 1992; Luoma and Carter 1993). This method is one of the least complicated and most economical because it brings the testing into the familiar aquatic toxicity testing arena. Common methods of porewater extraction include centrifugation (Edmunds and Bath 1976; Carignan et al. 1985; Ankley et al. 1990; Saager et al. 1990), squeezing (Presley et al. 1967; Bender et al. 1987), pressure (Jahnke 1988), vacuum (Winger and Lasier 1991); and various types of *in-situ* porewater sampling methods (Sayles 1976; Carignan et al. 1985; Mitchell et al. 1989; Whitman 1989). However, many methods have been limited to laboratory use and often produce only small amounts of sediment porewater for analysis.

The objective of this study was to develop and evaluate an easy to use porewater extraction method that would allow us to collect large volumes of sediment porewater from sediment samples in the laboratory or in the field for chemical and toxicity analyses, while maintaining the precision and accuracy of each individual analysis. Through the use of an electric vacuum pump, we modified the conventional vacuum porewater extraction methods to allow us to extract larger volumes of porewater samples either *in-situ* from sediment sampling devices or in the laboratory from sediment collection containers. This method was evaluated to determine if the toxicity of extracted porewaters was comparable to the toxicity of porewater using a standard method. We also evaluated the comparability of replicate samples (samples collected in close proximity) to determine spatial variability and the effect of toxicity on this variability.

EXPERIMENTAL METHOD

Collection/Extraction

Sediment samples were collected from an inland lake in northwest Michigan from areas of intrusion by groundwater contaminated by both metals and organic constituents. Sediment was collected using an Eckman dredge (233 cm^2) and placed in washed polyurethane buckets (19 L). Lake water in the sampler was decanted before transfer to the sample container to reduce dilution of sediment porewater. Samples were placed on ice after collection and stored at 4°C until analysis. Time between collection and analysis was less than 14 days for toxicity tests and less than two days for analytical tests. The dredge was decontaminated between each sample site using both 10% nitric acid and 100% acetone to prevent cross contamination of samples.

Prior to extraction, sediment samples were homogenized in the sample buckets for ten minutes using an electric stirrer. Three aquarium grade air stones (15 cm long) were submersed in the sediment at equal distances and attached to a vacuum flask using aquarium tubing. Vacuum pressure (5-15 psi) was applied to the air stones and the porewater extracted into a glass flask until the desired volume of porewater was extracted. On average, it took approximately seven hours to extract the four liters necessary to conduct the toxicological and analytical tests. Because there was a breakthrough of finer sediment when extraction was first initiated, the first 100 mL of extracted porewater was discarded. During extraction, the air stones were periodically scraped to remove accumulated sediment and transferred to a different (i.e. wetter) location in the bucket. The extracted porewater was stored at 4°C until analysis and the maximum storage time between extraction and analysis was three days.

For centrifuged sediment, a 250 mL aliquot of sediment was first mixed by slow rotation for about an hour. Samples were then centrifuged for 20 minutes and the porewater was decanted into a sample container. Each 250 mL aliquot yielded about 60 mL of porewater.

hemical Analysis

Chemical analysis focused on priority pollutant metals and onventional parameters using standard EPA methods because of the uspected type of contamination. Chemical analyses were conducted on uplicate and replicate vacuum extracted sediment porewater to determine he precision of each analysis using the vacuum extraction method. No hemical analyses were used to compare differences between the vacuum xtraction and centrifugation methods. Chemical analyses for nine onventional parameters (BOD, COD, color, hardness, TDS, TOC, TSS, lkalinity, sulfate and chloride) and four metals (barium, iron, aqnesium and manganese) were performed on duplicate samples (samples ollected from the same location) to determine reproducibility. eplicate samples (samples collected in close proximity) were analyzed or the same conventional parameters and metals, along with three dditional metals (arsenic, potassium, and sodium) to determine spatial ariability. Duplicate samples were collected in the uncontaminated rea (control) of the lake and replicate samples were collected in both he control area and the area of suspected contamination. Samples for etals analysis were filtered (0.2 μm) prior to shipment.

oxicity Testing

Porewater samples were also used to conduct acute (48-h) and hronic (7 days) toxicity testing with *Ceriodaphnia dubia*. Acute and hronic *C. dubia* toxicity tests were conducted concurrently with uplicate samples collected using this vacuum extraction method. In ddition, acute toxicity tests were conducted on duplicate samples using wo different techniques, vacuum and centrifugation extraction, using orewaters extracted from contaminated lake sediment and from porewater xtracted from a reference sediment. Reference sediment was econstituted by adding DI water to a laboratory reference soil from outh central Michigan. The median lethal toxicant concentration (LC_{50}) as calculated from the acute toxicity tests. The no-observed-effect-oncentration (NOEC) and impairment concentration (IC_{25}) were calculated rom the chronic toxicity tests. The LC_{50}, NOEC, and IC_{25} values are all xpressed as percent porewater.

ESULTS

xtraction

The vacuum extraction method produced sufficient amounts of ediment porewater for chemical and toxicity analyses and was rapid, imple and economical. The average rate of extraction of porewater from he sediment was 9.7 mL/min and the sediment yielded about 25% porewater y volume. The lake sediment was relatively homogeneous throughout the tudy area and was composed of fine sand (37%), silt (37%) and clay 26%) in the control area and fine sand (34%), silt (47%) and clay (19%) n the area of contamination. The mean extraction rate (mL/min) and 95% onfidence interval for the control area sediment (N=8) and contaminated rea sediment (N=8) was 11.5±2 and 7.8±4, respectfully. The effect of ediment composition on the rate and amount of porewater extracted was ot evaluated, but the extraction rate will vary depending on sediment haracteristics such as particle grain size and percent moisture. The stimated rate of porewater extraction using centrifugation was about 3 L/min; this estimated rate includes the time needed to prepare the 250 L aliquot for centrifugation.

Chemical Analysis

Percent similarity of duplicate chemical analyses ranged from 67 to 100% (mean value of 88%) for conventional parameters and 90 to 99% (mean value of 95%) for metals; eleven of the 14 variables had a percent similarity equal to or greater than 90% (Table 1). Biological Oxygen Demand (BOD) had the lowest percent similarity of 67%, followed by chloride at 71% and color at 79%.

Chemical variability of replicate samples was higher than that of duplicate samples, and variability increased in contaminated sediment (Table 1). Control area sediment had the lowest contamination levels when compared to the impacted area. Percent similarity of replicate samples from the control area not impacted by contaminated groundwater ranged from 33 to 98% (mean value of 75%) for conventional parameters and 62 to 97% (mean value of 82%) for metals. In the zone of suspected groundwater contamination, mean percent similarity ranged from 4 to 93% (mean value of 33%) for conventional parameters and 1 to 80% (mean value of 36%) for metals. For both duplicate and replicate samples, percent similarity was consistently higher for metals than for conventional parameters. No chemical analyses were used to compare differences between the two extraction methods.

Toxicity Testing

Acute and chronic C. dubia toxicity tests were conducted on duplicate porewater samples collected by vacuum extraction (Table 2). The LC_{50} values for four duplicate acute toxicity tests were 38, 35, 35, and 35% (percent similarity of 96). The IC_{25} values for the duplicate chronic toxicity tests using the same porewater sample as that used for the acute tests were 43 and 33% (percent similarity of 77) and the NOEC values for the chronic tests were the same (25.0%, percent similarity of 100).

Variability in chronic toxicity of replicate samples increased in the areas of suspected groundwater contamination (Table 2). The IC_{25} values from replicate chronic toxicity tests of porewater from the control area were 100 and 86 (percent similarity of 86). For samples collected in the area of suspected groundwater contamination, IC_{25} values for three replicate chronic toxicity tests were as follows: 34 and 55 (percent similarity of 62), 15 and 50 (percent similarity of 30) and 4 and 8 (percent similarity of 50). Variability was also evident by grouping all samples from the two zones. In the control area, the mean IC_{25} was 81±22, in the area of suspected of groundwater contamination the mean IC_{25} value was 23±21.

Acute toxicity test results were also similar for the tests comparing the two extraction techniques (Table 2). The LC_{50} values for contaminated porewater were 69% for vacuum extraction and 58% for centrifugation (percent similarity of 84). The LC_{50} values using reference porewater were the same (>100%). Chronic toxicity tests were not used for the methods comparison.

DISCUSSION

Porewater extraction using the vacuum extraction methodology was faster and less labor intensive than previously reported techniques. Using the electric vacuum pump, 9.7 mL/min were extracted, versus 2.5 mL/min using the hand operated pump; an increase in efficiency of about 75%. Because a sediment of similar consistency was used, high variability in extraction rates was not observed. However, other studies using the vacuum extraction technique have reported that the extraction rate will vary depending on partial grain size and percent moisture (Winger and Lasier 1991).

TABLE 1--Conventional and Metal Analysis for Duplicate and Replicate Sediment Porewater Samples Collected in a Control Area and in Areas of Suspected Intrusion of Contaminated Groundwater.

Parameter	Duplicate (Dup) Control Area			Replicate (Rep) Control Area			Replicate (Rep) Impacted Area		
	Dup 1	Dup 2	Percent Similarity	Rep 1	Rep 2	Percent Similarity	Rep 1	Rep 2	Percent Similarity
				CONVENTIONAL (mg/L)					
BOD	2	3	67	6	2	33	28	69	41
COD	34	33	97	49	41	84	60	1,600	4
Color (SU)	260	330	79	380	1,000	38	670	9,300	7
Hardness	210	210	100	200	240	83	250	280	89
TDS	250	250	100	260	270	96	340	2,500	14
TOC	12	13	92	16	13	81	23	790	3
TSS	21	19	90	40	39	98	40	43	93
Alkalinity	190	190	100	190	230	83	230	1,300	18
Chloride	17	12	71	16	20	80	18	60	30
Percent Similarity (Conventional)			88			75			33
				METALS (µg/L)					
Arsenic	9.7	NT	NA	6.8	5.8	85	5.1	33.6	15
Barium	34	36	94	32	37	86	29.2	2,930	1
Iron	6,440	6,530	99	7,390	12,000	62	8,370	10,500	80
Magnesium	15,000	14,700	98	14,300	17,000	84	16,800	22,700	74
Manganese	920	832	90	830	1,200	69	779	496	64
Potassium	893	NT	NA	1,010	984	97	1,140	6,300	18
Sodium	8,140	NT	NA	8,180	8,670	94	18,500	837,000	2
Percent Similarity (Metals)			95			82			36

NT = Not Detectable; NA = Not Available

TABLE 2--Acute and Chronic Toxicity Results for Duplicate (Dup) an
Replicate (Rep) Sediment Porewater Samples Collected in a Control Are
and in Areas of Suspected Intrusion of Contaminated Groundwater.

SAMPLE AREA	END POINT	ACUTE TOXICITY		
		DUP 1	DUP 2	% SIMILARITY
CONTAMINATED	IC_{25}	38	35	92
CONTAMINATED	IC_{25}	35	35	100
		VACUUM	CENTRIFUGE	% SIMILARITY
CONTAMINATED	LC_{50}	69	58	84
CONTROL	LC_{50}	100	100	100
		CHRONIC TOXICITY		
		DUP 1	DUP 2	% SIMILARITY
CONTAMINATED	IC_{25}	43	33	77
CONTAMINATED	NOEC	25	25	100
		REP 1	REP 2	% SIMILARITY
CONTROL	IC_{25}	100	86	86
CONTAMINATED	IC_{25}	34	55	62
CONTAMINATED	IC_{25}	15	20	30
CONTAMINATED	IC_{25}	4	8	50

IC_{25} = impairment concentration; LC_{50} = median lethal toxicant
concentration; NOEC = no-observed-effect-concentration

Maintenance of this technique is minimal after initial setup.
Because of the turbidity associated with the initial porewater
extraction, it is necessary to discard the first 100 mL. This initial
turbidity associated with vacuum extraction was also observed in other
studies (Mitchell et al. 1989; Winger and Lasier 1991). After the
initial extraction, finer sediments were trapped in the pores of the ai
stones and acted as a filter for the finer sediment. Periodic
monitoring of the declining rate of extraction will determine when the
air stones should be scraped clean and placed in a wetter location in
the bucket. Turbid porewater does not appear after each cleaning
because the finer sediment remains entrapped in the air stones. For
sediment used in this study, this technique was relatively maintenance
free and allowed for the extraction of a large volume of porewater over
a short period of time with a minimal labor investment.

Chemical and toxicological analyses of duplicate samples were
similar. Percent similarity decreased for replicate samples collected
in areas that were more toxic (areas of suspected groundwater
intrusion). Because of the nature of the contamination (i.e.
groundwater intrusion into a lake) spatial variability was expected.
Groundwater would not uniformly enter a lake but would enter in select
areas, following geologic formations and the path of least resistance.
Spatial variability of sediment quality is important and increased
replication of samples may be necessary to reduce this variability
(Stemmer and Burton 1990).

The type of extraction technique selected would most likely have
an effect on the chemical characteristics of the porewater, but this
comparison was beyond the scope of this study. Comparison of acute

toxicity in relation to the type of extraction technique (vacuum versus centrifugation) indicated close similarity. Some level of variability in the chemical and toxicological characteristics of sediment porewater would be expected considering the complexity of the sediment matrix and its reaction to different manipulations. Future work should be conducted comparing these two techniques on different samples.

Standardization of sediment toxicity assessments is critical because of the inherent complexity. At present, there are a variety of sub-matrices tested from a single matrix (sediment), including whole sediment, sediment porewater and sediment elutriate. Different organisms can be tested from each of these submatrices. Numerous studies have been conducted to determine which of these sub-matrices and test organisms are the best indicators of sediment toxicity (Giesy et al. 1988, 1990; Hoke et al. 1990, 1993; Green et al. 1993; Harkey et al. 1994). All sub-matrices and test organisms were able to detect toxicity in sediments but selecting a test that is the best indicator of sediment toxicity is not possible. The use of C. dubia in toxicity testing of sediment porewater as a screening tool, along with a more integrated approach at selected stations may be the best and most cost effective approach (Ross et al. 1992). This integrated approach would include toxicity testing using all three sub-matrices along with traditional chemical and biological studies. The biological portion of this integrated approach would include an assessment of the resident benthic community (Malueg et al. 1984; Rosiu et al. 1989; Watzin et al. 1994). The key is to be consistent in the methodology employed at a specific study area; comparison of sediment toxicity with other sites using other techniques will be difficult until standardized approaches are adopted.

REFERENCES

Ankley, G. T., Katko, A., and Arthur, J. W., 1990, "Identification of Ammonia as an Important Sediment-Associated Toxicant in the Lower Fox River and Green Bay, Wisconsin," Environmental Toxicology and Chemistry Vol. 9, pp 1313-1322.

Ankley, G. T., and 14 others, 1992, "Integrated Assessment of Contaminated Sediments in the Lower Fox River and Green Bay, Wisconsin," Ecotoxocology and Environmental Safety, Vol. 23, pp 46-63.

Bender, M., Martin, W., Hess, J., Sayler, F., Ball, L., and Lambert, C., 1987, "A Whole Core Squeezer for Interfacial Porewater Sampling," Limnology and Oceanography, Vol. 32, pp 1214-1225.

Carignan, R., Rapin, F., and Tessier, A., 1985, "Sediment Porewater Sampling for Metal Analysis: a Comparison of Techniques," Geochimica et Cosmochimica Acta, Vol. 49, pp 2493-2497.

Edmunds, W. M. and Bath, A. H., 1976, "Centrifuge Extraction and Chemical Analysis of Interstitial Waters," Environmental Science and Technology, Vol. 10, No. 5, pp 467-472.

Giesy, J. P., Graney, R. L., Newsted, J. L., Rosiu, C. J., Benda, A., Kreis, R. G., and Horvath, F. J., 1988, "Comparison of Three Sediment Bioassay Methods Using Detroit River Sediments," Environmental Toxicology and Chemistry, Vol. 7, pp 483-498.

Giesy, J. P. and Hoke, R. A., 1989, "Freshwater Sediment Toxicity Bioassessment: Rational for Species Selection and Test Design," Journal of Great Lakes Research, Vol. 15, No. 4, pp 539-569.

Giesy, J. P., Rosiu, C. J., Graney, R. L., and Henry, M. G., 1990, "Benthic Invertebrate Bioassays with Toxic Sediment and Pore Water," Environmental Toxicology and Chemistry, Vol. 9, pp 233-248.

Green, A. S., Chandler, G. T., and Blood, E. R., 1993, "Aqueous-, Porewater-, and Sediment-Phase, Cadmium: Toxicity Relationships for Meiobenthic Copepod," Environmental Toxicology and Chemistry, Vol. 12, pp 1497-1506.

Harkey, G. A., Landrum, P. F., and Klaine, S. J., 1994, "Comparison of Whole-Sediment, Elutriate and Porewater Exposures for Use in Assessing Sediment-Associated Organic Contaminants in Bioassays," Environmental Toxicology and Chemistry, Vol. 13, pp 1315-1329.

Hoke, R. A., Giesy, J. P., Ankley, G. T., Newsted, J. L., and Adams, J. R., 1990, "Toxicity of Sediments from Western Lake Erie and the Maumee River at Toledo, Ohio, 1987: Implications for Current Dredged Material Disposal Practices," Journal of Great Lakes Research, Vol. 16, No. 3, p 457-470.

Hoke, R. A., Giesy, J. P., Zabik, M., and Unger, M., 1993, "Toxicity of Sediments and Sediment Pore Waters from the Grand Calumet River - Indiana Harbor, Indiana Area of Concern," Ecotoxicology and Environmental Safety, Vol. 26, pp 86-112.

Jahnke, R. A., 1988, "A Simple, Reliable, and Inexpensive Porewater Sampler," Limnology and Oceanography, Vol. 33, No. 3, pp 483-487.

Luoma, S. N. and Carter, J. L., 1993, "Understanding the Toxicity of Contaminants in Sediments: Beyond the Bioassay-Based Paradigm," Environmental Toxicology and Chemistry, Vol. 12, pp 793-796.

Malueg, K. W., Schuytema, G. S., Krawczyk, D. F., and Gakstatter, J. H. 1984, "Laboratory Sediment Toxicity Tests, Sediment Chemistry and Distribution of Benthic Macroinvertabrates in Sediments from the Keweenaw Waterway, Michigan," Environmental Toxicology and Chemistry, Vol. 3, pp 233-242.

Mitchell, D. F., Wagner, K. J., Monagle, W. J., and Beluzo, G. A., 1989 "A Littoral Interstitial Porewater (LIP) Sampler and its Use in Studyin Groundwater Quality Entering a Lake," Lake and Reservoir Management, Vol. 5, No. 1, pp 121-128.

Presley, B. J., Brooks, R. R., and Kappel, H. M., 1967, "A Simple Squeezer for Removal of Interstitial Water from Ocean Sediments," Journal of Marine Research, Vol. 25, pp 355-357.

Rosiu, C. J., Giesy, J. P., and Kreis, R. G., Jr, 1989, "Toxicity of Vertical Sediments in the Trenton Channel, Detroit River, Michigan, to Chironomus tentans (Insecta: Chironomidae)," International Association of Great Lakes Research, Vol 15, No. 4, pp 570-580.

Ross, P. E., and 12 others, 1992, "Assessment of Sediment Contamination at Great Lakes Areas of Concern: the ARCS Program Toxicity-Chemistry Work Group Strategy," Journal of Aquatic Ecosystem Health, Vol. 1, pp 193-200.

Saager, P. M., Sweerts, J. P., and Ellermeijer, H. J., 1990, "A Simple Porewater Sampler for Coarse, Sandy Sediments of Low Porosity," Limnology and Oceanography, Vol. 35, No. 3, pp 747-751.

Sayles, F. L., Mangelsdorf, P. C., Jr., Wilson, T. R. S., and Hume D. N., 1976, "A Sampler for In Situ Collection of Marine Sedimentary Pore Waters," Deep-Sea Research, Vol. 22, pp 259-264.

Stemmer, B. L. Burton, G. A., Jr., and Sasson-Brickson G., 1990, "Effec of Sediment Spatial Variance and Collection Method on Cladoceran

oxicity and Indigenous Microbial Activity Determinations,"
nvironmental Toxicology and Chemistry, Vol. 9, pp 1035-1044.

atzin, M. C., Roscigno, P. F., and Burke, W. D., 1994, "Community-
evel Field Method for Testing the Toxicity of Contaminated Sediments in
stuaries," Environmental Toxicology and Chemistry, Vol. 13, pp 1187-
193.

nitman, R. L., 1989, "A New Sampler for Collection of Interstitial
ater from Sandy Sediments," Hydrobiologia, Vol. 176/177, pp 531-533.

inger, P. V. and Lasier, P. J., 1991, "A Vacuum-Oporated Porewater
ntractor for Estuarine and Freshwater Sediments," Archives of
nvironmental Contamination and Toxicology, Vol. 21, pp 321-324.

Joshua Lipton[1], Edward E. Little[2], John C.A. Marr[3], Aaron J. DeLonay[4]

USE OF BEHAVIORAL AVOIDANCE TESTING IN NATURAL RESOURCE DAMAGE ASSESSMENT

REFERENCE: Lipton, J., Little, E. E., Marr, J. C. A., and DeLonay, A. J., **"Use of Behavioral Avoidance Testing in Natural Resource Damage Assessment,"** *Environmental Toxicology and Risk Assessment: Biomarkers and Risk Assessment—Fifth Volume, ASTM STP 1306,* David A. Bengtson and Diane S. Henshel, Eds., American Society for Testing and Materials, 1996.

ABSTRACT: Natural Resource Damage Assessment (NRDA) provisions established under federal and state statutes enable natural resource trustees to recover compensation from responsible parties to restore injured natural resources. Behavioral avoidance testing with fish has been used in NRDAs to determine injuries to natural resources and to establish restoration thresholds. In this manuscript we evaluate the use of avoidance testing to NRDA. Specifically, we discuss potential "acceptance criteria" to evaluate the applicability and relevance of avoidance testing. These acceptance criteria include: (1) regulatory relevance, (2) reproducibility of testing, (3) ecological significance, (4) quality assurance/quality control, and (5) relevance to restoration. We discuss each of these criteria with respect to avoidance testing. Overall, we conclude that avoidance testing can be an appropriate, defensible, and desirable aspect of an NRDA.

KEYWORDS: behavior, avoidance, natural resource damage assessment, NRDA, restoration

Natural resource damage assessment provisions established under various federal (e.g., the Comprehensive Environmental Response, Compensation and Liability Act (CERCLA), the Oil Pollution Act (OPA)) and state statutes enable public trustees for natural resources to recover compensation to restore natural resources injured by

[1]Director and senior scientist, Hagler Bailly Consulting Inc., Boulder, CO 80306

[2]General Biologist, National Biological Service, Midwest Science Center, Columbia, MO 65201.

[3]Senior Associate, Hagler Bailly Consulting Inc., Boulder, CO 80306

[4]General Ecologist, NBS, Midwest Science Center, Columbia, MO 65201.

discharges or releases of oil and hazardous substances. "Injury" is a regulatory term of art that means that natural resources are adversely affected by the oil or hazardous substances released by the responsible party. Under NRDA regulations established by the Department of Interior (DOI) for NRDAs performed under the aegis of CERCLA (43 CFR Part 11), behavioral avoidance is recognized as an injury for fish. NRDA regulations developed for OPA do not specifically identify avoidance testing as an accepted procedure for determining injuries.

Behavioral avoidance testing may be an appropriate procedure to use in NRDAs. However, the approach has relatively little precedent in litigated or administrative proceedings. Therefore, we have developed several "acceptance criteria" to evaluate the use of avoidance testing in NRDAs. These acceptance criteria include: (1) regulatory relevance, (2) reproducibility of testing, (3) ecological significance, (4) quality assurance/quality control, and (5) relevance to restoration. We do not intend these acceptance criteria to serve as a comprehensive list of "necessary conditions". Rather, the criteria represent our analysis of a series of conditions that can be used to evaluate the appropriateness of avoidance testing in NRDA. A similar list of questions could be developed to evaluate other sublethal endpoints in toxicity testing (e.g., reduced growth, tissue residues, biomarkers).

METHODS

In this manuscript we address each of our "acceptance criteria" in terms of applicability to behavioral avoidance testing. As examples, we refer to avoidance testing performed at two NRDA sites: the Clark Fork River, MT, and the Blackbird Mine, ID. The Clark Fork River is a site highly contaminated with a mixture of metals (Cd, Cu, Pb, and Zn) from mining and mineral processing operations in the vicinity of Butte, MT. The specific methodologies and results of testing performed for this NRDA are described in Woodward et al. (1995), Lipton et al. (1995), and DeLonay et al. (1995). The Blackbird Mine site, located in the Salmon River drainage in north-central Idaho, is highly contaminated with copper and cobalt. The specific methodologies and results of testing performed for this NRDA can be found in Marr et al. (1995).

REGULATORY RELEVANCE

As noted above, under NRDA regulations established by DOI for CERCLA assessments, behavioral avoidance is recognized as an accepted injury to fish [43 CFR § 11.62(f)(4)(iii)(B)]. As a result, behavioral avoidance injuries and testing have standing in NRDAs performed in compliance with DOI regulations. Moreover, trustees that perform NRDAs in compliance with these regulations obtain a rebuttable presumption of validity. Regulations proposed by the National Oceanic and Atmospheric Administration (NOAA) for NRDAs performed under OPA do not specifically identify behavioral effects -- or other adverse responses -- as accepted injuries. Rather, these regulations provide that injuries are measurable adverse responses caused by a discharge of oil. State statutes vary in their degree of specificity on accepted injuries. Behavioral avoidance testing, therefore, is directly relevant to NRDAs performed under the DOI regulations. NRDAs performed under other statutory authorities may not specifically include avoidance testing as a regulatory measure of injury.

REPRODUCIBILITY

An important aspect of laboratory testing in NRDAs relates to the reproducibility of the testing methodology. This reproducibility can include both intra-laboratory reproducibility (similar to the concept of analytical precision) and inter-laboratory reproducibility.

Reproducibility of data on contaminant-avoidance behavior depends on a number of factors including the calibration and stability of the apparatus to produce stable contaminant gradient while minimizing other sensory cues, such as temperature, flow, light or disturbance that may bias spatial selection of the fish. It also requires that the test organism be in good health, and acclimated from handling to ensure that they are responsive in the test system (ASTM 1994). In our studies (see Woodward et al. 1995; DeLonay et al. 1995; Marr et al. 1995), we have used dye tests to confirm that counter current avoidance testing chambers provided a stable contaminant gradient with well-defined margins between contaminated and uncontaminated areas of the apparatus (Fig. 1). The formation of the gradient was highly predictable, and the rinsing regime was sufficiently rigorous to ensure that biasing metal residues were absent in control areas of the apparatus. Similarly, other variables such as light, temperature, flow and depth were held constant in control and test areas of the apparatus to minimize potentially biasing stimuli.

Inter-laboratory test comparisons were completed as part of the Clark Fork River NRDA (DeLonay et al. 1995). The results of testing performed at the Midwest Science Center-Columbia, MO and at the Midwest Science Center-Jackson, WY showed extremely close agreement for testing performed with both brown and rainbow trout (Fig. 2). Statistical analysis of the two datasets (least significant difference test, $\alpha = 0.05$, Snedecor and Cochran 1980) demonstrated that avoidance of the metals mixture was not significantly different in the inter-laboratory tests. As a result, we conclude that behavioral avoidance testing can be highly reproducible.

ECOLOGICAL SIGNIFICANCE

To be of relevance to NRDA, behavioral avoidance as an endpoint should have ecological significance. The impairment of behavioral function can have immediate consequences for fish populations, including contributing as directly to their limitation or elimination as reproductive failure or mortality. The avoidance of contaminants can lead to emigration of fish from impacted areas and result in

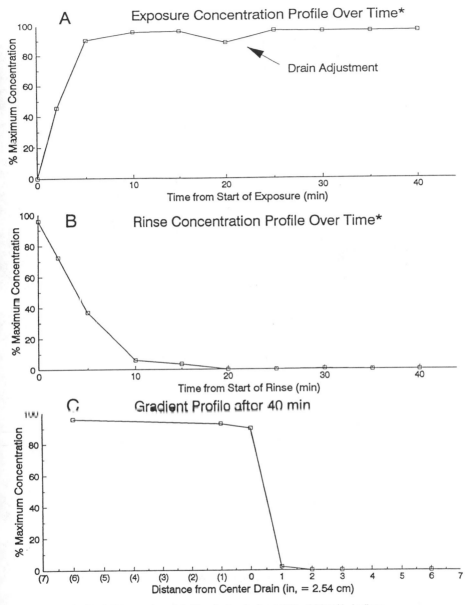

* Measured 2/3 of distance from inlet to center drain at 750 - 800 ml/min flow.

FIG. 1--Observations of dye concentration in counter-current avoidance chamber: (A) during onset of dye release in chamber (note effect of drain malfunction); (B) during rinse period; and (C) showing dye concentration across the length of the chamber.

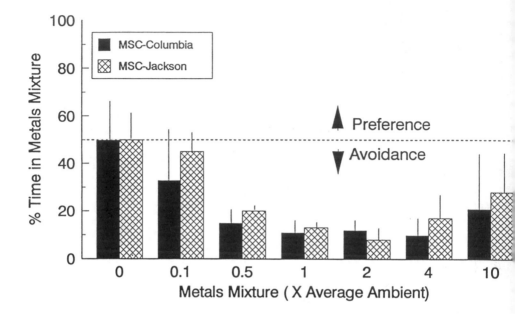

FIG. 2--Comparison of brown trout avoidance reaction to metals mixture characteristic of the Clark Fork River, Montana, measured at Midwest Science Center laboratories in Columbia, MO (MSC-Columbia) and Jackson, WY (MSC-Jackson). Vertical lines above bars represent 1 SD of the mean.

population declines. Persistent avoidance of contaminated areas thus represent a loss of habitat for that species.

Fish movements during migration can also be interrupted by the avoidance of contaminant gradients encountered along the migratory route. For example, releases of copper and zinc have been observed to inhibit upstream Atlantic salmon migration because of behavioral avoidance (Saunders and Sprague 1967), and the spawning migration of coho salmon halted when fish encountered effluents of kraft mill (Brett and MacKinnon 1954). Impaired downstream or seaward migrations could also be similarly blocked or inhibited as fish encounter contaminated areas.

In addition to direct avoidance of contaminants, migrations can also be blocked by physiological impairments arising from contaminant exposure. For example, exposure to metals during early development has been found to affect the smoltification process which includes osmoregulatory adaptations for life in seawater as well as negative rheotaxic orientation to water flow that will orient fish toward the sea and trigger preference for saline waters. Additionally, studies by Lorz and McPherson (1976) have shown that coho salmon fail to develop physiological osmoregulatory capacity to survive in sea water. Fish exposed to copper and zinc (Lorz and McPherson 1976), arsenic (Nichols et al. 1984), and selenium (Hamilton et al. 1986) failed to exhibit seaward migration. The consequences of the failure to migrate would be insufficient growth for survival and reproduction. The consequences of the inability to osmoregulate could be death (Davis and Shand 1978; Clarke 1982).

Fig. 3 presents a hypothetical description of potential behavioral avoidance mechanisms at a contaminated site. Returning anadromous adults (designated as (A) in Fig. 3) may avoid both contaminated spawning habitats and uncontaminated upstream habitats, effectively decreasing the available amount of spawning habitat utilized. Outmigrating anadromous juveniles (e.g., salmon smolts; designated as (B) in Figure 3) produced in uncontaminated waters may avoid contaminated stream segments, thus precluding or delaying outmigration, ultimately causing reduced survival or outmigrants. Juveniles of anadromous and resident fish seeking larger size rearing habitats (designated as (C) in Figure 3) may avoid moving downstream into contaminated stream segments. This may effectively reduce the amount of available rearing habitat. This could also reduce migration of resident fish populations between the mainstem and tributaries, potentially resulting in less-resistant or resilient meta-populations in tributaries.

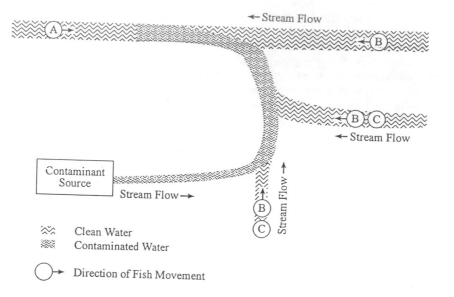

FIG. 3--Hypothetical example depicting behavioral responses to surface water contamination by returning anadromous adults (A), outmigrating anadromous juveniles (B), and anadromous and resident juveniles moving to rearing habitat (C).

We conclude, therefore, that behavioral avoidance has ecological relevance in terms of potentially affecting survival, reproduction, and habitat availability. As a result, it represents an appropriate injury endpoint for NRDAs.

QUALITY ASSURANCE/QUALITY CONTROL (QA/QC)

QA/QC is a potentially important aspect of studies performed in support of NRDAs, particularly when litigation is involved. QA/QC measures help ensure that data are collected in a systematic manner, and assist in the overall defensibility of avoidance studies.

Methodological issues that merit consideration in QA plans include: (1) variables that bias spatial selection by fish, (2) abnormal behavior that limits or alters the responsiveness of test organisms, including maintaining test organisms in good condition, (3) establishment/maintenance of a stable contaminant gradient to facilitate interpretation of test results, and (4) rigorous identification of data and samples, including both analytical QC and, potentially, chain-of-custody over data.

Variables that Can Bias Spatial Selection

It is important that the testing apparatus be appropriately calibrated to ensure that potentially biasing stimuli such as temperature, flow, light, or disturbance do not influence spatial selection of the fish. This requires measuring flow rates entering and leaving each end of the chamber (this is important both to ensure the stability of the contaminant concentration gradient, and because water flow provides a sensory cue that may influence the spatial selection of the fish), as well as other variables such as temperature, dissolved oxygen, pH, hardness, light intensity. For example, temperature differences of greater than 0.4° C have been shown to influence avoidance thresholds (Kleerekoper 1973).

Maze bias is normally controlled for by randomizing the end of the avoidance chamber receiving the toxic substance. In addition to monitoring water flow, contaminant gradient, temperature, water quality, and light, bias can be measured by comparing responses to different ends of the testing apparatus during application of uncontaminated water. During tests by DeLonay et al. (1995), brown trout and rainbow trout resumed normal activity within the allotted habituation or preexposure period and did not exhibit any signs of abnormal behavior or heightened aggression during the testing procedure. Under ideal conditions, with no apparatus biases or directing stimuli (i.e., contaminants), fish should randomly distribute themselves and spend approximately the same amount of time on each end of the apparatus. Also in the tests by DeLonay et al. (1995), the distribution over time of both species in the control tests was very near this expected 50% distribution (see Figure 2).

Test Organisms

Responsiveness of the test organisms is also important. The test organism should be in good health. They should be fully acclimated ($\geq$ 14-d acclimation period) to the dilution water used during the test to ensure that responses observed are not confounded by physiological adjustments or habituation stresses. The test regime should allow sufficient time for the test organism to recover from handling and to be habituated to the test chamber before testing to ensure that they are responsive. An organism stressed by changes in water quality, alarmed by handling, or inhibited by an unfamiliar test environment may freeze, become hyperactive and unresponsive to contaminant cues, or exhibit skewed spatial selection to the extent that reactions to contaminant gradients will be obscured or inhibited. Although there is no single indicator of "normal" responsiveness, the resumption of movement within the apparatus is generally used as an indication of recovery from handling (Little and DeLonay 1995). Alternatively a reduction in speed and frequency of movement indicates recovery among fish whose initial response is hyperactive fright reactions. Recovery may also be indicated by a return to normal coloration or posture. Recovery times may vary with species and age of fish, and must be considered when developing the test regime.

Whether fish are tested in pairs or small groups, it is important to ensure that there are no aggressive interactions that may bias spatial selection among individuals. The occurrence of nips, nudges, or chases could trigger criteria for rejecting a test. During an avoidance test it is particularly important to monitor the frequency of gradient crossing. A criterion can be created to ensure that the fish are sufficiently active to explore and make contact with the contaminant. Spatial bias should also be monitored during the preexposure period. Gross behavioral form and posture should be monitored to ensure that the fish are not injured or impaired by the contaminant exposure. Behavioral activity levels should also be monitored to ensure that the fish have recovered from handling, are sufficiently active to explore the gradient, but not impaired by contaminant exposure. Schooling and aggressive behaviors should also be examined to ensure that the response of the fish are not altered by an aggressive individual.

Stable Concentration Gradient

In avoidance testing it is especially critical that the test apparatus produce consistent stable contaminant gradients. Both dye tests and chemical analysis of water quality were used in Marr et al. (1995) to demonstrate that the counter current chamber provided a highly stable contaminant gradient with well defined margins between contaminated and uncontaminated areas of the apparatus.

Data Collection: Summary

Table 1 summarizes data that can be collected to demonstrate appropriate QA/QC in behavioral avoidance testing. It should be recognized that not all of these variables may require measurement for all tests. However, the table provides a summary of the types of data that could be collected to ensure appropriate data quality.

RELEVANCE TO RESTORATION

For NRDAs performed under both CERCLA and OPA, restoration of injured natural resources is the ultimate objective. Therefore, injury testing should have relevance to the development of restoration goals, objectives, and approaches. This relevance can include: (1) determining the nature and extent of any injuries to natural resources, including determining what resources (including both species and habitats) are injured

TABLE 1--Examples of QA/QC data for avoidance testing.

▸ Variables to Control for Spatial Bias	▸ water flow rate ▸ temperature ▸ water quality (e.g., dissolved oxygen, pH, hardness) ▸ contaminant gradient ▸ outside disturbance ▸ light
▸ Behavioral variables	▸ frequency of gradient crossing ▸ gross behavioral form and posture ▸ activity levels ▸ schooling/aggressive behavioral interactions
▸ Analytical variables	▸ purity of source water ▸ confirm chemical composition of test/control water ▸ removal of contaminant after rinsing ▸ standard analytical QA/QC

and the spatial and temporal extent of those injuries, and (2) determining the appropriate "level" of restoration (e.g., setting cleanup thresholds).

As depicted above in Figure 3, avoidance responses can differentially affect the various species, life stages, and habitats present at a site. Behavioral avoidance testing can, in conjunction with population survey and site water quality monitoring programs, identify injured species and life stages, as well as quantifying the spatial extent of avoidance injuries. Such information is important in scaling restoration programs. Moreover, behavioral responses can be important components of identifying restoration cleanup thresholds because avoidance thresholds often are substantially lower than acutely lethal levels. For example, in the Blackbird Mine NRDA, Marr et al. (1995) demonstrated that salmonids avoided Cu and Co concentrations as low as 3 and 180 μg/L, respectively, whereas acute lethality thresholds for Cu and Co were on the order of 10 and 250 μg/L, respectively. Therefore, restoration of this site to prevent acute lethality would not be sufficiently protective of avoidance injuries.

SUMMARY AND CONCLUSIONS

In summary, we conclude that behavioral avoidance testing is an appropriate endpoint for use in NRDAs. Specifically, behavioral avoidance testing:

1.   has been recognized by the DOI as an accepted injury for NRDAs performed under CERCLA;

2.   is reproducible, showing both high inter- and intra-laboratory reproducibility;

3.   is ecologically significant, potentially affecting survival, reproduction, and habitat availability;

4.   is amenable to quality assurance/quality control measures, thereby generating defensible data;

5.   is of relevance to NRDA restoration programs, including both scaling the nature and extent of restoration, as well as determining appropriate restoration cleanup thresholds.

ACKNOWLEDGMENTS

The authors wish to acknowledge Dan Woodward and Jim Hansen for collection of MSC-Jackson avoidance data, and Chris Ingersoll and Edmund Smith for manuscript review.

REFERENCES

ASTM, 1994, "Standard guide for behavioral testing in aquatic toxicology," E1604-94, American Society for Testing and Materials, Philadelphia, Vol 11.04 pp. 1510-1517.

Brett, J.R., and MacKinnon, D., 1954, "Some aspects of olfactory perception in migrating adult coho and spring salmon," Journal of the Fisheries Research Board of Canada, Vol. 11, pp. 310-318.

Clarke, W.C., 1982, "Evaluation of the seawater challenge test as an index of marine survival," Aquaculture, Vol. 28, pp. 177-183.

Davis, J.C., and Shand, I.G., 1978, "Acute and sublethal copper sensitivity, growth, and saltwater survival in young Babine Lake sockeye salmon," Fisheries Marine Service Technical Report 847, Department of Fisheries and the Environment, Vancouver, BC, Canada.

DeLonay, A.J., Little, E.E., Lipton, J., Woodward, D.F., and Hansen, J.A., "Behavioral avoidance as evidence of injury to fishery resources: Applications to natural resource damage assessments," Environmental Toxicology and Risk Assessment: Fourth Volume, ASTM STP 1262, Thomas W. LaPoint, Fred T. Price, and Edward E. Little, Eds., American Society for Testing and Materials, Philadelphia, 1995.

Hamilton, S., Palmisano, A., Wedemeyer, G.A., and Yatsutake, W.T., 1986, "Impacts of selenium on early lifestages and smoltification of fall chinook salmon," Transactions of the 51st Wildlife & Natural Resources Conference, pp. 343-356.

Kleerekoper, H., Waxman, J.B., and Matis, J., 1973, "Interaction of temperature and copper ions as mediating stimuli in the locomotor behavior of the goldfish, Carassius auratus," Journal of the Fisheries Research Board of Canada, Vol. 30, pp. 725-728.

Lipton, J., Beltman, D., Bergman, H.L., Chapman, D., Hillman, T., Kerr, M., Moore, J., and Woodward, D.F., 1995, Aquatic Resources Injury Assessment Report. Upper Clark Fork River Basin, Report to State of Montana, Natural Resource Damage Litigation Program, Helena, MT. January, 1995.

Little, E.E., and DeLonay, A.J., 1995, "Measures of fish behavior as indicators of sublethal toxicosis during standard toxicity tests," Environmental Toxicology and Risk Assessment: Fourth Volume, ASTP STP 1262, T.W. LaPoint, F.T. Price, and E.E. Little, Eds., American Society for Testing and Materials, Philadelphia. In Press.

Lorz, H.W., and McPherson, B.P., 1976, "Effects of copper or zinc in fresh water on the adaptation to sea water and ATPase activity, and the effects of copper on migratory disposition of coho salmon (Oncorhynchus kisutch)," Journal of the Fisheries Research Board of Canada, Vol. 33, pp. 2023-2030.

Marr, J., Lipton, J., Cacela, D., Bergman, H.L., Hansen, J., Meyer, J.S., and MacRae, R., 1995, Fisheries Toxicity Injury Studies. Blackbird Mine Site, Idaho, Report prepared for the National Oceanic and Atmospheric Administration, Washington, DC. February, 1995.

Nichols, J.W., Wedemeyer, G.A., Mayer, F.L., Dickhoff, W.W., Gregory, S.V., Yatsutake, W.T., and Smith, S.D., 1984, "Effects of freshwater exposure to arsenic trioxide on the parr-smolt transformation of coho salmon (Oncorhynchus kisutch)," Environmental Toxicology and Chemistry, Vol. 3, pp. 143-149.

Saunders, R.L., and Sprague, J.B., 1967, "Effects of copper-zinc mining pollution on a spawning migration of atlantic salmon," Water Research, Vol. 1, pp. 419-432.

Snedecor, G.W., and W.G. Cochran. 1980. Statistical Methods. The Iowa State University Press, Ames, IA.

Woodward, D.F., Hansen, J.A., Bergman, H.L., Little, E.E., and DeLonay, A.J., 1995, "Brown trout avoidance of metals in water characteristic of the Clark Fork River, Montana," <u>Canadian Journal of Fisheries and Aquatic Sciences</u>, Vol. 52, No. 9, In Press.

Valentin A. Nepomnyashchikh[1], Aaron J. DeLonay[2], and Edward E. Little[2]

BEHAVIORAL STUDIES OF CONTAMINANT EFFECTS ON AQUATIC INVERTEBRATES: A REVIEW OF RUSSIAN INVESTIGATIONS

REFERENCE: Nepomnyashchikh, V. A., DeLonay, A. J., and Little, E. E., "**Behavioral Studies of Contaminant Effects on Aquatic Invertebrates: A Review of Russian Investigations.**" *Environmental Toxicology and Risk Assessment: Biomarkers and Risk Assessment—Fifth Volume, ASTM STP 1306,* David A. Bengtson and Diane S. Henshel, Eds., American Society for Testing and Materials, 1996.

ABSTRACT: Studies by Russian scientists have documented significant alterations and impairment of critical behavioral functions in aquatic organisms following exposure to environmental contaminants. Behavioral responses disrupted by sublethal exposure to toxicants are intimately involved in habitat selection, foraging, competition, predator-prey relationships, and reproduction, and are essential to survival. Behavioral responses of benthic invertebrates have received considerable study in Russia. A range of invertebrate taxa have been studied, including leeches, insects, molluscs, plankton, and crustaceans. In addition, aquatic invertebrates exhibit a large number of behavioral responses which are sensitive to contaminant exposure and are easily quantified. Standardized behavioral methodologies for measuring contaminant effects are being developed.

KEYWORDS: behavior, behavioral methods, benthic invertebrates

Behavioral responses of aquatic invertebrates exposed to sublethal levels of environmental contaminants have received considerable attention in Russia. Aquatic

[1]Head of Behavioral Ecology Research Group, Institute for Biology of Inland Waters, Russian Academy of Sciences, 152742 Borok, Nekouz, Yaroslavl, Russia.

[2]Ecologist and General Biologist, respectively, National Biological Service, Midwest Science Center, Columbia, MO 65201.

invertebrates are easily obtainable, readily cultured, and frequently inhabit the interface between contaminated water and sediment. Invertebrates possess a rich repertoire of behavioral responses that can be readily observed and measured effectively to characterize the consequences of sublethal exposure to a range of chemical stressors. Alteration of critical behavioral functions such as habitat selection, foraging, competition, predator-prey relationships, and reproduction are indicative of probable deleterious effects that would be detrimental to individual survival in the environment and may be predictive of impacts to populations. In addition, methods that measure behavioral changes during toxicity tests may be effective as rapid indicators of water quality, or may aid in contaminant identification. This paper describes the Russian research previously conducted on a wide range of invertebrate taxa, and the diverse array of behavioral responses that have been evaluated (Table 1).

LEECHES

Leeches have frequently been used in water pollution tests in Russia. Although they are less sensitive than standard test species such as daphnids, they are easily handled, often occur in highly polluted water and are effective in contaminant screening tests. The leech *Hirudo medicinalis* is the most studied test subject in Russia. Leeches of different age groups can be used in such studies, but newly hatched and unfed juveniles are most sensitive to water pollutants. A number of simple and complex behavioral responses to contaminant exposure have been observed in the leech, including impaired reflex responses, alterations in locomotory activity, avoidance, and depressed or disrupted feeding.

Simple reflex behavior is frequently used to indicate the effect of exposure on neuromuscular integration. Commonly, the induction or cessation of movement (startle response) in adult *H. medicinalis* can be induced by weak electric currents (Baraeva 1987). The threshold of startle reaction is determined by applying a weak electric current and gradually increasing the electric current intensity until the response occurs. The response thresholds increased among organisms sublethally exposed to copper sulphate (10 μmol/L) or methyl parathion (1 μmol/L) for 24 h. Thus sublethal exposure to contaminants impaired the leeches' ability to produce effective "startle responses" to external stimuli.

Exposure to some contaminants elicits specific clinical behavioral responses that are often characteristic or symptomatic of the class of contaminant. Lapkina and Flerov (1979; 1980) found that some chemicals cause specific symptoms of poisoning in *H. medicinalis* during the first few hours of exposure at relatively high chemical concentrations (about 48-h LC_{50} level). The symptoms of organophosphate exposure include ventral twisting of body segments, spiral twisting of the whole body, progressive contraction of body, and eventually edema. Ventral twisting of anterior segments and convulsions were observed among leeches exposed to PCB. Potentially, these specific symptoms may be used diagnostically to identify classes of toxicants.

TABLE 1--Contaminant concentration and exposure duration that cause a behavioral response in aquatic invertebrates.

Organisms	Contaminant	Behaviorally Effective Exposure Conc. (mg/L)	Exposure Duration	Lethal Conc. (mg/L)	Behavioral Response
1	2	3	4	5	6
BENTHOS					
Hirundinea, Hirudinidae					
Hirudo medicinalis (juveniles)	$CuSO_4$	0.01	15 min.	0.25 (48-h LC_{50})	locomotor[a] activity
	$HgCL_2$	0.01	- " -	0.3 (48-h LC_{50})	- " -
	$KMnO_4$	0.5	- " -	5.0 (48-h LC_{50})	- " -
	$Al(NO_3)_3$	1.0	- " -	40 (48-h LC_{50})	- " -
	iodine (5% alcohol solution)	0.05	- " -	0.5 (48-h LC_{50})	- " -
	KBr	0.5	- " -	100 (48-h LC_{50})	- " -
	hydroquinone	0.5	- " -	1.0 (48-h LC_{50})	- " -
	phenol	50	- " -	950 (48-h LC_{50})	- " -
	strobane	0.5	- " -	1.0 (48-h LC_{50})	- " -
	DDVP	1.0	- " -	0.1 (48-h LC_{50})	- " -
	dylox	no response at 10 (mg/L)	- " -	0.45 (48-h LC_{50})	- " -
	methyl parathion	1.0	- " -	1.0 (48-h LC_{50})	- " -
	paraoxon	10	- " -	1.2 (48-h LC_{50})	- " -

TABLE 1--Continued.

1	2	3	4	5	6
	malathion	10	- " -	10 (48-h LC$_{50}$)	- " -
	sevin	0.05	- " -	13 (48-h LC$_{50}$)	- " -
H. medicinalis (adults)	"Lotos-71"	1	10 min	190 (48-h LC$_{50}$)	avoidance[b]
	phenol	50	- " -	290 (48-h LC$_{50}$)	- " -
	strobane	5	- " -	5 (48-h LC$_{50}$)	- " -
	dylox	no response at 0.6 mg/L	- " -	0.3 (48-h LC$_{50}$)	- " -
	- " -	0.1	- " -	- " -	preference
	CuSO$_4$	0.01	24 h	--	response[c] to electric current
	methyl parathion	0.001	- " -	--	- " -
	dylox	0.0005	30 d	no death for 40 d at 0.005 mg/L	sequence[d] of behavior
	CuSO$_4$	0.05	50 min	no death for 48 h at 0.5 mg/L	- " -
	dylox	0.6	6 h	0.3 (48-h LC$_{50}$)	posterior[e,f] segment twisting

TABLE 1--Continued.

1	2	3	4	5	6
	malathion	11	6 h	11 (48-h LC$_{50}$)	anterior segment twisting
Glossiphoniidae					
Hemiclepsis marginata	dylox	0.05	18 h	5 (24-h max. tolerated conc.)	feeding[g]
Isopoda					
Asellus aquaticus	"Lotos-71"	0.1	30 min	220 (48-h LC$_{50}$)	preference[h]
	-"-	1	-"-	-'-	avoidance
	phenol	0.01	-"-	75 (48-h LC$_{50}$)	preference
	-"-	1	-"-	-"-	avoidance
	strobane	0.1	-"-	0.02 (48-h LC$_{50}$)	preference
	-"-	1	-"-	-"-	avoidance
	dylox	10	-"-	0.13 (48-h LC$_{50}$)	preference
	-"-	100	-"-	-"-	avoidance
Amphipoda					
Streptocephalus torvicornis	"Lotos-71"	no response at 20 mg/L	30 min	12 (48-h LC$_{50}$)	avoidance[i]
	phenol	10	-"-	30 (48-h LC$_{50}$)	-"-
	strobane	no response at 0.25 mg/L	-"-	0.17 (48-h LC$_{50}$)	-"-

TABLE 1--Continued.

1	2	3	4	5	6
	dylox	10	-"-	0.04 (48-h LC$_{50}$)	-"-
Eulimnogammarus verrucosus	resorcinol	0.01	2-3 h	--	preference[j]
	phenol	1	-"-	--	avoidance
	pyrocatechol	1	-"-	--	-"-
	ethyl mercaptan	1	-"-	--	preference
	hydroquinone	10	-"-	--	avoidance
	pyrogallol	10	-"-	--	-"-
Decapoda					
Astacus sp.	phenol	0.1	24 h	--	response to[k] electric current
	hydroquinone	2	-"-	--	-"-
	-"-	0.02	48 h	--	-"-
Insecta					
Trichoptera, Limnephylidae					
Chaetopteryx villosa	methyl parathion	0.00001	48 h	0.0001 (48-h max. tolerated conc.)	speed of[l] case building

TABLE 1--Continued.

1	2	3	4	5	6
	dylox	0.0001	24 h	0.0001 (24-h LC_{50})	sequence[n] of behavior
Phryganeidae					
Phryganea sp.	Cu^{++}	0.1	24 h	—	response[c] to electric current
Aeschna sp.	Cu^{++}	0.1	24 h	—	- " -
	methyl parathion	0.01	- " -	—	- " -
Diptera					
Chironomus plumosus	NaCl	0.0001	2 min	—	speed of[n] locomotion
	- " -	0.001	6 min	—	phototaxis
	$CuCl_2$	0.000001	2 min	—	speed of locomotion
	- " -	0.001	6 min	—	phototaxis
	$CaCl_2$	no response at 0.001 mg/L	2 min	—	speed of locomotion
	- " -	0.001	6 min	—	phototaxis
	$NiCl_2$	0.001	2 min	—	speed of locomotion

TABLE 1--Continued.

1	2	3	4	5	6
	KNO_3	$1\cdot10^{-7}$	-"-	--	-"-
	$NaNO_3$	$1\cdot10^{-7}$	-"-	--	-"-
Mollusca					
Bivalvia					
Unio pictorum	ethyl mercaptan	10	48 h	--	filtration[o] activity
	phenol	10	-"-	--	-"-
	hydroquinone	10	-"-	--	-"-
	pyrogallol	10	-"-	--	-"-
	phenol	0.0001	24 h	--	valve[p] movement
	hydroquinone	0.01	-"-	--	-"-
	dimethyl sulfide	0.005	-"-	--	-"-
Mizuhopecten yessoensis	decrease of salinity	to 26-22‰	9 h	--	valve[q] movement and jumps
	decrease of dissolved oxygen	to 1 mL/L	24 h	--	-"-
	"Dela"	1	instant response	--	-"-
	"Triton X-100"	0.1	-"-	--	-"-

TABLE 1--Continued.

1	2	3	4	5	6
Crenomytilus greyanus	Cu^{++}	0.05	-"-	--	closure[r] of valves
	decrease of salinity	to 23‰	12 h	--	frequency of valve[q] movement
	-"-	to 22-1‰	6 h	--	-"-
	decrease of dissolved oxygen	to 2 mL/L	6 h	--	-"-
	"Triton X-100"	0.1	instant response	--	-"-
Gastropoda					
Viviparus viviparus	phenol	50	15 min	—	avoidance[s]
	-"-	200	45 min	—	mucous excretion
Planorbis corneus	phenol	100	30 min	--	avoidance
	-"-	50	36 h	--	mucous excretion
PERIPHYTON					
Ciliata					
Vorticella microstoma	$Zn(CH_3COO)_2$	0.0008%	1 h	--	feeding[t]
	-"-	-"-	72 h	--	vacuole pulsations

TABLE 1--Continued.

1	2	3	4	5	6
V. convallaria	Zn(CH$_3$COO)$_2$	0.002%	1 h	--	feeding and free swimming
	- " -	- " -	72 h	--	vacuole pulsation
PLANKTON					
Rotatoria					
Brachionus plicatilis	HgCl$_2$	0.025 (EC$_{50}$)	24 h	0.045 (24-h LC$_{50}$)	phototaxis[u]
	CdSO$_4$	5 (EC$_{50}$)	- " -	35 (24-h LC$_{50}$)	- " -
	dylox	0.5 (EC$_{50}$)	- " -	50 (24-h LC$_{50}$)	- " -
Cladocera					
Daphnia magna	phenol	0.1	1 h	--	respiratory[v] movements

[a]Lapkina et al. 1987, [b]Flerov and Lapkina 1976, [c]Baraeva 1987, [d]Nepomnyashchikh et al. 1988, [e]Lapkina and Flerov 1979, [f]Lapkina and Flerov 1980, [g]Nepomnyashchikh and Eljakova 1987, [h]Tagunov and Flerov 1978, [i]Flerov and Tagunov 1978, [j]Volkova 1986, [k]Baraeva 1988, [l]Nepomnyashchikh et al. 1988, [m]Nepomnyashchikh and Valjushok 1989, [n]Orlov and Kokneva pers. comm., [o]Kiseleva 1983, [p]Hrefjeva pers. comm., [q]Karpenko and Tjurin 1987, [r]Tjurin 1987, [s]Stadnichenko et al. 1983, [t]Barausova 1983, [u]Grozdov 1986, [v]Kolupaev 1988.

The locomotory activity of leeches has been examined in numerous studies with toxicants (Lapkina and Flerov 1979; 1980; Lapkina et al. 1987), and assays which measure changes in activity of leeches have been recommended for use in the rapid assessment of industrial effluents in Russia. Commonly, this behavior is measured by counting the number of active and resting individuals that have been placed in different toxicant solutions. The observations begin within 3 to 7 min of exposure and continue at 1 min intervals for 10 to 15 min. The locomotory activity is affected by metals, phenolic compounds, halogens, and carbaryl at concentrations of 1 to 10 % of the 48-h LC_{50}. Organophosphates, on the other hand, only evoke responses at concentrations approximating the LC_{50} or greater (Lapkina et al. 1987; Flerov et al. 1988). Differing sites of toxicant activity or modes of action may account for the varying behavioral sensitivities observed. Metals at low exposure concentrations, for example, may act on the skin surfaces and membranes as a general irritant, whereas organophosphates and high concentrations of metals may cause behavioral effects by impairing or disrupting the physiological function of cells and tissues.

Heightened locomotory activity is often correlated with avoidance behavior (Lapkina et al. 1987). Avoidance reactions provide protection from the harmful effects of contaminants, yet also drive organisms from preferred habitats into areas that may be less suitable for survival. Avoidance responses were studied using a test chamber which received contaminated water at one end and uncontaminated water at the other to form a sharp gradient in the center where the apparatus drained (Flerov and Lapkina 1976). Measures of average time spent in the contaminated area, and the exploratory movements at the boundary of the gradient revealed that leeches successfully avoided sublethal concentrations of anionic detergent and phenol considerably below the incipient lethal concentration (Figure 1). PCBs were avoided at concentrations in excess of the 48-h LC_{50} which indicates that leeches are unlikely to avoid concentrations inducing lethality. The organochlorine, Dylox, was not avoided at concentrations up to 0.6 mg/L, twice the LC_{50} concentration. Leeches seldom penetrated gradients of phenol or detergent, but were not so strongly repelled by PCB. The duration of time spent in areas contaminated with PCBs, detergent, or phenol was negatively correlated with increasing log concentrations of those chemicals.

Complex behaviors such as feeding are readily disrupted by exposure to contaminants and thus can serve as sensitive measures of contaminant effect. Complex behavioral responses can be assessed through an analysis of the sequential components of the behavior. Feeding behavior in leeches consists of a series of simple behaviors, each of which may be carried out only upon the completion of the preceding response. Thus contaminant effects on each behavior will decrease the probability of the successful completion of the whole pattern of response (Nepomnyashchikh and Flerov 1988). Feeding behavior of the leech *Hemmiclepsis marginata* was studied during sublethal exposure using this approach. After some period of exposure, the initial food-searching stages of feeding behavior in the absence of prey were recorded at 10 min intervals for 1 h. Subsequently, an immobilized carp was placed into each chamber and the behavior of leeches was again recorded for 4 h. Leeches failed to accomplish the last stages of feeding behavior (attachment to the fish and blood sucking) after sublethal 18-h exposure to dylox; the initial stages of the sequence (scanning and crawling) were disrupted to a lesser degree (Nepomnyashchikh and Eljakova 1987).

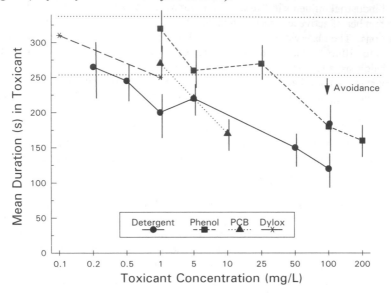

FIGURE 1--Avoidance reactions of the leech, *Hirudo medicinalis* shown as cumulative mean duration of time (with standard deviation bars) spent in areas of the chamber receiving solutions of an anionic detergent, phenol, PCB, or an insecticide, dylox. Dashed lines indicate the 95% confidence interval of response when no substance is present in the chamber. From Flerov and Lapkina (1976).

Prey-searching behavior of the medicinal leech was also assessed using a similar sequential analysis. Behaviors and their duration were recorded during observations of individual leeches in open field tests. The behaviors included swimming (characterized as continuous locomotion in the water column); resting (not moving on the bottom with attachment on substrate); searching (the protrusion, retraction, and side to side movements of the elevated anterior body with stationary attached posterior); and crawling (a non-swimming motion on substrate with sequential anterior protrusion, anterior attachment, release of posterior, and forward movement of posterior). These independent behaviors occur in different combinations. Different contaminants disrupt different stages of prey-searching, providing a mechanistic examination of contaminant effects. For example, sublethal exposure to chlorophos decreased resting intervals after crawl-search. In contrast, copper sulfate increased the frequency of rest units after crawl-search combinations. Thus the effect of contaminants disrupts the sequence of behavioral activity.

CRUSTACEANS

Simple reflex responses are also useful for examining toxicant effects in crustaceans. Exposure of crayfish (*Astacus sp.*) to sublethal concentrations of phenol and hydroquinone resulted in a reduced ability to produce startle reflexes in response to a noxious external stimuli (Baraeva 1988), using methods previously described for measuring the neuromuscular integration of leeches (Baraeva 1987).

Behavioral toxicological investigations of crustaceans have largely focused on preference/avoidance reactions to contaminants. The intent of these investigations is to assess the extent of which the harmful effects of exposure are minimized by avoidance responses, or enhanced by attraction to contaminated areas. Methods for such studies involve testing previously unexposed organisms in a Y maze. Uncontaminated water and toxic solutions are alternately added to the right and left arms of the Y maze to control biasing stimuli and position preferences of the test organisms. The number of organisms entering each arm are counted every 2 min during the 30 min test.

Isopods (*Asellus aquaticus*) significantly avoided detergents and sublethal levels of phenol (Figure 2). Chlorophos and PCB were only avoided at lethal concentrations, however intermediate sublethal concentrations of these chemicals were attractive to *A. aquaticus* (Tagunov and Flerov 1978). Similarly the amphipod, *Streptocephalus torvicornis*, avoided phenol at the maximum tolerated concentration, and chlorophos at the lethal concentration, while the detergent and PCB evoked no response (Flerov and Tagunov 1978). Subsequent studies showed that amphipods failed to avoid phenol following a short (30 min) exposure to either PCBs or the detergent solution suggesting that these contaminants may damage chemoreceptors, preventing avoidance and further impairing the ability of these organisms to respond to other external stimuli.

Another method for determining preference-avoidance responses involves the use of a counter-current chamber, in which uncontaminated and contaminated water are added to either end of the chamber to form a steep gradient at the center where the water drains from the chamber. The test was conducted for 2 to 3 h and the number of animals in opposite halves of the chamber were counted. This method was used to study the effect of individual components of waste waters of a Baikal paper mill (resorcinol, phenol, pyrocatchol, ethyl mercaptan, hydroquinone, and pyrogallol) on another amphipod, *Eulimnogammarus verrucosus*. Concentrations tested were 0.01, 1.00 and 10.00 mg/L. At the least concentration, there were no responses to any chemical, with the exception of a preference response to resorcinol. At the intermediate concentration, phenol and hydroxibenzol were avoided, hydroquinone and pyrogallol caused no response, and resorcinol and ethyl mercaptan were preferred to clean water. At the greatest concentration, only resorcinol and ethyl mercaptan caused no response (Volkov 1986).

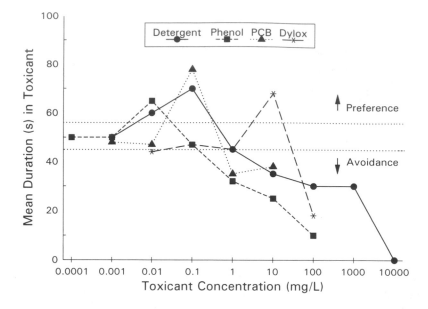

FIGURE 2--Avoidance and preference reactions of the isopod, *Asellus aquaticus* shown as cumulative mean duration of time spent in the area of the test chamber areas receiving solutions of an anionic detergent, phenol, PCB, and an insecticide, dylox. Dashed lines indicate the 95% confidence interval of response when no substance is present in the chamber. From Tagunov and Flerov (1978).

INSECTS

Simple reflex behaviors in insects, such as the withdrawal response of caddisfly larvae (Trichoptera) into its tube or displacement behavior in dragonflies (Odonata), can be used to assess the effect of a contaminant on neuromuscular integration. Invertebrates are typically exposed to some concentration of a contaminant and the threshold of an external stimulus (e.g., an electrical current) required to induce the reflexive reaction is determined (Baraeva 1987). For example, a 24 h exposure to copper and methyl parathion increased the threshold for the reflexive withdrawal of the caddisfly (*Phryganea sp.*) into its case. Copper decreased the threshold required to induce a displacement behavior of the dragonfly (*Aeshna sp.*), mask grooming, whereas methyl parathion increased the threshold (Baraeva 1987).

Phototaxis and locomotory behavior are commonly studied behavioral responses in contaminant-exposed insects. In studies with the chironomid, *Chironomus plumosus L.* speed and distance of movement and phototactic responses were examined following exposure to a number of chloride and nitrate metal salts. The trajectory traveled was traced onto semi-transparent paper during 2 min observation. Phototaxis was measured

TABLE 2--The sensitivity and tolerance to different metal concentrations in *Hirudo medicinalis* juveniles (after Lapkina et al. 1987).

Compound	Metal ion concentration (mg/L)	Mean number of leeches moved (9 animals in experiment)	The duration of time (h) before effect is displayed in animals		
			Avoidance	Pathologic Twisting	Death
CuSO$_4$	0.01	3.7	2.0	30.0	96.0
	0.1	8.7	0.7	15.0	72.0
	1.0	9.0	0.17	3.0	20.0
	10.0	9.0	0.1	0.5	12.0
HgCl$_2$	0.01	2.5	absent	48.0	--
	0.1	7.3	3.0	30.0	--
	1.0	9.0	0.8	1.0	14.0
	10.0	9.0	0.05	0.05	5.0
Al(NO$_3$)$_3$	1.0	2.4	absent	30.0	--
	10.0	4.6	3.0	30.0	96.0
	100.0	9.0	0.05	3.0	18.0

TABLE 3--The effect of chlorides and nitrates on the swimming speed of *Chironomus plumosus* larvae (Orlov and Korneva pers. comm.).

Concentration (mol/L)	Chlorides						Nitrates			
	K$^+$	Na$^+$	Cu^{+2}	Ca^{+2}	Ni^{+2}	Cd^{+2}	K$^+$	Na$^+$	Cd^{+2}	Ni^{+2}
1·10^{-7}	...	-	...	...	-	-	f	f	f	f
1·10^{-6}	...	-	s	...	-	-	f	f	f	f
1·10^{-5}	...	-	s	...	-	-	f	f	f	f
1·10^{-4}	...	s	s	...	-	-	f	f	f	f
1·10^{-3}	-	s	s	-	s	-	f	-	-	f

s - Slower speed in the experiment than in the control
f - Faster speed than in the control
- - No difference between experiment and control

by placing animals into half-covered Petri dishes and counting the number of larvae in the dark half of dishes during a 6 min experiment. Most compounds tested (Table 3) affected distance and speed, metal nitrates causing greater effect than chlorides. Both nitrates and chlorides increased negative phototaxis. Phototaxis and swimming speed were independently affected by exposure (Orlov and Korneva, pers. comm.).

The influence of sublethal contaminant exposure on complex patterns of insect behavior has been intensively studied. (Nepomnyashchikh and Flerov 1988). Some caddis fly species build elaborate cases of sand particles (Limnephilidae). Larvae were pushed out of their cases and placed in dishes containing a bottom layer of sand. Periodic observations were made during the 48-h test, and the stage of case building (anchor, tube, cutting off anchor, and completion of the tube) was recorded. Exposure to methyl parathion at concentrations as low as 0.05 µg/l disrupted critical phases of the construction process. The building process was slower. Tube construction of exposed organisms lagged behind that of controls with progressively earlier delays being apparent as the concentration increased (Nepomnyashchikh et al. 1988).

Another method was used to study the effect of chlorophos on the tube-repairing behavior of this species. In this case the tubes were partially destroyed and the observation included measuring the duration and sequence of tube repair activities of larvae exposed to chlorophos solutions (from 0 to 0.05 μg/L) for 24 h. During the 1-h observation a typical sequence of behaviors, which was repeated until the tube was repaired, included the larva's searching for sand, inspection of individual sand particles, attachment of particles to the tube, and internal inspections of tubes. Chlorophos affected the sequence of behavioral acts at all concentrations. The largest changes were noted in the frequency of transition from gluing to internal inspection and from internal inspection to particle inspection. Such changes in the sequence of behaviors were more sensitive indicators of water quality than the cumulative frequencies and durations of each phase. For example, the sum quantity of particles attached to the tube during a given period of time, was not significantly affected at low concentrations (Nepomnyashchikh and Valjushok 1989). However, at higher concentrations the case building was significantly altered.

MOLLUSCS

Filtration activity is a commonly measured response to contaminant effects on bivalve molluscs. To perform such measures, *Unio pictorum* were exposed to toxicants in the laboratory for 48 h. They were then taken to the field where they were suspended in net funnels 25 to 30 cm above the river bottom. Particles carried by the molluscs' respiratory stream accumulated in a sampler at the bottom of the funnel net which was later weighed to provide a measure of filtration activity over a period of 4 h. The toxicants, ethyl mercaptan, phenol, hydroquinone, and trihydroxybenzol (paper mill waste), reduced particulate filtration between 32 and 64% at 10 mg/L each (Kiseleva 1983).

Valve movement and closure are also affected by exposure and are readily monitored using inexpensive, automated recording techniques. The movements are recorded automatically with the help of a chart recorder connected to one valve with a thread. Toxicant effect was measured as the decrease in duration of periods when valves moved. Altered valve movement or complete valve closure occurred during exposure to metals, detergents, low dissolved oxygen, increased salinity, and paper mill effluents.

Phenol, hydroquinone and dimethyl sulphide affect valve movements in *Unio pictorum* (Arefjova 1983). The number of valve movements per time period and the duration of periods of closed valves were measured in *Mizuhopecten yessoensis* and *Crenomytilus greyanus* in response to reductions in salinity (32 to 17‰), decreased dissolved oxygen (5.5 to 1.0 mL/L), and the presence of the detergents (1.0 mg/L) (Karpenko and Tjurin 1987). The number of movements initiated by *M. yessoensis* decreased when salinity was reduced to 26‰, and increased at low dissolved oxygen (1.0 mL/L). Detergents also caused increased movement. These changes in water quality also caused a jumping response which may have been an attempt to avoid these conditions. Valve closure was also induced in this species by 50 μg/L copper (Tjurin 1985). The frequency of valve movements of *C. greyanus* increased when salinity decreased to 23‰, whereas further reductions in salinity induced prolonged periods of closed valves. *Crenomytilus greyanus* closed valves in response to detergent and to reduced dissolved oxygen (2.0 mL/L).

Gastropod molluscs may alter activity patterns and exhibit avoidance behavior in the presence of contaminants. *Viviparus viviparus* avoided phenol at 50 mg/L. *Lymnaea fulva* and *Planorbis corneus* avoided phenol at 100 mg/L by climbing the aquaria walls and settling above the water surface. The velocity of movement increased significantly with increasing concentration (Stadnichenko et al. 1983). Prolonged exposure also caused mucus secretion in *L. fulva* and *P. corneus*, which may have been a protective reaction to the toxin.

PERIPHYTON

Phagocytosis and the formation of vacuoles was reduced in sedentary ciliates *Vorticella microstoma* and *V. convallaria* during sublethal exposures to zinc (Barausova 1983). Aqueous exposure to zinc also induced swimming behavior in the normally sedentary *V. convallaria*, forcing them from the sediment. In spite of reduced activity of the contractile vacuoles evident after day 3 of exposure, growth was not affected by these sublethal concentrations.

PLANKTON

Phototaxis in the plankton rotifer *Brachionus plicatilis* was affected by sublethal concentrations of several chemicals including mercury chloride, cadmium sulfate and dylox. The response was measured by noting the rotifers' movement across a grid in response to lateral light stimulus. The chemical concentration which caused a 50 % decrease in phototaxis relative to controls (EC50) ranged from 1 to 10 % of the 24-h LC_{50} (Grozdov 1986).

The frequency of respiratory movements and heart rate of the planktonic cladoceran, *Daphnia magna*, decreased by sublethal exposure to phenol at concentrations of 0.1 mg/L and greater. Daphnids were placed in capillary tubes filled with clean water for 1 h, then the responses were measured during the next hour every 5 to 10 min using a microscope. Then test solution was piped into the tube and the response was recorded again in the same manner (Kolupaev 1988).

CONCLUSIONS

The data described are by no means the complete information on the current state of aquatic behavioral toxicology in Russia. Most publications on the topic are printed as brief abstracts in different local periodicals published by various department laboratories. In addition, there are no special publications in the field of water quality protection and as a consequence, no standard form of publications. We have selected only detailed articles for this review.

Benthic invertebrates are among the most widely used test species in Russia. Medicinal leeches and bivalve molluscs are most studied. Rapid detection (leeches and molluscs) and automated methods (molluscs) have been developed using these species. The use of the species and methods to control the quality of effluents and natural water is highly probable during the next few years in Russia. Industries in Russia are presently obligated to monitor effluents. These monitoring efforts includes measurements of mortality in various organisms, and in cell cultures, and certain behavioral responses reported here. However, there is still no nation-wide program for bioassay development. Tests such as the *Ceriodaphnia* toxicity tests (ASTM, E1295) are being used in Russia and other ASTM procedures are being adapted for use in Russian monitoring efforts.

Most methods are based on the use of simple and easily observable behavioral responses. The development of more complicated methods, such as behavioral act sequence analysis, are now being initiated because of the availability of digital processors, however, such methods are still not available for routine monitoring.

There is no widely accepted general approach to the study of behavioral responses to water pollution. Flerov and coworkers (1988) have suggested that the study of pollution effects on fixed action patterns (FAP) is critically important for ecological monitoring since these are crucial behaviors which provide the animals' feeding, defense, reproduction, and other needs. They are governed mainly by internal factors and are resistant to changes in the animals environment. It is highly probable that toxicants which eliminate FAP in laboratory experiments will cause the same effect under natural

:onditions. For this viewpoint, some results cited above may be used in ecological prognoses.

ACKNOWLEDGMENTS

Support for this review was made possible through scientific linkage grant #950428 from the North Atlantic Treaty Organization (NATO), Scientific and Environmental Affairs Division.

REFERENCES

Arefjeva, T.V., 1983, "The effects of low concentrations of chemicals on valve movements in molluscs: Reports on comparative physiology and adaptation to environmental abiotic factors in animals," Jaroslavl State University, pp. 43-46.

Baraeva, T.V., 1987, "The effect of chemicals on the behavior of various aquatic animals in constant electric current: The problem of comparative physiology and water toxicology," Jaroslavl State University, Jaroslavl, pp. 50-56.

Baraeva, T.V., 1988, "The effect of phenols on crayfish behavior in constant electric current: The physiology and toxicology of aquatic organisms," Jaroslavl State University, Jaroslavl, pp. 136-141.

Barausova, O.M., 1983, "Behavioral response of Vorticella to high zinc concentrations: Aquatic invertebrate behavior," 4th All Union Symposium, Borok, USSR Academy of Sciences, Leningrad, pp. 33-37.

Flerov, B.A., Kozlovskaya, V.I., Nepomnyashchikh, V.A., 1988, "The evaluation of an ecological danger of pollutants using physiological and behavioral responses in aquatic animals: Ecotoxicology and environmental protection," Urmala Republic Conference, USSR Academy of Sciences, Riga, pp. 195-197.

Flerov, B.A. and Lapkina, L.N., 1976, "The avoidance of solutions of some toxic substances in the medicinal leech," Biology of Inland Waters Information Bulletin, No. 30, Nauka Publishers, Leningrad, pp 48-52.

Flerov, B.A. and Tagunov,V.B., 1978, "The analysis of avoidance response to toxic substances in Streptocephalus torvicornis (Waga)," Biology of Inland Waters Information Bulletin, No. 40, Nauka Publishers, Leningrad, pp. 68-71.

Grozdov, A.O., 1986, "Phototaxis as a test response for bioassays," Hydrobiological Magazine, Vol. 22, pp. 68-71.

Karpenko, A.A. and Tjurin, A.N., 1987, "Behavioral adaptation to environmental stress in *Mizuhopecten yessoensis* and *Crenomytilus greyanus*," Physiology and Biochemistry of aquatic organisms. Jaroslavl State University, Jaroslavl, pp. 18-31.

Kiseleva, O.A., 1983, "The influence of abiotic factors on the filtration in molluscs in a natural waterbody," Reports on Comparative physiology and adaptation to environmental abiotic factors in animals. Jaroslavl State University, Jaroslavl, pp. 37-42.

Kolupaev, B.I., 1988, "The method of biotesting using changes of respiration and heart beats in Daphnia," Water Bioassay Methods. Chernogolovka, USSR Academy of Sciences pp. 103-104.

Lapkina, L.N., and Flerov, B.A., 1979, "The study of leech poisoning with some toxic substances," Physiology and parasitology of freshwater animals. Nauka Publishers, Leningrad, pp. 50-59.

Lapkina, L.N., and Flerov, B.A., 1980, "The use of leeches for pesticide identification in water," Hydrobiological Magazine, Vol. 16, pp.113-119.

Lapkina, L.N., Flerov, B.A., Chalova, I.V., and Jakovleva, I.I., 1987, "The use of behavioral responses in *Hirudo medicinalis* juveniles for bioassays," The problems of comparative physiology and water toxicology. Jaroslavl State University, Jaroslavl, pp. 11-17.

Nepomnyashchikh, V.A., and Eljakova, N.B., 1987, "The comparison of sensitivity to dylox of the simple and complex behavior in the leech *Hemiclepsis marginata*," Biology of Inland Waters Information Bulletin No. 74, pp. 42-45.

Nepomnyashchikh, V.A., Flerov, B.A., and Henry, M.G., 1988, "The effect of methyl parathion on the building behavior in the caddisfly *Chaetopteryx villosa* larvae," Nauchnye doclady vysshei shkoly:Biologicheskie nayki. No. 9 pp. 70-73.

Nepomnyashchikh, V.A., and Flerov, B.A., 1988, "Biotesting of aquatic environments based on the behavioral reactions of aquatic animals," In Protection of River Basins, Lakes, and Estuaries R.C. Ryans (editor) American Fisheries Society, Bethesda, Maryland pp. 147- 157.

Stadnichenko, A.P., Aleksejchuk, A.P., Voloshenko, A.V., Blotskaja, N.F., Kotkatskaja, V.V., Labunets, N.V., Shimanovitch, S.A., 1983, "The effect of phenol pollution on fast behavioral responses in freshwater molluscs," In: Applied Ethology: Proceedings of 3rd All-Union Conference on Animal Behavior, Vol. 3, pp. 149-151.

Tagunov, V.B., and Flerov, B.A., 1978, "The avoidance response in Asellus aquaticus," Biology of Inland Waters Information Bulletin, No. 39, pp. 80-84.

Tjurin, A.N., 1985, "Using bivalve molluscs for bioassays," In: D.A. Sakcharov, editor, Simple Nervous System. Vol. 2, Kazan State University, Kazan pp. 94-98.

Volkov, V.M., 1986, "The study of the avoidance of some components of waste waters in the Baikal gammarus," In: V.G. Gagarin, editor, Behavior of Aquatic Invertebrates:Proceedings of the 4th All-Union Symposium. Institute of Biology of Inland Waters p. 100-102.

Raj Misra,[1] John Antonelli,[1] Kiran Misra,[1] Craig Steele,[1,2] and Carol Skinner[1]

SUBLETHAL EXPOSURE TO CADMIUM INTERFERES WITH COVER SEEKING BEHAVIOR OF JUVENILE CRAYFISH, PROCAMBARUS CLARKII (GIRARD).

REFERENCE: Misra, R., Antonelli, J., Misra, K., Steele, C., and Skinner, C., "Sublethal Exposure to Cadmium Interferes with Cover-seeking Behavior of Juvenile Crayfish, *Procambarus clarkii* (Girard)," *Environmental Toxicology and Risk Assessment: Biomarkers and Risk Assessment—Fifth Volume, ASTM STP 1306,* David A. Bengtson and Diane S. Henshel, Eds., American Society for Testing and Materials, 1996.

ABSTRACT: The behavioral effects of heavy metals on crayfishes may significantly affect their survival in the environment. Changes in their ability to remain under cover could substantially decrease their survivorship due to increased predation. The effect of sublethal cadmium exposure on the ability of juvenile crayfish to remain in cover was evaluated. Four different treatment groups were used (N=11 juveniles each): a control group (not exposed to cadmium), and three experimental groups exposed to 1, 2, or 3 mg Cd/L for 7 d. Crayfish were placed, individually, into glass aquaria containing 3 L of laboratory water pre-treated to detoxify all heavy metals, with continuous aeration. Each crayfish was provided with a dark, thigmotactic shelter. Cadmium was introduced into the aquaria on days 1 and 4 to maintain the nominal concentrations. Beginning on day 5 and continuing through day 7, observations were taken on each crayfish five times per day with a minimum of 30 minutes between observations. Crayfish position was recorded as in cover or in the open area of an aquarium. Juveniles in the control groups were in cover 78.3% of the observations. Over the 3 d of observations, juveniles in the 1 mg Cd/L exposure groups used cover 72.1%. Those in the 2 and 3 mg Cd/L groups used cover 53.9% and 60.0%, respectively, indicating hyperactivity induced by cadmium exposure. Examining the daily results, however, those juveniles in the 1 mg Cd/L group were in cover only 60.0% of the time by day 7, indicating a latency to produce hyperactivity at this concentration. Those in the 2 mg Cd/L group were using the covers similarly to the controls by day 7 of exposure, indicating habituation to the cadmium or "exhaustion" of the animals by hyperactivity. Those in the 3 mg Cd/L group behaved similarly to controls on day 5, but beginning on day 2 and continuing into day 3 of the observations spent progressively fewer of the observations in cover, suggesting that initial hyperactivity occurred prior to the beginning of observations, and "exhausted" the animals, or that they were severely traumatized by the exposure to 3 mg Cd/L and required time to recover before exhibiting hyperactive behavior.

KEYWORDS: cadmium, sublethal exposure, behavior, behavioral toxicity

[1]Department of Biology and Health Services, Edinboro University, Edinboro, PA 16444.

[2]To whom correspondence should be addressed.

The red swamp crayfish, Procambarus clarkii, was introduced into Ohio at the London State Fish Hatchery in 1975 along with minnows purchased from Arkansas (Tim Nagel, pers. comm.). By 1983, the species had reached the Akron State Fish Hatchery in northeastern Ohio and the Sandusky Bay area in northern Ohio (Norrosky 1983; more current information on P. clarkii range extension is not available, Norrosky, pers. com.). This species is reducing or eliminating native Orconectes species of crayfishes in Ohio and could reach the Erie, Pennsylvania, area in the not-so-distant future. Our interest in P. clarkii thus stems from its ability to out-compete and replace Orconectes species Orconectes rusticus is the only species of crayfish in our area) and its classification as a pest" in some places where it has been introduced (Huner et al. 1991).

Cadmium is important in many industrial processes, especially in the manufacture of paints and automobile fuels (Merian 1990). It is a heavy-metal pollutant of increasing environmental concern because it is a common component of industrial effluents discharged into receiving waters and of auto exhaust discharged onto roadside plants and drainage ditches (Friberg et al. 1971; Merian 1990). It also appears to have no biological uses (is nonessential) and is generally regarded as highly toxic (Hiatt and Huff 1975; Mirenda 1986; Merian 1990). Cadmium, like other heavy metals, is not decayed by natural processes and accumulates in organic and inorganic material (Lindquist and Block 1994; Klüttgen and Ratte 1994). Crayfish accumulate and retain cadmium in their gills and viscera (Anderson and Brower 1978; Dickson, et al. 1982). Because cadmium is not regulated by crayfishes, sublethal concentrations of cadmium become a cumulative poison which may affect crayfish behavior (Bryan 1976; Gillespie et al. 1977; Dickson, et al. 1982). As a result, the behavioral effects of heavy metals on crayfishes may significantly affect their survival in the environment. Changes in their ability to remain under cover could substantially decrease their survivorship due to increased predation.

Our objectives in evaluating the behavioral toxicity of sublethal cadmium exposure on juvenile P. clarkii using cover-seeking behavior as the bioassay were to evaluate its potential as a behavioral endpoint and to provide data to develop the hypothesis that resistance to pollutants by juveniles may be a factor in promoting the spread of introduced P. clarkii.

METHODS

Four treatment groups (N=11, each) of juvenile (≤3 cm carapace length; Nagayama et al. 1986) P. clarkii crayfish were used in this study: a control group (not exposed to cadmium), and three experimental groups exposed to 1, 2, or 3 mg Cd/L for 7 d. These concentrations used reflect the reported 7-day LC50s and 95% confidence limits for Orconectes adults (1.8 [1.5-2.3] mg Cd/L; Mirenda 1986; Thorp and Gloss 1986).

Juveniles were placed, individually, into glass aquaria containing 3 L of continuously aerated laboratory water which was pre-treated with NovAqua Tapwater Conditioner (Kordon Division of Novalek, Inc.) to detoxify all heavy metals, remove chlorine, and buffer the water (pH 7.0-7.5). Water temperature was a consistent 23±1°C. Other water quality parameters measured were: total hardness, 232.6 mg $CaCO_3$/L; total alkalinity, 146.4 mg $CaCO_3$/L. Windows in the laboratory provided seasonal summer photoperiod. Illumination in the aquaria varied between 269-323 lx (25-30 fc; GE Type 214 light meter) during photophase.

Each aquarium contained a dark, thigmotactic shelter, which has been shown to be the preferred shelter of juvenile P. clarkii (Antonelli 1996). Illumination in the shelter was below detection limit of the light meter (<10 lx [<1 fc]). Cadmium was introduced into the aquaria on days 1 and 4 (two "pulse injections" to produce and to restore the nominal concentrations used). Nominal concentrations were used to evaluate the potential of the

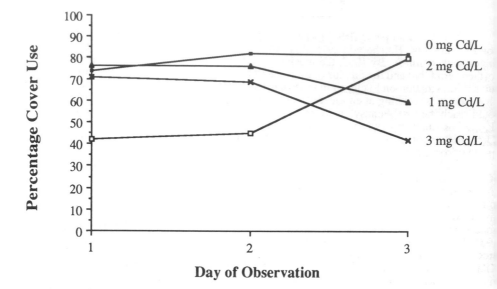

FIG. 1--Daily cover use by juvenile Procambarus clarkii crayfish in four treatment groups.

behavior as an endpoint for further bioassay refinement and development of a more definitive test. The crayfish were fed TetraMin® fish flakes daily, ad libitum, but not fed after the second "pulse" of cadmium.

Beginning on day 5 and continuing through day 7, observations were taken (from behind a black plastic "blind") on each crayfish five times per day, with a minimum of 30 minutes between observations (15 observations per crayfish). The position of a crayfish was recorded as in cover or in the open area of an aquarium. Data were analyzed by one-way repeated measures ANOVA, using Statview 512+ software (Abacus Concepts, Inc.).

RESULTS AND DISCUSSION

Juveniles in the control groups were in the covers 78.3% of the observations. Over the 3 d of observations, juveniles in the 1 mg Cd/L exposure groups were in cover 72.1% of the observations (not significantly different from controls). Juveniles in the 2 mg Cd/L and 3 mg Cd/L groups used the cover 53.9% and 60.0% of the observations over the 3 d, respectively, indicating hyperactivity induced by cadmium exposure (although only the results of the 2 mg/L group were significantly different from the controls: $F_{1,21}=4.5$; $P \leq 0.05$).

From the daily results (Fig. 1), however, juveniles in the 1 mg Cd/L group were in cover only 60.0% of the observations by day 7 of exposure (day 3, observations); those in the 2 mg Cd/L group were using the covers similarly to the controls by day 7 (day 3, observations); those in the 3 mg Cd/L group behaved similarly to controls on day 5 (day 1, observations), but beginning on day 2 and continuing into day 3 of the observations (days 5 and 7 of exposure, respectively) were found progressively less often in cover. Only one juvenile P. clarkii died at this exposure concentration (on day 7 [day 3, observations]).

Future studies will focus on increasing the sample sizes to compensate for the natural variability of behavior among animals, on refining the exposure concentrations of cadmium used, and on repeating this bioassay with juveniles of native Orconectes spp. to compare their resistance to that of juvenile P. clarkii.

SUMMARY

Exposure of juvenile P. clarkii to nominal concentrations of 2 mg Cd/L and 3 mg Cd/L induced hyperactivity in these crayfish. Such hyperactivity (as evidenced by a concomitant decrease in cover-use) in a natural situation could expose them to increased predation. Lack of significance of the data of the 3 mg Cd/L exposure from the control data may be due to the variability in behavior among the animals; increased sample sizes should be used in future studies.

The daily data on cover-use by juveniles in the 1 mg Cd/L exposure group indicate a latency to produce hyperactivity at this concentration of cadmium.

The daily data on cover-use by juveniles in the 2 mg Cd/L group suggest habituation to the cadmium and/or "exhaustion" of the animals due to hyperactivity.

The daily data on cover-use by juveniles in the 3 mg Cd/L group suggest that initial hyperactivity may have occurred prior to the beginning of the observations, which "exhausted" the animals (a situation often reported in behavioral toxicity studies of heavy metals with fishes; e.g. see review in Steele 1985), or that they were severely traumatized by the high exposure concentration (>LC50 for Orconectes adults), and that they required time to recover before exhibiting hyperactive behavior.

REFERENCES

Anderson, R.V. and Brower, J.E., 1978, "Patterns of Trace Metal Accumulation in Crayfish Populations," Bulletin of Environmental Contamination and Toxicology, Vol. 20, pp. 120-127.

Antonelli, J., 1996, "Cover-seeking Behavior in Adult and Juvenile Procambarus clarkii," M.S. thesis, Edinboro University, Edinboro, Pennsylvania.

Bryan, G.W., 1976, "Some Aspects of Heavy Metal Tolerance in Aquatic Organisms," Effects of Pollutants on Aquatic Organisms, 2nd Volume, A.P.M. Lockwood, Ed., Cambridge University Press, Cambridge, U.K., pp. 7-34.

Dickson, G.W., Giesy, J.P. and Briese, L.A., 1982, "The Effect of Chronic Cadmium Exposure on Phosphoadenylate Concentrations and Adenylate Energy Charge of Gills and Dorsal Muscle Tissue of Crayfish," Environmental Toxicology and Chemistry, Vol. 1, pp. 147-156.

Friberg, L., Piscator, M. and Nordberg, G., 1971, Cadmium in the Environment, CRC Press, Cleveland, Ohio.

Gillespie, R., Reisine, T. and Massaro, E.J., 1977, "Cadmium Uptake by the Crayfish, Orconectes propinquus propinquus (Girard)," Environmental Research, Vol. 13, pp. 364-368.

Hiatt, V. and Huff, J.E., 1975, "The Environmental Impact of Cadmium: An Overview," International Journal of Environmental Studies, Vol. 7, pp. 277-285.

Huner, J.V., Barr, J.E. and Coleman, E.B., 1991, Red Swamp Crawfish: Biology and Exploitation, Sea Grant Publication No. LSU-T-80-001.

Klüttgen, B. and Ratte, H.T., 1994, "Effects of Different Food Doses on Cadmium Toxicity to Daphnia magna," Environmental Toxicology and Chemistry, Vol. 13, pp. 1619-1627.

Lindquist, L. and Block, M., 1994, "Excretion of Cadmium and Zinc During Moulting in the Grasshopper Omocestus viridulus (Orthoptera)," Environmental Toxicology and Chemistry, Vol. 13, pp. 1669-1672.

Merian, E., 1990, "Environmental Chemistry and Biological Effects of Cadmium Compounds," Toxicological and Environmental Chemistry, Vol. 26, pp. 27-44.

Mirenda, R.J., 1986, "Toxicity and Accumulation of Cadmium in the Crayfish, Orconectes virilis (Hagen)," Archives of Environmental Toxicology and Chemistry, Vol. 15, pp. 401-407.

Nagayama, T., Takahata, M. and Hisada, M., 1986, "Behavioral Transition of the Crayfish Avoidance Reaction in Response to Uropod Stimulation," Experimental Biology, Vol. 46, pp. 75-82.

Norrosky, M.J., 1983, "Procambarus (Scapulicambarus) clarkii (Girard, 1852): The Red Swamp Crayfish in Ohio," Ohio Journal of Science, Vol. 83, pp. 271-273.

Steele, C.W., 1985, "Latent Behavioural Toxicity of Copper to Sea Catfish, Arius felis, and Sheepshead, Archosargus probatocephalus," Journal of Fish Biology, Vol. 27, pp. 643-654.

Thorp, J.H. and Gloss, S.P., 1986, "Field and Laboratory Tests on Acute Toxicity of Cadmium to Freshwater Crayfish," Bulletin of Environmental Contamination and Toxicology, Vol. 37, pp. 355-361.

Michael C. Harrass[1] and Donald J. Klemm[2]

QUALITY ASSURANCE GUIDANCE FOR
LABORATORIES PERFORMING AQUATIC TOXICITY TESTS[3]

REFERENCE: Harrass, M. C. and Klemm, D. J., "Quality Assurance Guidance for
Laboratories Performing Aquatic Toxicity Tests," *Environmental Toxicology and Risk
Assessment: Biomarkers and Risk Assessment—Fifth Volume, ASTM STP 1306,* David A.
Bengtson and Diane S. Henshel, Eds., American Society for Testing and Materials, 1996.

ABSTRACT: Satisfactory laboratory performance is critical to the use of aquatic
toxicity tests in regulatory, industrial and research applications. Quality Assurance
and Quality Control (QA/QC) practices are fundamental to demonstrating satisfactory
performance. Laboratory aquatic toxicity test procedural and performance criteria can
help a potential client decide that an aquatic toxicity laboratory will meet a need, as
well as help an outside reviewer determine that test results are valid. Laboratory
practices to assure and control quality include training staff, using standard
procedures, and keeping valid records, but also include evaluating and improving
performance. These components echo several widely used quality management
principles. The costs of poor quality (lost time, lost production and lost image) touch
both the laboratory and the laboratory's customers. While the level of quality should
reflect the use of the study, higher quality work provides for better control, better
data and better service, benefits ultimately shared by both the suppliers and users of
aquatic toxicity data.

KEYWORDS: aquatic toxicity tests, quality assurance, quality control, performance
criteria, whole effluent testing

[1]Environmental toxicologist, Environment, Health and Safety Department, Amoco
Corporation, 130 E. Randolph Dr., Chicago, IL 60601.

[2]Research Aquatic Biologist, Ecosystem Research Branch, Ecological Exposure
Research Division, National Exposure Research Laboratory, U.S. Environmental
Protection Agency, 26 W. Martin Luther King Drive, Cincinnati, OH 45268

[3]This article has been reviewed by the Ecological Exposure Research Division,
National Exposure Research Laboratory, USEPA, and approved for publication. The
mention of trade names or commercial products does not constitute endorsement or
recommendation for use.

Quality issues are part of all products and services in today's environment. Aquatic toxicity tests are appropriately seen as products or services and so quality issues are part of the picture. Further, quality issues must be addressed to achieve the goal of standardization. Quality issues are also critical to the use of aquatic toxicity testing results for stewardship and compliance.

Results from biomonitoring tests of a refinery effluent by two laboratories illustrate the importance of the last point (Table 1). The test was the *Ceriodaphnia dubia* 7 day test which monitors survival and reproduction (USEPA 1989b, c; 1994a). The effluent sample was split and tests were conducted by two laboratories (Lab A and Lab B). Lab A reported that the effluent was relatively toxic, with 16 chronic toxicity units (TU$_c$) relative to survival. Lab B reported much less toxicity, 4 TU$_c$, for both survival and reproduction.

A number of quality issues are problematic in the Lab A report: *Ceriodaphnia* reproduction was marginally above the acceptance criterion, and no data were provided about the number of broods per adult. No raw data (e.g., no bench sheets or no record of daily young production) were provided, just means (with standard deviations) for each treatment. There was no mention of test results with standard reference toxicants. An arithmetically impossible result was reported, but the report provided no way to determine if this was a typographical error or something else. Both laboratory reports were signed by a "QC Coordinator."

Which laboratory was correct? Would an outside reviewer conclude that the refinery effluent exhibited high chronic toxicity or not? Suppose that the refinery's wastewater discharge permit specified that chronic toxicity above 8 TUc was a permit violation. Was the refinery effluent in violation of such a specification? Quality issues are clearly central to resolving such questions.

GOALS OF A QUALITY ASSURANCE (QA) PROGRAM

There are at least three explicit goals of a QA program in the aquatic toxicity lab: (1) to demonstrate adherence to a protocol or standard, (2) to characterize the background conditions during the work and (3) to provide tools to objectively evaluate the "quality" of a lab test. Practitioners of aquatic ecotoxicology are probably very familiar with the first two of these goals. For example, typical QA practices provide for describing the competence of staff, demonstrating the performance of equipment and organisms, and detailing the protocol used. Consideration of the technical aspects, however, may not fully consider how to evaluate "quality" itself.

Methods of establishing quality will vary. Students of quality control or quality management have developed numerous different tracks, but the concepts proposed by

Table 1. Comparison of Chronic Toxicity Tests for *Ceriodaphnia dubia*

Split samples of a refinery effluent were provided to the laboratories.
Reported test results are compared with the USEPA criteria for acceptance,
where appropriate.

	Criterion	LAB A	LAB B
Control Group Performance			
Control Survival	80%	90%	90%
Neonates (mean)	≥ 15	15.44	32.8
Adults with			
3 broods or more	$\geq 60\%$	Not reported	90%
Reference Toxicant			
Test of a standard	Recommended	None	Summary
chemical	to show control	noted	included
Test Report			
Raw data	Should be included	Not reported	Reported
Anomalous data	Should be	"67%" mortality reported	Explan-
	explained	at one concentration,	ation
		but with 10 organisms per	given
		concentration, this is an	when
		arithmetic impossibility	needed
Endpoints			
7 day LC50		9.6%	40.6%
TU_c-survival		16	4
TU_c-reproduction		> 31.95 (estimated)	4
NOEC-survival		6.25%	25%
NOEC-reproduction		$< 6.25\%$	25%

Deming, Juran and others (Juran 1974; USEPA 1978; Walton 1990) are widely known, e.g., "Total Quality Management" (TQM). Therefore, it may be useful in this context to point out the overlap between these approaches and the QA/QC elements that are specific to laboratory aquatic toxicity tests.

As used in this review, Quality Assurance (QA) includes all those planned and systematic actions necessary to provide adequate confidence that a product or service will satisfy given requirements for quality. Quality Control (QC) refers to the operational techniques and activities that are used to fulfill requirements for quality aimed both at monitoring a process and at eliminating causes of unsatisfactory performance. These definitions follow the ISO 9000 guidance (ISO 1987a, b, c, d).

A paradigm in business relationships is to see a supplier-customer chain in the development and use of a product or service. A useful definition of a customer is anyone who benefits from or uses a product or service from another individual or group (Clemmer 1992). We quickly recognize that each of us acts as both supplier and customer within our organizations and outside them. If we are the source of the product or service, we are the supplier. If others are the source, we are the customer. One modification of this concept is to add a distributor (supplier-distributor-customer), or the infamous "middleman." The role of the distributor is to pass along a product or service, essentially unchanged, but in a manner so as to get the right product or service passed along at the right time. The right product or service is the one that meets the customer's needs, and quality is one of those needs.

Part of recognizing quality as one part of the customer's needs is recognizing that not every customer needs the same quality. Consequently, it is not surprising to note that laboratory aquatic toxicity tests currently have different levels of performance. A test submitted for registering a new chemical might meet Good Laboratory Practice (GLP) levels of performance. A test done to demonstrate compliance with a wastewater permit would meet specific procedural and performance criteria different from GLP requirements. And, a test done for research might be evaluated on entirely different acceptability criteria.

We write from the perspective of customers of aquatic toxicity tests, or perhaps as distributors of aquatic toxicity test results to other customers. Viewed this way, QA issues become a business issue for private sector laboratories, the suppliers of many aquatic toxicity test results. For both private and public sector labs, QA issues become a comparative benchmark for evaluating present status and future improvements.

Uses of the QA program

Both private and public organizations are coming under increasing pressure to have add value and to eliminate unnecessary actions. The QA program therefore will be scrutinized internally and externally for what value it adds and the following uses make clear some of these values.

1. Provide for confident use by customer.

The uses of a QA program have traditionally emphasized things that permit outside review of the validity of a lab test. For example, if a company wants to report aquatic toxicity information on its Material Safety Data Sheet (MSDS), it sees QA as a way to establish that the reported information is reliable and accurate. If a regulatory agency wants to determine compliance or set regulatory criteria, QA provides a way to evaluate whether the conditions of testing are acceptable. USEPA Order 5360.1, for example, stated the USEPA objective to collect data of "known and documented quality that is adequate for its intended use" (USEPA 1984). The dimensions of the "known and documented quality" include precision, accuracy, completeness, comparability, and representativeness.

Consistent with this perspective is the recognition that one size QA program does not fit all needs. A prescriptive approach to QA might serve some specific needs. For example, labs doing testing in the context of regulatory compliance under the NPDES program, i.e., whole effluent testing (WET), generally use USEPA's guidance for lab evaluations (USEPA 1991a). This guidance contains specific criteria, including checklists, which focus attention on aspects of testing deemed critical for conducting accurate effluent tests. However, even the checklist focuses on whether a program element is in place, more than on whether a program element matches, dimension by dimension, an ideal program.

2. Facilitates self-evaluation and improvement.

A second use for the QA program is to provide lab managers and staff with a tool for self-evaluation and control of performance. This aspect has also been called "internal quality assurance" and is described as those activities aimed at providing confidence to the management of an organization that the intended quality is being achieved (ISO 1987a, 1990).

Consistent with this perspective is the recognition that quality issues contribute to improvement in any organization for any type of aquatic toxicity project. Excessive reliance on a static, one-size-fits-all approach to QA would stifle innovation by fostering a mindset that, once a QA program is in place, the work is done. Recognizing the competitive nature of quality issues instead leads to using QA results and programs as a way to identify the next step to meeting customer needs.

3. Meeting customer needs.

A third use for the QA program is to convince current customers or potential customers to use a specific supplier. Using this perspective, a laboratory can easily see QA a competitive issue, not just a compliance issue, or a cost of doing business. If the supplier envisions the QA program as a potential advantage in securing new customers and retaining old customers, then QA issues may make more sense to managers seeking to grow a business.

Activities aimed at providing confidence to the customer that the supplier's quality system will provide a product or service that will satisfy the customer's stated quality requirements are often called "external quality assurance" (ISO 1987a). Standards are a way of establishing the specifications or requirements of a test and quality is one dimension that can be specified. To quote the business literature, "specifications should define what it takes to satisfy the customer" (Peters 1987).

Quality is one of the dimensions necessary for customer satisfaction, and so is a critical component of an aquatic toxicity test. For example, several WET reports from an Amoco facility were received that noted the failure of the test on the front page summary. Although these did not constitute a compliance issue, the reported failures understandably upset Amoco managers. Upon reading the text, it was clear that the test had failed to meet the acceptance criteria, not that the effluent sampled had exhibited excess toxicity. It should surprise no one that Amoco considered this supplier to have unacceptable quality in two ways: the capacity to conduct reliable tests and an appropriate way to report test quality.

The development of data quality objectives (DQOs) provides a tool to describe what "known and documented quality" means in the context of a specific aquatic toxicity project. DQOs are qualitative and quantitative descriptors of the completeness, type and amount of error that are expected and are acceptable in a data set (USEPA 1993b). DQOs are not necessarily the same as the acceptance criteria for a test, but should be viewed as target values. Because DQOs provide the best guidance about what levels of performance the supplier will seek to achieve, DQOs should reflect the customers' needs. For example, regulatory enforcement actions require different DQOs than would an exploratory study. Clearly, the development of DQOs should be part of the planning stages of a project so that expectations are shared by all participants and resources properly allocated.

COMPONENTS OF A QA PROGRAM IN Aquatic toxicity LABORATORIES

A review of USEPA evaluation guidance (USEPA 1991a) and of several QA manuals from laboratories conducting different aquatic toxicity tests suggests that there are common components of these QA programs. As illustrations, sections from three different documents are shown.

Elements of a QA program that are recommended for laboratories testing effluents (Table 2) may be worded as performance criteria, i.e., they specify elements of the program that need to be addressed in rather general terms.

Table 2. USEPA-recommended Elements of QA
for an Effluent testing Laboratory

The following elements are summarized from USEPA (1991a) Section 9, "Quality Assurance and Data Handling."

1. Maintain a written QA plan and QA program
2. Consider sampling, handling, and preservation of test material
3. Establish the health of the test organisms
4. Document instrument and equipment performance, calibration, and maintenance.
5. Document the methods and procedures used, including SOPs
6. Maintain data integrity
7. Review data evaluation procedures
8. Use reference toxicants and control charts
9. Document the entire testing process properly

Several QA elements are recognizable in section headings from a chapter on QA from the SOP manual (Table 3) of an aquatic toxicity testing laboratory that works primarily with effluents, such as whole effluent testing (WET) and toxicity identification evaluations (TIE). The components are consistent with the items in Table 2, but emphasize the details of the testing as developed for the specific laboratory.

Similarly, QA elements are illustrated by chapter titles from the QA manual of a laboratory that primarily tests chemical products, not wastewater effluents (Table 4). This type of laboratory often must comply with Good Laboratory Practice (GLP) regulations which require slightly different documentation and practices than are needed in wastewater effluent testing. Nevertheless, they address similar items.

In general, all the QA programs addressed the following eight components:
- capabilities and quality in past work
- staff development
- consistency in culture and test methods
- specific performance criteria
- standard operating procedures
- correct sample handling and custody practices
- accurate data collection and management
- search for improvement

Description of typical components of a QA program

1. Capabilities and quality in past work
Documentation to demonstrate the capabilities and quality of past work is typically contained in organizational histories, QA plans, descriptions of activities, lists of clients categorized by type of work done, and statements of capabilities. This information seeks to provide the customer with an acceptable level of confidence that the unit can meet the customer's needs, whether for demonstrating compliance with regulations or to support a product stewardship statement. This component can be expressed as a data quality objective: the customer needs to be very certain that the laboratory has demonstrated capability to produce acceptable test results.

An organizational history should demonstrate that the laboratory has an active testing program sufficient that the staff maintains expertise. In stating its capabilities, the laboratory should identify what types of testing it has conducted. Because of the variety of aquatic toxicity protocols in use, the laboratory should specify what methods or standard methods are used, what kinds of materials are tested, and what test organisms are used. Lists of clients can be useful in demonstrating past successes, but their use should not conflict with client's wishes for confidentiality. An organizational chart showing staffing and general responsibilities helps to convey the types of expertise within the organization. Use of subcontractors, for example, to conduct advanced chemical analyses, should be noted.

QA plans identify the expected and systematic actions necessary to provide adequate confidence that a product or service will satisfy given requirements for quality. A QA plan may address the management of an entire facility, e.g., the testing laboratory, or may be more limited in scope, focussing on a specific project, e.g., a QA project plan (USEPA 1993c; 1995a). A QA plan should be written and should cover all aspects of the laboratory's activity, including sampling, sample handling, test conditions, equipment, methods, record-keeping, data evaluation and reporting (USEPA 1991a). Training and improvement issues should also be considered in a QA plan. Guidance in QA plans and programs has been prepared by USEPA (1978, 1980, 1989a, 1991a) and by the American Society for Quality Control (ASQC 1991).

2. Staff development

Documentation of the development and maintenance of staff capabilities is typically provided in the form of position descriptions that state the functional responsibilities, combined with resumes or profiles of the training and experience of the technical staff. This information seeks to provide the customer with confidence about the precision, accuracy and comparability of the data.

The laboratory organization is responsible for establishing personnel qualifications and training requirements for all positions. The structure, functional responsibilities, levels of authority and job descriptions for activities should be documented. Each member of the organization must possess the education, training, technical knowledge, and experience, to perform the assigned functions. Personnel qualifications should be documented in terms of education, experience and training. Each member of the organization should have a clear understanding of her or his duties and the relationship of those responsibilities to the total effort. One person may cover more than one organizational function.

A laboratory staff organization typically is headed by a manager who bears the responsibility for the overall performance of the laboratory and establishes policy for the unit, including quality assurance. To properly supervise an aquatic toxicity and QA program, the manager must have sufficient training and experience. This often is interpreted to mean academic degree(s) in biological science plus a year or more experience in the conduct of aquatic toxicity testing, e.g., culturing, testing, analysis and interpretation.

A professional level person is responsible for the specific performance of a test or suite of tests. Position titles include principal investigator, project leader, and professional biologist. For larger projects, the principal investigator may supervise and coordinate several tasks performed by others. This person should be able to perform toxicological tests and the associated activities with no or minimal supervision. Preparation of reports, including analysis of the data and interpretation of the results, is also the responsibility of the principal investigator or project leader. Adequate training and experience usually includes an academic degree in biological science plus training and experience in aquatic toxicity testing. This level of experience is generally equivalent to the "professional biologist" level described by USEPA (1991a).

A technician is the person who conducts the aquatic toxicity testing and organism culture under supervision. The technician should be able to follow SOPs and collect reliable data generated by such methods. Minimum training and experience usually includes a high school education, supplemented by training in testing and culturing.

Training should be provided for all staff as necessary, so they can properly perform their functions. Training opportunities in toxicity testing include those offered by academic institutions, short courses offered by Federal or State agencies or through professional organizations, and practical training (on-the-job). Training descriptions should be included on the resumes of staff to document the improved competencies so acquired.

3. Consistency in culture and test methods

For standardized toxicity testing, customers expect the laboratory to follow methods that are widely accepted and practiced, i.e., standards, such as those established by ASTM or regulatory agencies. In other instances, technically justified modifications of standard methods are appropriate and necessary. In either situation, consistency is the key to adequate quality. To achieve consistency, the laboratory should demonstrate the consistency of the procedures (e.g., use of SOPs as discussed in a separate point) and the consistency of the materials and conditions of testing. This information provides the customer with high confidence that the results will have the maximum precision and accuracy associated with the method, and that the results can confidently be compared with data obtained previously or elsewhere using the standardized method.

In order to achieve consistency, appropriate and adequate equipment and facilities must be available. The laboratory facilities should provide a working environment that is clean, comfortable, and safe. The instrumentation and equipment must be suitable for the operational needs of the laboratory. The specific instrumentation, equipment, materials, and supplies needed for the performance of a standard test method are usually described in the written standard (e.g., aquatic toxicity test methods in the Annual Book of ASTM Standards, (ASTM 1994)).

The laboratory should be kept as free from environmental contamination as possible in order to protect cultured organisms, instrumentation, and test materials. Separation of areas for culture, testing, cleaning, storage, and chemical analyses is strongly recommended in order to avoid contamination of samples, cultures or tests, each of which can affect the precision, accuracy and comparability of test results.

Production of valid data requires maintaining samples as closely as possible to their original condition through careful handling and storage. Recommended or required procedures for collecting, transporting, handling and storage of test materials are described in the relevant standard methods (e.g., ASTM 1994).

A safe work environment is conducive to high quality work. Appropriate safety measures must be used, especially for handling wet materials and hazardous or potentially hazardous materials. Typical measures include the use of chemical hoods, floor mats, eye-wash and first-aid stations, and personal safety devices such as gloves, glasses, aprons, coats, or masks. Disposal of materials must be appropriate and comply with all applicable regulations, such as described in ASTM D 5283.

Production of consistent test organisms requires attention to the biological requirements and attributes of the species. The laboratory should monitor the health and productivity of the stock cultures used. The time and source of stock cultures, including species identification should be recorded. Foods used should be consistent in nutritional value and contaminant levels. If purchased or field-collected organisms are used, the laboratory should have procedures to ascertain and document the health and condition of these organisms.

Consistent methodology requires attention to maintenance and calibration of instrumentation and equipment, as well as their proper operation. The laboratory should have operating manuals available and provide for routine maintenance and calibration as needed. All maintenance and calibration activities should be recorded.

4. Specific performance criteria

Tests of laboratory performance involve testing a reference toxicant, analyzing control organism performance, and similar measurements to establish that the data were generated "in control," that is, systems were behaving as expected. This information provides confidence that the precision, accuracy, and comparability of the data are acceptable.

Performance of the laboratory must be related to criteria that permit determination of whether a procedure is being performed as expected. However, materials tested for aquatic toxicity may be unique, variable or unstable, such as a complex effluent that reflects the upstream operations, the effectiveness of wastewater treatment, and the matrix of a particular combination of materials from a discharger. Consequently, sample volume may be limited and its composition may be variable over time, preventing extensive repeated testing. Consequently, performance measures for aquatic toxicity tests use measurements or test materials that may be less direct measures than used in equivalent chemical analytical procedures, e.g., ASTM D 3856.

Commonly used performance measures for aquatic toxicity testing include: periodic testing of a reference toxicant, evaluation of control organism performance, and use of a simultaneous positive control (USEPA 1991a, b; EPS 1990). Periodic testing of a reference toxicant is accomplished by conducting a full-scale toxicity test using a pure chemical of known quality. Periodic tests of standard toxicants validate the accuracy of the method used and assure that the procedure is under control. A reference toxicant test also tests the condition of the test species when the test is conducted at the same time as a test on an effluent or product. By using the same toxicant, tested at the same concentrations in the same dilution water and analyzed by the same data analysis, sufficient data are generated to depict the expected range of results.

The results of repeated testing can be graphically displayed as a control chart that displays the test endpoint, such as an EC50, and upper and lower 95% confidence limits (often approximated as two standard deviations above and below the endpoint) over time (USEPA 1991a, 1993a). The endpoint ± two standard deviations can also be calculated for all accumulated data and plotted on the same control chart. Subsequent tests of the reference toxicant are judged to be "in control" if they yield endpoints within the upper and lower ranges of the cumulative data.

Long-term changes in the sensitivity of the test can be observed by evaluating the running average of the endpoint, e.g., the average of the three most recent tests. Changes in the precision of the test, reflecting the variability of the data, can be observed by evaluating the range between the upper and lower confidence limits--as laboratory experience removes sources of variability, the range should decrease. For a laboratory with substantial history in conducting tests, a control chart may document that relatively little has changed (Figure 1, used with permission of The Advent Group).

Control organism performance compares the observations made during the test with either absolute standards or historic standards. For example, whole effluent tests with *Ceriodaphnia* done using the USEPA protocol (USEPA 1993a) must demonstrate at least 90% survival of the control organisms during the acute (4 day) test. In whole effluent tests to evaluate chronic effects, control survival must be at least 80%, with an average of 15 young per surviving adult (USEPA 1989b, c; 1994a). The similar ASTM protocol (ASTM E 1295) requires that control survival must be at least 80%, that there be an average of 15 young per surviving adult, that the number of young per brood increase with each successive brood, and that young production start within 8 days of test initiation. All of the above performance criteria are absolute standards. However, some laboratories develop standards determined from their experience. For example, a laboratory may find that the *Ceriodaphnia* routinely produce 30 or more

Figure 1. **Ceriodaphnia dubia**
ACUTE REFERENCE TOXICANT TESTING
SODIUM CHLORIDE (NaCl) 1994-1995

(Used by permission of The Advent Group, Inc.)

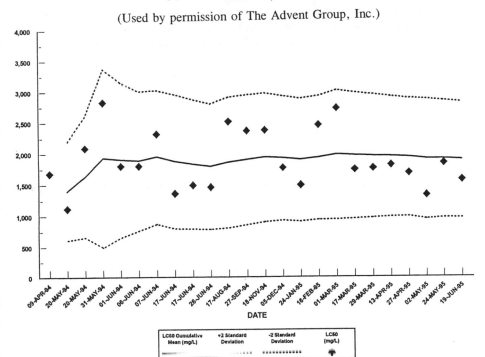

Table 3. QA Section of Standard Operating Procedure Manual

The section headings shown below are from a chapter on QA, part of the Standard Operating Procedure (SOP) manual for an aquatic toxicity testing laboratory that works primarily with effluents. (Used with permission.)

Water Sampling and Handling
Test Organisms
Culture Health - reference toxicants
    and control charts
Facilities, Equipment and
    Test Chambers
Analytical Methods

Calibration and Standardization
Dilution Water
Test Conditions
Test Acceptability
Documentation and Record
    Keeping

young per female in their chronic bioassays. For that laboratory, control performance of less than 30 young may mean that their system is out-of-control as regards their historical performance.

The use of a simultaneous positive control has been advocated as another tool to demonstrate the accuracy and comparability of test results (Henebry 1993). A positive control test group is treated by exposure to the concentration of the reference toxicant associated with the average endpoint as derived for the control chart. A test is accepted if the response of the positive control is reasonably similar to the average control chart endpoint. For example, if the EC50 is used as the endpoint, a positive control group would be exposed to a concentration equal to the average EC50. If this positive control shows partial effects, e.g., 30% or 70% response, then the performance is judged acceptable. Lack of any response suggests the test organisms were somewhat less sensitive than expected, while overwhelming response would suggest that the test organisms were more sensitive than expected. Henebry (1993) has used this approach with effluent toxicity tests using algae, *Ceriodaphnia* and fathead minnows.

Acceptance criteria can include the above items plus other data that suggest that test data might not be of suitable quality. These may include lack of adequate environmental controls, (e.g., temperature excursions beyond normal ranges), the presence of confounding, stressful conditions (e.g., low oxygen concentrations, pH variations), excessive differences in test material concentrations between replicate systems (e.g., measured concentrations ranging over two-fold among the same treatment group), the lack of replication, or the significant failure to observe the conditions of the protocol. Acceptance criteria are typically included in standard methods, e.g., ASTM E 729, ASTM E 1295, USEPA 1988a, 1989b, 1991b, 1993a, 1994a, b, 1995b.

5. Standard operating procedures
A SOP is a written procedure and is necessary to insure that a method is conducted consistently. This information provides confidence about the comparability and representativeness of the data.

The laboratory should have written SOPs for all procedures performed routinely that affect data quality. Because any equipment that comes in contact with the test organisms or test materials may reasonably affect data quality, SOPs are needed for virtually every routine procedure in the aquatic toxicity testing laboratory (USEPA 1991a). Table 4 provides an illustration of topics subject to SOP development.

Corrective actions are an important part of SOPs. Corrective actions are the procedures used to identify and correct deficiencies or variations from the SOP. The SOP should specify how a problem will be identified (e.g., definition of a deviation),

Table 4. QA Manual from Ecotoxicology Testing Lab.

Shown are the chapter titles from the QA manual of a laboratory that conducts aquatic ecotoxicology testing primarily on products, not wastewater effluents. (Used with permission.)

1. QA system description and policy
2. QA Manual
3. Organization and Management
4. Personnel
5. Environmental control and safety
6. Documentation and data control
7. Reports
8. Purchasing and contracts
9. Sample control
10. Test Equipment and methods
11. QC Practices
12. QA audits and inspections
13. Customer relations
14. Continuous improvement

what steps will be taken to correct the problem, and how to determine that the problem has been successfully resolved (e.g., validation of the correction).

Preparation of the SOP represents just one part of their appropriate use. SOPs must be readily available in the laboratory and the staff must be familiar with them. Staff training and updating the SOPs should be part of the laboratory's ongoing QA program.

6. Correct sample handling and custody practices

Test material may need specific handling or storage conditions to maintain stability, or materials may need to be tested in a timely manner, such as for compliance with NPDES permits (USEPA 1988b). In addition, legal enforcement actions may require special chain-of-custody procedures. Information about handling and custody provides confidence that the data are accurate and complete, and representative of the intended test material.

The requirements for sample handling and custody will vary with the test material and the intent of the aquatic toxicity test protocol, i.e., appropriate quality for these components must reflect the needs of the customer. Testing of pure substances, such as for product registration or stewardship will typically require appropriate chemical analyses to verify that the material was handled correctly and was in fact the intended material. Testing of effluents, such as for NPDES compliance, requires sampling, handling and custody procedures that meet the conditions of the NPDES permit. These are described in general terms by USEPA (1991a) but are detailed in the permit for a facility. Issues of concern include traceability of the sample, time from sampling to testing, holding conditions, and avoidance of any potential for contamination.

7. Accurate data collection and management

The procedures and tools used to record, transfer, manipulate, calculate, analyze and store data should be documented as part of the QA program. This information provides confidence that the data, especially as summarized and reported, are accurate and representative of the intended test material.

Basic aquatic toxicity data is most often recorded on data sheets and in bound laboratory notebooks. Instrumental data, such as produced in analytical methods, may be generated in computerized formats. The QA program should address how such original data are treated in the generation of summary statistics and report tables, as well as how the original data are maintained and archived. As laboratories make increased use of automated procedures for data collection and handling, such as Laboratory Information Management Systems (LIMS) and Good Automated Laboratory Practices (GALP), procedures to validate computer software and system security should be considered (USEPA 1990). Short and long-term storage of data and supporting information should be considered as well.

Procedures for entering, checking, and correcting data should be addressed. For best accuracy, data should be checked thoroughly during the test for outliers and gross mistakes, to permit early corrective actions or to avoid compounding errors. Transfers of data from worksheets to permanent logs or to computer files should be checked for accuracy. Corrections should clearly identify both the original entry and correction, as well as document the reason for correction and the person making the correction.

Procedures that transform data or calculate summary statistics should be validated using data sets with known results. Changes to the procedures or tools used (e.g., updated software versions) should be re-validated. Statistical programs used should follow any recommendations associated with the test design.

8. Search for improvement
    A basic tenet of ISO 9000 programs and similar quality management programs is the continuous improvement of the product or service (ISO 1987a, 1990). Consistent with this is the use of facility inspections and visits by outsiders (including customers), programmed self-evaluations, and accreditation by third-party organizations. Participation in round-robin or interlaboratory comparative testing is often part of these activities. This information provides confidence that the data have the best accuracy and precision attainable, and that results are comparable to data obtained previously or elsewhere.

Given the customer's interest in quality, site visits are often part of selecting a test laboratory. If the visitor is familiar with aquatic toxicity testing, then technical comments can be useful to the laboratory staff and management by helping identify oversights or problem areas. Even non-technical comments can be helpful. For example, one laboratory displayed test results in its facility, apparently to illustrate their capabilities. However, the presence of the customer's name on the results might be objectionable to some clients, as was realized by a visitor's comment. More formal inspections may be needed to evaluate some requirements, such as Good Laboratory Practices (GLP), or to audit past work.

An on-going effort at self-evaluation provides a means for managers and staff to consider recommendations and improvements. In general, the persons most capable of identifying opportunities are those directly involved in conducting aquatic toxicity testing, so this component ensures that this source is encouraged.

Accreditation is another means by which the quality of a laboratory can be evaluated (Royal and Jop 1993). While there may be no federal system for accrediting aquatic toxicity laboratories, USEPA has provided materials for performance testing in laboratories conducting NPDES effluent tests (USEPA 1991a). Some state certification programs exist, such as South Carolina's. Many state programs provide an endorsement for whole effluent testing for municipalities subject to state permits.

QUALITY MANAGEMENT AND THE AQUATIC TOXICOLOGY LABORATORY

The laboratory QA program has a number of features that echo TQM principles. Recognizing these helps encourage the business perspective noted in an earlier section. For example, W. Edwards Deming repeatedly emphasized 14 points for quality management (Walton 1990). While some of the statements are broadly worded, the overlap between Deming's quality management principles and the QA components is evident. Staff training is mentioned in principle 6 ("Institute training") and principle 13 ("Institute a vigorous program of education and training.") Principle 5 ("Improve constantly and forever the system of production and service") reflects the need for continuous improvement through inspections, visits, self-evaluations and accreditation. Principle 12 ("Remove barriers to the pride of workmanship") captures some observations made at past visits to testing laboratories: small touches in the laboratory evidenced the pride that staff had in their work, and this appeared more clearly in quality organizations. This suggests that the QA program can be an ongoing, internally-driven process.

A management concern about costs is frequently encountered with actions driven by QA. However, the cost of unacceptable tests and delayed regulatory action should be considered as part of the cost of bad quality. According to one report about toxicity studies submitted with pesticide registrations, rejected studies could cost industry about $600 to $1,200 million for repeated studies, and require about 97,800 additional USEPA review hours (Anon. 1995). While not the only cause for rejection, study quality is one factor cited for rejection. Unacceptable tests for effluents require repeated sampling as well as testing, meaning additional costs both for the supplier of the test (the laboratory) and the customer (who must provide the sample).

Discussions of the cost of quality are included in many business reviews (Lundvall and Juran 1974; Walton 1990; Peters 1987; Clemmer 1992). If we apply this concept to aquatic toxicity testing, several costs become visible. The expense of conducting an acute toxicity test is not especially large: current prices are in the $1000 to $2500 range for the basic tests. However, suppose that an effluent test needed to be repeated because it failed to meet acceptance criteria. Additional costs to the supplier would include (1) time and materials to repeat the test, (2) time and materials to investigate the cause of the lack of control and remedy it, (3) possible loss of the customer, and (4) possible loss of other customers or potential customers.

Business studies report that unhappy customers typically share their bad experiences with 9 or 10 other people (Clemmer 1992). So one way to estimate the cost of bad quality might be to presume that one lost customer represents 10 years of business with that customer plus 10 years of business with 9 other customers. If effluent tests were done quarterly, one lost customer might represent a loss of $400,000 (4 tests per year x $1,000 per test x 10 customers x 10 years). Few business ventures can afford such losses.

Additional costs to the customer would include: (1) staff time to decide if the work should be repeated by the same laboratory or contracted to another laboratory, (2) facility staff time to provide another sample, and (3) staff time to discuss the problematic results internally and with any regulatory agencies involved. If there were a product registration involved, as in the pesticide registrations discussed above, then delays in approval would mean lost sales revenue during the delay and possibly a permanent loss of market share as competitive products get a better start. Even if there are no registration issues, and the test is done to support product stewardship, i.e., provide accurate information to customers, a delay can adversely affect market position and perceived responsiveness to public or customer concern.

Finally, one sensitive aspect of many current organization structures is the creation of a QA officer. This position is often highly visible on the organization chart, frequently represented by a box to the side, like a flag hanging from the pole that extends from the director to the laboratory staff. While such a position emphasizes the autonomy of the QA function, it may simultaneously emphasize the concept of the "QA police," or subtly suggest that quality is the responsibility of this branch, not of management nor of operations. One observer described the problem with such a concept: quality is not something that the top can tell the middle to do to the bottom (Clemmer 1992). All organizational levels, including management must participate in quality programs.

CONCLUSIONS

Quality Assurance should be an integral part of aquatic toxicity testing. QA provides a tool by which the supplier, distributor and customer of aquatic toxicity services can gain confidence in the test results. QA provides a tool to evaluate and control performance in the aquatic toxicity laboratory. QA also provides a basis for supplier-customer discussion of the data quality necessary for a project. While the details of QA programs and requirements differ among laboratories doing aquatic toxicity testing, there are a number of common components addressed: the laboratory's past work, staff capabilities, culture and testing methods, evaluating performance against standards, use of SOPs, sample handling and custody, data collection and management, and improvement through evaluations from within and outside the organization. QA issues can have real impacts on the business success of the supplier and the customer, if total costs of quality are assessed. Poor quality work results in lost time, lost production and lost image, costs which ultimately are shared by the supplier and the customer. High quality work provides for better control, quicker responses and enhanced image, again ultimately shared by the supplier and the customer.

Acknowledgements

The authors thank Scott Hall and Erika Godwin-Saad of The Advent Group, Inc. for the information they provided and acknowledge the help from another laboratory that wished to remain anonymous. We also thank Loys P. Parrish and Lora S. Johnson of USEPA for their helpful review of the manuscript.

REFERENCES

Anonymous, 1995, "Ecological Effects Rejection Rate Still Too High, EPA Says." February 15, 1995, Pesticide & Toxic Chemical News, pp. 23-24.

ASQC (American Society for Quality Control), 1991. "Quality Assurance Program Requirements for Environmental Programs." ANSI/ASQC-E4. Milwaukee.

ASTM (American Society for Testing and Materials), 1994, Annual Book of ASTM Standards, Volumes 11.01, 11.02, 11.04. American Society for Testing and Materials, Philadelphia.

ASTM D 3856 "Standard Guide for Good Laboratory Practices in Laboratories Engaged in Sampling and Analysis of Water" Annual Book of ASTM Standards, Vol. 11.04. American Society for Testing and Materials, Philadelphia.

ASTM D 5283 "Standard Practice for Generation of Environmental Data Related to Waste Management Activities: Quality Assurance and Quality Control Planning and Implementation" Annual Book of ASTM Standards, Vol. 11.04. American Society for Testing and Materials, Philadelphia.

ASTM E 729 "Standard Guide for Conducting Acute Toxicity Tests with Fishes, Macroinvertebrates, and Amphibians," Annual Book of ASTM Standards, Vol. 11.04. American Society for Testing and Materials, Philadelphia.

ASTM E 1295 "Standard Guide for Conducting Three-brood, Renewal Toxicity Tests with Ceriodaphnia dubia," Annual Book of ASTM Standards, Vol. 11.04. American Society for Testing and Materials, Philadelphia.

Clemmer, J., 1992. Firing on All Cylinders: the Service/Quality System for High-Powered Corporate Performance. Irwin Professional Publ., Burr Ridge, Illinois. p. 131.

EPS, 1990. "Guidance document on control of toxicity test precision using reference toxicants." Environmental Protection Conservation and Protection Environmental Canada, Ottawa, Ontario, Environmental Protection Series, Report EPS 1/RM/12 August 1990.

Henebry, M., 1993. "Corrective Action Plans: Definitive Reference Toxicant Tests and Positive Control Reference Toxicant Tests (Draft)." Division of Laboratories, Illinois Environmental Protection Agency, Springfield, Illinois.

ISO, 1987a. "ISO 9000: Quality management and quality assurance standards--Guidelines for selection and use." International Organization for Standardization, Geneva, Switzerland.

ISO, 1987b. "ISO 9001: Quality systems -- Model for quality assurance in design/development, production, installation and servicing." International Organization for Standardization, Geneva, Switzerland.

ISO, 1987c. "ISO 9002: Quality systems -- Model for quality assurance in production and installation." International Organization for Standardization, Geneva, Switzerland.

ISO, 1987d. "ISO 9003: Quality systems -- Model for quality assurance in final inspection and test." International Organization for Standardization, Geneva, Switzerland.

ISO, 1990. "ISO Guide 25: General requirements for the competence of calibration and testing laboratories." 3rd Edition. International Organization for Standardization, Geneva, Switzerland.

Juran, J.M. 1974. Quality Control Handbook. 3rd. Edition, McGraw-Hill, Inc. NY. pp. 1-1 to 48A-10.

Lundvall, D.M. and J.M. Juran. 1974. "Quality Costs." In: J.M. Juran, Quality Control Handbook, McGraw-Hill, Inc., NY. pp. 5-1 to 5-22.

Peters, T , 1987 Thriving on Chaos; Handbook for a Management Revolution. Harper & Row, New York. 101 pp..

Royal, P.D. and K.M. Jop, 1993. "Quality assurance in programs regulated by the U.S. Environmental Protection Agency." Environmental Toxicology and Risk Assessment: 2nd Volume, ASTM STP 1216, J.W. Gorsuch, F.J. Dwyer, C.G. Ingersoll and T.W. LaPoint (Eds.) American Society for Testing and Materials, Philadelphia.

USEPA, 1978. Environmental monitoring series, Quality Assurance Guidelines for biological testing. Environmental Monitoring and Support Laboratory, Las Vegas, NV. EPA-600/4-78-043.

USEPA, 1980. "Guidelines and specifications for preparing quality assurance project plans." Report No. QAMS-005/80. Office of Monitoring and Quality Assurance, Office of Research and Development, U.S. Environmental Protection Agency, Washington DC.

USEPA, 1984. "Policy and program requirements to implement the quality assurance program." EPA Order 5360.1. U.S. Environmental Protection Agency, Washington, DC.

USEPA, 1988a. "Short-term methods for estimating the chronic toxicity of effluents and receiving waters to marine and estuarine organisms." C.I. Weber, W.B. Horning II, D.J. Klemm, T.W. Neiheisel, P.A. Lewis, E.L. Robinson, J. Mendedick, and F.A. Kessler (Eds.). Environmental Monitoring Systems Laboratory, U.S. Environmental Protection Agency, Cincinnati, OH. EPA/600/4-87/028.

USEPA, 1988b. "NPDES Compliance Inspection Manual," Office of Water Enforcement and Permits, U.S. Environmental Protection Agency, Washington, DC.

USEPA, 1989a. "Preparing perfect project plans. A pocket guide for the preparation of quality assurance project plans." U.S. Environmental Protection Agency, Office of Research and Development, Risk Reduction Engineering Laboratory, Cincinnati, OH 45268. EPA/600/9-89/087.

USEPA, 1989b. "Short-term methods for estimating the chronic toxicity of effluents and surface waters to freshwater organisms." 2nd Edition. C.I. Weber, W.H. Peltier, T.J. Norberg-King, W.B. Horning II, F.A. Kessler, J.R. Mendedick, T.W. Neiheisel, P.A. Lewis, D.J. Klemm, Q.H. Pickering, E.L. Robinson, J.M. Lazorchak, L.J. Wymer, and R.W. Freyberg (Eds.). Environmental Monitoring Systems Laboratory, U.S. Environmental Protection Agency, Cincinnati, OH. EPA/600/4-89/001.

USEPA, 1989c. "Supplement to Short-term methods for estimating the chronic toxicity of effluents and surface waters to freshwater organisms (EPA/600/4-89/001)." Environmental Monitoring Systems Laboratory, U.S. Environmental Protection Agency, Cincinnati, OH 45268.

USEPA, 1990. "Good automated laboratory practices." Office of Information Resources Management, U.S. Environmental Protection Agency, Research Triangle Park, NC (Draft).

USEPA, 1991a. "Manual for the evaluation of laboratories performing aquatic toxicity tests." D.J. Klemm, L.B. Lobring, and W.H. Horning II. Environmental Monitoring Systems Laboratory, U.S. Environmental Protection Agency, Cincinnati, OH 45268 EPA/600/1-90/001.

USEPA, 1991b. "Technical Support Document for Water Quality-based Toxics Control." Office of Water, U.S. Environmental Protection Agency, Washington, DC. EPA/505/2-90-001 (NTIS Order No. PB91-127415).

USEPA, 1993a. "Methods for measuring the acute toxicity of effluents and receiving waters to freshwater and marine organisms." 4th Edition. C.I. Weber (Ed.). Environmental Monitoring Systems Laboratory, U.S. Environmental Protection Agency, Cincinnati, OH 45268. EPA/600/4-90/027F.

USEPA, 1993b. "Fish Field and Laboratory Methods for evaluating the biological integrity of surface waters." D. J. Klemm, Q.J. Stober, and J.M. Lazorchak. Environmental Monitoring Systems Laboratory, U.S. Environmental Protection Agency, Cincinnati, OH 45268. EPA/600/R-92/111.

USEPA, 1993c (Draft). "EPA requirements for quality assurance project plans for environmental data operations." EPA QA/R5. U.S. Environmental Protection Agency, Quality Assurance Management Staff, Washington, DC.

USEPA, 1994a. "Short-term methods for estimating the chronic toxicity of effluents and surface waters to freshwater organisms" 3rd Edition. P.A. Lewis, D.J. Klemm, J.M. Lazorchak, T.J. Norberg-King, W.H. Peltier, and M.A. Heber (Eds.). Environmental Monitoring Systems Laboratory, U.S. Environmental Protection Agency, Cincinnati, OH 45268. EPA/600/4-91/002.

USEPA, 1994b. "Short-term methods for estimating the chronic toxicity of effluents and receiving waters to marine and estuarine organisms" 2nd Edition. D.J. Klemm, G.E. Morrison, J.M. Lazorchak, T.J. Norberg-King, W.H. Peltier, and M.A. Heber (Eds.). Environmental Monitoring Systems Laboratory, U.S. Environmental Protection Agency, Cincinnati, OH 45268. EPA/600/4-91/003.

USEPA, 1995a "Generic quality assurance project plan guidance for programs using community level biological assessment in wadable streams and rivers." Assessment and Watershed Protection Division, Monitoring Branch, Office of Water, U.S. Environmental Protection Agency, Washington, DC 20460 EPA 841-B-95-004.

USEPA 1995b. "Short-term methods for estimating the chronic toxicity of effluents and receiving waters to west coast marine and estuarine organisms." G.A. Chapman, D.L. Denton, and J.M. Lazorchak (eds). National Exposure Research Laboratory, U.S. Environmental Protection Agency, Cincinnati, OH 45268. EPA/600/R-95-136.

Walton, M., 1990. Deming Management at Work. Perigee Books, New York. 249 pp.

W. Scott Hall[1]

A REVIEW OF LABORATORY TOXICITY IDENTIFICATION PROCEDURES-INVESTIGATIVE AND APPLIED APPROACHES

REFERENCE: Hall, W. S., "A Review of Laboratory Toxicity Identification Procedures-Investigative and Applied Approaches," *Environmental Toxicology and Risk Assessment: Biomarkers and Risk Assessment—Fifth Volume, ASTM STP 1306,* David A. Bengtson and Diane S. Henshel, Eds., American Society for Testing and Materials, 1996.

ABSTRACT: This paper reviews some of the laboratory Toxicity Identification Evaluation (TIE) protocols published to date. A history of the development of these techniques and their application in effluents is presented. Also presented are examples of applications of these techniques, a review of selected techniques, a summary of individual techniques and the chemicals they remove or render nontoxic, and case studies. Many laboratory TIE techniques are available beyond those published by USEPA, and a myriad of techniques have been successfully applied. The published techniques were found to be generally "investigative" or "applied" in nature. It is concluded from this review that the generally chemical-specific investigative techniques and the applied techniques, which do not emphasize the identification of specific toxicants, can both be useful under various conditions. However, it is recommended that as a means to preliminarily evaluate full-scale wastewater treatment options and possibly identify specific toxicants amenable to "upstream" control, laboratory TIE methodologies combining both approaches be used.

KEYWORDS: Toxicity Identification Evaluation, TIE, Toxicity Reduction Evaluation, TRE, Aquatic Toxicity, Toxicity Characterization, Fractionation, Wastewater Treatment

[1] Manager, Ecotoxicology Group, The ADVENT Group, Inc. Brentwood, TN 37027.

INTRODUCTION

In recent years dischargers have increasingly been required to reduce or eliminate whole effluent toxicity (WET) to aquatic organisms. These requirements often call for the reduction of acute toxicity, but regulatory agencies are increasingly concerned about and requiring the control of chronic effluent toxicity. Inherent to any toxicity control program is the process of appropriately documenting effluent toxicity, identifying the cause of toxicity, and subsequently identifying and applying the most cost-effective measures to achieve toxicity compliance. Laboratory Toxicity Identification Evaluation (TIE) methodologies have received increased attention and have been incorporated in the United States Environmental Protection Agency's (USEPA) approach to identifying and controlling WET (Burkhard and Ankley 1989). Most of the work in this area has been done with freshwater effluents.

Laboratory TIE History

Some of the earliest work done to separate the components of a mixture having biological effects was done with cigarette smoke (Swain et al. 1969). Similar "fractionation" techniques were applied to evaluate the carcinogenic and mutagenic effects of different components of synthetic crude oils (Rubin et al. 1989). Some of the first aquatic toxicity identification or "fractionation" protocols were published by Parkhurst et al. (1979) and Walsh and Garnas (1983). Walsh also briefly presented this protocol in an early USEPA acute toxicity testing manual (USEPA 1985a).

Wide-spread interest in laboratory TIE procedures rapidly developed with the initial release of USEPA's "Phase I" (USEPA 1988). "Phase II" (USEPA 1989a) and "Phase III" (USEPA 1989b) documents. The Phase I, II, and III documents provide methodologies for the characterization, identification, and confirmation, respectively, of the acutely toxic constituents in freshwater effluents. These procedures received wide-spread application in efforts to identify the specific cause of effluent toxicity, and were suggested for use in toxicity reduction protocols published by USEPA for industrial (USEPA 1989c) and municipal (USEPA 1989d) effluent toxicity control. More recently, the USEPA has published revised toxicity characterization protocols primarily for acutely toxic effluents (USEPA 1989e) as well as protocols specifically designed to characterize the source of toxicity in chronically toxic effluents (USEPA 1991). In 1993, USEPA published protocols designed to identify (USEPA 1993a) and confirm (USEPA 1993b) the sources of toxicity in effluents exhibiting acute and chronic toxicity. In 1994, USEPA released a guidance document for conducting TIEs in marine settings (USEPA 1994). Throughout this time others have developed various laboratory TIE protocols, and some investigators have begun research to automate laboratory TIE procedures (Fort et al. 1995). The use of laboratory TIE procedures in Toxicity Reduction Evaluations (TREs) has been discussed by Hall and Mirenda (1990), and Backus and DiGiano (1994), and has been reviewed by others in various texts (Lankford and Eckenfelder 1990, Ford 1992).

Purpose

Despite the cost-effectiveness and increased emphasis on laboratory TIE procedures, there has to date been no review of available methods for conducting laboratory TIE studies. Much of the work in this area has essentially utilized the widely popular methods published by USEPA. Although very useful "investigative" tools for identifying the specific chemical(s) possibly causing effluent toxicity, many treatment steps in the USEPA protocols are not amenable to full-scale application in wastewater treatment facilities. Other protocols utilize a more "applied" approach, developing data useful in preliminary evaluations of possible wastewater treatment technologies.

This paper reviews some of the investigative and applied laboratory TIE procedures published to date and discusses the applications of various investigative and applied techniques such that the benefits of each approach are evident. The goal of this paper is to provide an overview of the laboratory TIE protocols available, review their various applications, and provide examples of protocols which provide "screening level" data useful in identifying potentially applicable full-scale treatment technologies for toxicity control.

LABORATORY TOXICITY IDENTIFICATION PROCEDURES AND APPLICATIONS

One of the most cost-effective and expedient ways to identify the cause(s) of effluent toxicity is through the use of laboratory effluent "fractionation" or characterization protocols. These protocols utilize physical and chemical techniques to manipulate the effluent in such a way as to either separate the effluent components into major chemical groups (e.g., organic and inorganic) or reduce toxicity caused by specific groups of chemicals (e.g., metals, volatiles, etc.). Acute and/or chronic toxicity endpoints (e.g., LC_{50} Values, IC25 Values, respectively) in untreated effluent are compared to those for the same effluent sample treated in various ways so as to reduce the toxicity associated with various but specific groups of chemicals.

The term "fractionation" appeared in the early literature on these methods and is still used somewhat interchangeably with the terms TIE, and "toxicity characterization" to describe these techniques. As the USEPA methods evolved and were modified, other investigators developed methods to identify the chemical specifically responsible for effluent toxicity. Still other methods were developed which characterized the physical/chemical nature of the toxicant without emphasis on identifying the specific toxicant, but rather developing data useful in planning other studies of potentially successful full-scale treatment methodologies. In application, the chemical-specific/investigative techniques are best applied when identification of a specific toxicant(s) is likely to lend itself to more cost-effective "upstream" control of toxicants on a smaller volume basis (as compared to treating the whole effluent). The applied techniques are useful in screening for treatment technologies to be applied end-of-pipe or at key upstream locations. Selected examples of these techniques are provided below.

Investigative Techniques

The methods of Parkhurst *et al.* (1979) indicated that solvent extraction techniques were effective to separate the organic and inorganic components of synthetic fuels into their respective toxic components to *Daphnia magna*. Walsh and Garnas' (1983) protocol utilized techniques to first separate effluents into organic (acid, base, and neutral) and inorganic components, then additional techniques were utilized to further identify the causative toxicant(s). They utilized both freshwater and saltwater algae and crustaceans to evaluate the cause of toxicity in municipal and industrial effluents. More recently, the most up-to-date in the series of USEPA toxicity characterization (Phase I), identification (Phase II), and confirmation (Phase III) documents were released by the USEPA (USEPA 1989e, 1993a, 1993b, respectively), as were toxicity characterization protocols specifically for chronically toxic effluents (USEPA 1991).

The USEPA "Phase I" toxicity characterization procedures (USEPA 1989e) are designed to reduce or remove toxicity associated with different groups of chemicals (e.g., heavy metals, volatile or sorbable compounds, oxidants, etc.). Each step either removes a certain group of chemicals (e.g., via volatilization) or renders them biologically unavailable (e.g., metal chelation). The techniques rely heavily on the effect of pH on chemical form and toxicity and include: pH adjustment and filtration, pH adjustment and aeration, pH adjustment and C_{18} extraction, oxidant reduction with sodium thiosulfate, metal chelation with EDTA, and graduated pH testing for metals and ammonia toxicity evaluation.

The USEPA Phase II toxicity identification procedures have been less widely applied, but contain useful methodologies for further identifying and confirming suspected toxicants (USEPA 1993a). For example, in Phase II testing a useful procedure is presented for identifying non-polar organics. These compounds are removed from an effluent by sorption onto long chain (C_{18}) carbon resins, selectively removed with a solvent (typically methanol) tested for toxicity, and the specific chemical toxicants identified through HPLC or GC/MS methodologies.

Other methods for the identification of ammonia and toxic heavy metals are also presented. Confirmatory methods presented in the "Phase III" document (USEPA 1993b) include the evaluation of test species toxicity symptoms, evaluating differences in species sensitivity, spiking the effluent with the suspect toxicant, and other methodologies. These and similar techniques have been successfully applied to effluents and other media (e.g., sediments). The latest USEPA protocols are also often successfully combined with "before-and-after" chemical analyses to identify specific chemical toxicants. The USEPA techniques for identifying toxicants causing chronic toxicity (USEPA 1991) are very similar in methodology and application to the other USEPA procedures.

Specialized investigative methodologies have been published by Ankley et al. (1990) and Ankley and Burkhard (1990) for the identification of surfactants. Durhan et al. (1990, 1993) have published results specific to USEPA solid phase sorption/solvent extraction techniques which are very useful in identifying nonpolar organic toxicants. Some chemical-specific techniques have been published by Ankley et al. (1991), who used piperonyl butoxide to identify toxicity due to metabolically-activated organophosphate insecticides. Other techniques include the use of buffers to control pH to identify pH-altered toxicants (e.g., heavy metals, ammonia) as opposed to reducing test vessel head space for pH control as outlined in the various USEPA protocols.

Various derivations of the USEPA protocols coupled with chemical analyses have also successfully identified toxicants such as diazinon (Amato et al. 1992) and nonpolar organics (Burkhard et al. 1990). Methylparathion and carbofuran were identified as likely causes of toxicity in ambient waters using USEPA techniques and chemical analyses (Norberg-King et al. 1991). Finally, Burkhard and Jenson (1993) utilized USEPA Phase I, II, and III techniques as well as chemical testing in a toxicity identification study of a municipal effluent. Chromium, ammonia, and diazinon were identified as the causative toxicants.

Applied Techniques

Some of the more applied techniques (i.e., those integrating TIE methodologies with treatments potentially applicable in full-scale waste treatment operations) have typically been developed using effluents. For example, Reece and Burks (1985) published an early aquatic toxicity fractionation protocol which first separated refinery effluent components into volatile and non-volatile components (via steam stripping), then further characterized the toxicants with other treatments (e.g., organic carbon) and chemical analyses. Silica gel and ion exchange techniques were also applied, as were chemical analyses to assist in toxicant identification.

Gasith et al. (1988) also utilized activated carbon and ion exchange resins for toxicant identification in a complex wastewater. They used filtration and aeration in a protocol based on sequential physical/chemical separations. The approach of Doi and Grothe (1989) was based on the concepts utilized by Walsh and Garnas (1983), and utilized ion exchange resins, activated carbon, and silica gel to separate an effluent into its various organic and inorganic components. Building on the results with fractionation testing, Dorn et al. (1991) applied a hazard assessment and structure-activity approach to various organic toxicants present in a petrochemical plant effluent. Multiple species toxicity tests with individual chemicals and field validation studies were used to confirm results. Goodfellow et al. (1989) also used a multispecies fractionation approach in identifying toxicants. This study was conducted with a municipal effluent.

The toxicity characterization methods published by Hall and Mirenda (1990) expand and modify the USEPA Phase I methodologies in screening-level testing of technologies which could be applied in whole effluent or wastewater treatment scenarios (e.g., powdered carbon, pH adjustment and polymer addition, ion exchange). These techniques use smaller numbers of test organisms and batch bench-scale treatments to identify potentially promising effluent toxicity control technologies. Jop et al. (1991) utilized modified fractionation procedures such as filtration, nitrogen, purging, specialty resins, and zeolite, coupled with extensive chemical analyses in a TIE of a chemical plant effluent.

Other Applications and Endpoints

Whole effluent techniques have been applied to the identification of toxicants in hazardous waste site leachates and sediment pore waters, and toxicity endpoints other than those associated with regulatory effluent testing have been used. For example, Kuehl et al. (1990) and USEPA (1985b) have applied fractionation techniques to identify causative toxicants in hazardous waste site leachates. Ankley et al. (1992) have also applied or proposed the use of USEPA techniques to identify toxicants in sediment interstitial waters or dredged materials. Mutagenicity and teratogenicity have been utilized as endpoints in protocols published by Doreger et al. (1988), West et al. (1988), and Holmbom et al. (1983).

Review of Selected Treatment Steps

A list of selected toxicity identification/characterization techniques used in various media has been compiled from the above references. These methods are briefly discussed below as relates to the constituents removed or rendered biologically unavailable by each procedure. Some of the inherent limitations and caveats associated with some treatments are discussed. A distinction is made for each technique as to whether it is generally amenable to application on a full-scale basis for effluent toxicity control. Experimentally, a procedure is applied to a toxic effluent sample then compared to untreated effluent to assess toxicity reduction.

Air Stripping-Samples are vigorously air-stripped at the original effluent pH, and under highly acidic and basic conditions. Air stripping removes volatile and pH extractable organic chemicals as well as some inorganic chemicals (e.g., hydrogen sulfide and ammonia). Shifting the pH alters the form of some chemicals making them less ionic and hence more likely to air strip. Air stripping is a readily applicable wastewater treatment technique. "Sublimation" of chemicals during air stripping may give a false indication of the true mechanism of toxicity removal.

Nitrogen Stripping-Stripping with inert nitrogen gas is utilized when the true mechanism of removal must be verified in successful air stripping tests. Utilization of nitrogen controls for the possibility that air stripping tests were successful due to oxidation as opposed to volatilization of the chemicals removed.

C_{18} Adsorption-Long chain C_{18} resins are utilized to remove non-polar organic substances and some metal complexes. Varying pH levels are used to alter the form of chemicals in the effluent to convert them to less polar and hence more adsorbable forms. Elution with organic solvents such as methanol and subsequent chemical analysis is used to identify chemical toxicants. C_{18} resin would not be economically applied in effluent toxicity control programs.

Activated Carbon-Activated carbon treatments are typically conducted at ambient effluent pH, but can be conducted at varying pH as done in C_{18} testing. Activated carbon primarily removes organic chemicals by adsorption and pore entrapment, and some metals due to sorption and possibly ion exchange. Activated carbon removes a wide variety of chemicals and is readily applicable in effluent toxicity control programs.

Filtration-Sample filtration is typically conducted with a one-micron or smaller glass fiber filter to remove toxicity associated with particulate-bound toxicants. Sample pH adjustment can also be utilized to compare to unadjusted, filtered effluent. This may indicate that pH adjustment has altered the form of the toxic constituents such that they adsorb to particulates in the sample, or are precipitated at a different pH and are removed by filtration. Unless conducted under positive pressure, false indications of the mechanism of toxicity removal can occur with this technique if readily volatile toxicants are involved.

Filtration is readily applied in wastewater treatment programs and can be augmented with polymers prior to filtration. It should be cautioned, however, that polymers can be a cause of toxicity if "overdosed" beyond minimum levels needed for solids removal.

Zeolite Resin-Zeolite treatment is typically utilized in conjunction with high pH (11) air stripping and graduated pH tests to confirm or refute the presence of ammonia as the causative toxicant. Although zeolite possesses some ion exchange capacity and removes constituents other than ammonia (e.g., some metals), it is a useful step for comparison with the results of other tests designed to remove ammonia. Zeolite resins have some specific application in wastewater treatment programs.

Oxidant Reduction-Sodium thiosulfate is added to the effluent to reduce toxic oxidants such as chlorine. This step is very effective when oxidants are present. However, sodium thiosulfate can also reduce toxicity due to certain metals (e.g., copper). Other, more cost-effective oxidant reducers (e.g., bisulfite) are typically applied in wastewater treatment.

Metals Chelation-A chelating agent such as EDTA is added to the effluent to chelate toxic heavy metals. Many polyvalent, cationic heavy metals are chelated by EDTA, but anionic forms of heavy metals are not chelated (e.g., selenites, chromates). Other chelating agents such as nitrilotriacetic acid (NTA) have also been used successfully. These techniques are experimental in nature as they do not physically remove metals from solution and therefore do not achieve lower levels of effluent metals.

Ion Exchange-Cation and anion exchange resins have been used quite successfully to remove toxicity due to inorganics or to separate effluents into inorganic and organic components. These resins are typically applied to samples containing high levels of dissolved solids which are typically considered innocuous at lower levels (e.g., sodium, chlorides, etc.). The resins applied in succession are often successful at removing toxicity due to high levels of dissolved solids. These resins also remove toxic heavy metals either due to direct ion exchange (cation resin) or due to precipitation due to high pH in the case of hydroxide anion exchange resins. Ammonia is also readily removed by cation exchange resins. Ion exchange resins are applicable to full-scale effluents, and especially to highly concentrated, low-volume upstream wastes.

Graduated pH Testing-By testing the effluent under varying pH conditions within the physiologically tolerable range of the test organisms one can gain information on the type of toxicants present. For example, if toxicity is increased at pH 6 versus pH 8, one might suspect that metals are responsible for the observed toxicity due to increased solubility and hence toxicity of many metals. If toxicity is increased by an increase in pH, ammonia might be the causative toxicant due to the increased amount of the unionized, toxic form of ammonia with increased pH. These procedures are essentially only investigative in nature.

Chemical Oxidation-Rapid oxidation of chemicals with catalyzed hydrogen peroxide can degrade recalcitrant organic chemicals to non-toxic forms. This procedure represents a realistic pretreatment option. Ozone can also be utilized as a characterization step. Experimentally, one must be careful to reduce any remaining free oxidants which may cause toxicity.

Solvent Extraction-Extraction of organic chemicals with solvents has been successfully used in selected cases. However, problems with solvent toxicity often preclude the use of this procedure. Solvent extraction can also be used to separate an effluent into its organic and inorganic components. Solvent extraction is, however, a viable source control technology for wastes containing high concentrations of organic chemicals.

Molecular Sieves-Molecular sieves can be utilized to assess the toxicity of chemicals with different ranges of molecular weights. These procedures can be used to identify specific organic chemicals following tentative identification with more generic methods. This provides a useful investigative tool. However, the biocides used to preserve some of these sieves can cause sample toxicity if not properly leached prior to use.

Precipitation and Coagulation-High pH precipitation followed by polymer coagulation, alum/lime treatments, and sulfide treatments have been successfully used for the removal of some heavy metals. Appropriate controls must be run on these procedures due to the toxic nature of these additives if over dosed. Such techniques are readily applied in full-scale toxicity control programs.

Specialty Resins-Specialty treatment resins such as those designed to remove organic chemicals via pore entrapment and/or adsorption have been used quite successfully in selected applications. Specialty resins such as the XAD Amberlite® resins can be utilized to remove both polar and nonpolar organics. These resins can be effective in removing toxicity due to polar organics when other media are ineffective. Other resins such as "green sand" can also be used to remove inorganic constituents such as manganese.

Aging/Persistence Evaluation-The persistence of effluent toxicity can be evaluated through exposure of an uncovered effluent to light at room temperature for 24 to 48 hours. The necessary volume for a toxicity test is set aside and a toxicity test is conducted at the end of the aging period. Although not designed to identify toxicity due to any specific chemical group, results of the persistence evaluation may be used to support data generated from other fractionation steps.

CASE STUDIES

Case Study No. 1

Table 1 presents the results of a study with *Ceriodaphnia dubia* in which the fractionation of a moderately toxic effluent ($LC_{50} \approx 35$ percent) resulted in an increase in the LC_{50} value to >100 percent for several treatments. This is fairly common with effluents which are not highly toxic. Toxicity was reduced to the extent that an LC_{50} value could not be calculated (LC_{50}>100 percent) as a result of five different treatments:

- Nitrogen stripping at pH 11
- C_{18} treatment at the original sample pH
- Powdered carbon treatment
- Anion exchange
- Sodium thiosulfate addition

It should be noted that the confidence intervals of LC_{50} values overlapped. Due to the wide range of confidence intervals around LC_{50}s generated using the binomial method, it is very difficult to achieve statistical significance. However, the importance of the degree of toxicity removal by a treatment is obvious regardless of the lack of statistical significance. Other treatments which resulted in a clear increase in LC_{50} values included air stripping at pH 11 and cation exchange, which each raised the LC_{50} value of untreated effluent from 35.4 percent to greater than 70 percent. Removal of toxicity by powdered activated carbon (PAC) and C_{18} resin at the original sample pH may indicate that the chemical(s) responsible for toxicity are sorptive at near neutral pH. The fact that anion exchange and sodium thiosulfate treatment both removed toxicity indicates that an oxidant of some sort played a role in causing toxicity in the untreated sample. However, toxicity removal by nitrogen stripping at pH 11 and a large toxicity reduction by air stripping at pH 11 indicate that a base volatile compound was contributing to effluent toxicity. This is supported by the fact that toxicity was removed by cation exchange resin, since a cationic organic compound would be uncharged at pH 11 and hence volatile. The success of both air and N_2 stripping at pH 11 verifies that the mechanism of toxicity removal was volatilization and not oxidation during the pH 11 air stripping tests. The clear success of the anion exchange and high pH purging indicates a cationic toxicant, there were likely two different toxicants present in the untreated effluent. In order to resolve the actual sources of toxicity in this effluent, definitive analytical comparisons of before and after treatment samples would have to be conducted.

Case Study No. 2

Table 2 presents results of a fractionation study with *Daphnia pulex*. The effluent was moderately toxic and resulted in an LC_{50} of $\approx$ 52 percent. Treatments increasing the LC_{50} to > 100 percent were:

I.   Air stripping at pH 3
II.   Air stripping at pH 11
III. C_{18} treatment at pH 3
IV.   Zeolite resin treatment

Removal of toxicity by air stripping at pH 3 and pH 11 indicates that two toxicants were likely present, each of which is readily volatile under different pH conditions. The fact that C_{18} treatment at pH 3 removed toxicity indicates that a chemical was present which is also readily sorbed under low pH conditions. An organic chemical unionized at pH 3 should both sorb to C_{18} resin and be volatile. The results are thus in good agreement in this regard, and indicate that an acid-extractable compound was at least partially responsible for toxicity. The success of pH 11 air stripping can only be explained by the presence of a second toxicant of similar toxicity. The marginal success of both the cation and anion exchange resins further indicates the presence of two toxicants. Due to the success of the zeiolite resin treatment it is possible that ammonia is the other toxicant present in this effluent since ammonia would be removed by both zeolite and pH 11 air stripping.

Case Study No. 3.

Table 3 presents results of a fractionation study utilizing *D. pulex* and fathead minnows which compares toxicity removal for different species. The sample was very toxic to both *D. pulex* and the fathead minnow, with LC_{50} values of 0.12 and 1.2 percent respectively. Statistically significant increases in *D. pulex* LC_{50} values (reductions in toxicity) were achieved by PAC, and by pH 11 precipitation/filtration techniques. Although not statistically significant, the largest increase in the *D.* pulex LC_{50} value was achieved by a high level addition of EDTA. Other clear increases in *D. pulex* LC_{50} values were achieved by C_{18} treatment at pH 9 and by cation exchange, with the lower 95 percent confidence intervals for these treatments just bordering the upper 95 percent confidence intervals for the untreated effluent. Since pH 11 precipitation and filtration, high level EDTA treatment, and cation exchange all reduced toxicity, it is very likely that a heavy metal was responsible for toxicity to *D. pulex*. PAC can be expected to partially remove metals and the partial success of this treatment (although statistically significant) supports the hypothesis for metal toxicity. The success of the pH 9 C_{18} treatment also indicated metal toxicity since precipitation at pH 9 and physical removal (filtration) by the C_{18} resin bed also removes metals. The success of the anion exchange resin does not necessarily contradict the metals toxicity theory. Metals containing precipitated hydroxide forms, for example, are removed by the high pH, hydroxide anion exchange resin due to physical filtration.

The results of the fathead minnow fractionation with this same effluent also indicated that metals were the source of toxicity. The pH 9 C_{18} treatment, powdered carbon, cation exchange, anion exchange, zeolite, pH 11 precipitation and filtration, and high level EDTA treatment clearly reduced or removed effluent toxicity. Removal of toxicity ($LC_{50} > 100\%$) to the fathead minnow was achieved for all of these treatments except powdered carbon. Statistically significant increases in LC_{50} values were achieved by the high EDTA treatment, zeolite resin, pH 11 precipitation/filtration, and anion exchange. Removal of metals toxicity to fathead minnows would be achieved by these treatments as previously discussed for *D. pulex*. The pH 11 precipitation/filtration process was the only treatment resulting in statistically significant increases in the LC_{50} value for both species. This, coupled with the other results for both species (i.e., high EDTA treatments) solidifies the case for metal toxicity, supporting the metal toxicity theory.

An interesting result of this case study was the observed difference in species response to the treated and untreated effluents. None of the treatments removed toxicity to *D. pulex* to the extent that the LC_{50} value was > 100 percent, while five treatments accomplished this for the fathead minnow. This likely relates to the difference in sensitivity of *D. pulex* and *P. promelas* to heavy metals in general. Trace levels of heavy metals are often toxic to daphnids, while the fathead minnow is less sensitive to many metals. This finding illustrates the need to run tests with more than one species in preliminary fractionation studies.

Case Studies Summary

The case studies presented illustrate many of the previously discussed fractionation considerations. Most importantly, the results do not always clearly indicate the cause of toxicity. This is especially true for moderately or low toxicity effluents for which several treatments reduce toxicity. In these cases, the source of toxicity may be better defined by repeating fractionations until patterns develop. It cannot be emphasized enough that decisions on the source of toxicity should never be made based on the results of one fractionation study. Decisions on the source of toxicity and any control decisions should be based on multiple fractionations utilizing analytical support, and must consider specific conditions present at the facility. The "all or nothing" pattern of toxicity removal was observed for many of the treatments employed. This pattern is very common and has been observed for many other effluents studied, particularly when the effluent is not markedly toxic.

SUMMARY

All of the reviewed techniques can be used in a toxicity characterization or TIE study. These steps are intended to identify the likely group of chemicals responsible for toxicity. Although some are quite limited in their applicability in full-scale toxicity control programs, they provide data on the true mechanisms of toxicity control. Developing complementary data in a "weight-of-the-evidence" approach to identifying and controlling toxicity has been proposed by others. The author's experience has also shown that a combination of investigative and applied techniques is most useful. For example, EDTA and high pH filtration, as well as high pH air stripping and zeolite, are often used when toxicity due to heavy metals and ammonia, respectively, is suspected. Such an approach: 1) screens for potentially useful full-scale treatment technologies, 2) often provides confirmatory data as to the mechanisms of toxicity removal, and 3) determines whether further studies and supporting chemical analyses are required without *a priori* committing such resources. The experimental design in TIE studies must consider the investigative versus the applied nature of each potential technique, and several of these characterization studies must be conducted before a decision as to the likely cause of toxicity can be reached.

REFERENCES

Amato, J.R., Mount, D.I., Durhan, E.J., Lukasewycz, M.T., Ankley, G.T., and Roberts, E.D., 1992, "An example of the Identification of Diazinon as a Primary Toxicant in an Effluent," Env. Tox. and Chem., Vol. 11, pp 209-316.

Ankley, G.T., and Burkhard, L.P., 1990, "Identification of Surfactants as Toxicants in Primary Effluent," Env. Tox. Chem., Vol. 11, pp 1235-1248.

Ankley, G.T., Dierkes, J.R., Jensen, D.A., and Peterson, G.S., 1991, "Piperonyl Butoxide as a Tool in Aquatic Toxicological Research with Organophosphorus Insecticides," Ecotox. and Evn. Safety, Vol. 21, pp 226-274.

Ankley, G.T., Peterson, G.S., Lukasewycz, M.T., and Jensen, D.A., 1990, "Characteristics of Surfactants in Toxicity Identification Evaluations," Chemosphere, Vol. 21, No. 1-2, pp 3-12.

Ankley, G.T., Schubauer-Berigan, M.K., and Hoke, R.A., 1992, "Use of Toxicity Identification Evaluation Techniques to Identify Dredged Material Disposal Options: A Proposed Approach," Env. Mngt., Vol. 16, No. 1, pp 1-6.

Backus, P.M., and DiGiano, F.A., March 1994, "The Trouble with TREs," Water Env. & Tech., pp 57-60.

Burkhard, L.P., and Ankley, G.T., 1989, "Identifying Toxicants: NETAC's Toxicity-Based Approach," Env. Sci. Technol., Vol. 23, No. 12, pp 1438-1443.

Burkhard, L.P., and Jenson, J.J., 1993 "Identification of Ammonia, Chlorine and Diazinon as Toxicants in a Municipal Effluent," Arch. Env. Contam. Toxicol.. Vol. 25, pp 506-515.

Burkhard, L.P., Durhan, E.J., and Lukasewycz, M.T., 1990, "Identification of Nonpolar Toxicants in Effluents Using Toxicity-Based Fractionation with Gas Chromatography/Mass Spectrometry," Anal. Chem., Vol. 63, pp 277-283.

Doi, J., and Grothe, D.R., 1989, "Use of Fractionation and Chemical Analysis Schemes for Plant Effluent Toxicity Evaluations," Aquatic Toxicology and Environmental Fate, ASTM JSTP 1007, Suter and Lewis, Eds., American Society for Testing and Materials, Philadelphia, Vol. 11, pp 123-138.

Doreger, J.U., Meirer, J.R., Dubbs, R.A., Johnson, R.D., and Ankley, G.T., 1988, "Toxicity Reduction Evaluation at a Municipal Wastewater Treatment Plant Using Mutagenicity as an Endpoint," Arch. Environ. Contam. Toxicol., Vol. 22, pp 384-388.

Dorn, P.B., Van Compernolle, R., and Meyer C.L., 1991, "Aquatic Hazard Assessment of the Toxic Fraction of a Petrochemical Plant," Env. Toxicol. and Chem., Vol. 10, pp 691-703.

Durhan, E.J., Lukasewycz, M.T., and Amato, R., Jr., 1990, "Extraction and Concentration of Nonpolar Organic Toxicants from Effluents using Solid Phase Extraction," Env. Toxicol. and Chem., Vol 9, pp 463-466.

Durhan, E.J., Lukasewycz, M., and Baker, S., 1993, "Alternatives to Methanol-Water Elution of Solid-Phase Extraction Columns for the Fractionation of High Log K_{ow} Organic Compounds in Aqueous Environmental Samples," J. Chromatography, Vol. 629, pp 67-74.

Ford, D.L., 1992, Toxicity Reduction: Evaluation and Control, Technomic Publishing Company, Lancaster, PA.

Fort, D.J., Delphon, J., Powers, C.R., Helems, R., Gonzalez, R., and Stover, E.L., 1995, "Development of Automated Methods of Identifying Toxicants in the Environment," Bulletin of Environmental Contam. Toxicol., Vol. 54, pp 104-111.

Gasith, A., Jop, K.M., Dickson, K.L., Parkerton, T.F., and Kaczmarek, S.A., 1988, "Protocol for the Identification of Toxic Fractions in Industrial Wastewater Effluents," Aquatic Toxicology and Hazard Assessment, ASTM STP 971, Adams, Chapman, and Landis, Eds., American Society for Testing and Materials, Philadelphia, Vol. 10, pp 204-215.

Goodfellow, W.L. McCulloch, W.L., Jr., Botts, J.A., McDearmon, A.G., and Bishop, D.F., 1989, "Long-term Multispecies Toxicity and Effluent Fractionation Study at a Municipal Wastewater Treatment Plant," Aquatic Toxicology and Environmental Fate, ASTM STP 1007, Suter and Lewis, Eds., American Society for Testing and Materials, Philadelphia, Vol. 11, pp 135-158.

Hall, W.S., and Mirenda, R.J., 1990, "Toxicity Identification Evaluations," Toxicity Reduction in Industrial Effluents, P.W. Lankford and W.W. Eckenfelder, Jr., Eds., pp 35-59.

Holmbom, B., Voss, R.H., Mortimer, R.D., and Wong, A., 1983, "Fractionation, Isolation, and Characterization of Ames Mutagenic Compounds in Kraft Chlorination Effluents," Env. Sci. Technol., Vol. 18, No. 5, pp 333-337.

Jop, J.M., Kendall, T.Z., Askew, A.M., and Foster, R.B., 1991, "Use of Fractionation Procedures and Extensive Chemical Analysis for Toxicity Identification of a Chemical Plant Effluent," Env. Toxicol. and Chem., Vol. 10, pp 981-990.

Kuehl, D.W., Ankley, G.T., and Burkhard, L.P., 1990, "Bioassay Directed Characterization of the Acute Aquatic Toxicity of Creosote Leachate," Haz. Waste and Haz. Mtrls., Vol. 7, No. 3, pp 283-291.

Lankford, P.W., and Eckenfelder, W.W., Jr., 1990, (eds.), Toxicity Reduction in Industrial Effluents, Van Nostrand Reinhold, New York.

Norberg-King, T.S., Durhan, E.J., and Ankley, G.T., 1991, "Application of Toxicity Identification Evaluation Procedures to the Ambient Waters of the Cohusa Basin Drain, California," Env. Tox. and Chem, Vol. 10, pp 891-900.

Parkhurst, B.R., Gehrs, G.W., and Rubin, I.B., 1979, "Value of Chemical Fractionation for Identifying the Toxic Components of Complex Aqueous Effluents," Aquatic Toxicology, ASTM STP 667, Marking and Kimerle, Eds., American Society for Testing and Materials, Philadelphia, pp 122-130.

Reece, C.H., and Burks, S.L., 1985, "Isolation and Characterization of Petroleum Refinery Wastewater Fractions Acutely Lethal to Daphnia magna," Aquatic Toxicology and Hazard Assessment. Seventh Symposium, ASTM STP 854, Cardwell, Purdy, Bahner, Eds., American Society for Testing and Materials, Philadelphia, PA, pp 319-332.

Rubin, I.B., Guerin, M.R., Hardigree, A.A., and Epler, J.L., 1989, "Fractionation of Synthetic Crude Oils from Coal for Biological Testing," Env. Res., Vol. 12, pp 358-365.

Swain, A.P., Cooper, J.E., and Stedman, R.L., 1969, "Large Scale Fractionation of Cigarette Smoke Condensate for Chemical and Biological Evaluations," Cancer Res., Vol. 29, pp 579-583.

USEPA (US Environmental Protection Agency), 1985a, Methods for Measuring the Acute Toxicity of Effluents to Freshwater and Marine Organisms, Third Edition, EPA/600/4-85/013, Cincinnati, OH.

USEPA, 1985b, Application of Chemical Fractionation/Aquatic Bioassay Procedure to Hazardous Waste Site Monitoring, EPA 600/4-85/059, Las Vegas, NV.

USEPA, 1988, Methods for Aquatic Toxicity Identification Evaluations -Phase I Toxicity Characterization Procedures, EPA/600/3-88/034, Duluth, MN.

USEPA, 1989a, Methods for Aquatic Toxicity Identification Evaluations - Phase II Toxicity Identification Procedures, EPA/600/3-88/035, Duluth, MN.

USEPA, 1989b, Methods for Aquatic Toxicity Identification Evaluations - Phase III Toxicity Confirmation Procedures, EPA/600/3-88/036, Duluth, MN.

USEPA, 1989c, Generalized Methodology for Conducting Industrial Toxicity Reduction Evaluations (TREs), EPA/600/2-88/070, Cincinnati, OH.

USEPA, 1989d, Toxicity Reduction Evaluation Protocol for Municipal Wastewater Treatment Plants, EPA/600/2-88/062, Cincinnati, OH.

USEPA, 1989e, Methods for Aquatic Toxicity Identification Evaluations - Phase I Toxicity Characterization Procedures, Second Edition, EPA/600/6-91/003, Washington, D.C.

USEPA, 1991, Toxicity Identification Evaluation: Characterizing Chronically Toxic Effluents, Phase I, EPA/600/6-91/005, Washington, D.C.

USEPA, 1993a, Methods for Aquatic Toxicity Identification Evaluations - Phase II Toxicity Identification Evaluations for Samples Exhibiting Acute and Chronic Toxicity, EPA/600/R-92/080, Washington, D.C.

USEPA, 1993b, Methods for Aquatic Toxicity Identification Evaluations - Phase III Toxicity Confirmation Procedures for Samples Exhibiting Acute and Chronic Toxicity, EPA/600/R-92/080, Washington, D.C.

USEPA, 1994, Marine Toxicity Identification Evaluation (TIE) Guidance Document - Phase I, Draft. Env. Research Lab, Narraganset, RI.

Walsh, G.E., and Garnas, R.L., 1983, "Determination of Bioactivity of Chemical Fractions of Liquid Wastes Using Freshwater and Saltwater Algae and Crustaceans," Envir. Sci. Technol., Vol. 17, pp 180-182.

West, W.R., Smith, P.A., Booth, G.M., and Lee, M.L., 1988, "Isolation and Detection of Genotoxic Components in a Black River Sediment," Env. Sci. Technol., Vol. 22, No. 2, pp 224-228.

David M. Peterson[1] and Robert G. Knowlton, Jr.[2]

PRÉCIS - A Probabilistic Risk Assessment System

REFERENCE: Peterson, D. M. and Knowlton, R. G., Jr., **"PRÉCIS - A Probabilistic Risk Assessment System,"** *Environmental Toxicology and Risk Assessment: Biomarkers and Risk Assessment—Fifth Volume, ASTM STP 1306,* David A. Bengtson and Diane S. Henshel, Eds., American Society for Testing and Materials, 1996.

ABSTRACT: A series of computer tools has been developed to conduct the exposure assessment and risk characterization phases of human health risk assessments within a probabilistic framework. The tools are collectively referred to as the Probabilistic Risk Evaluation and Characterization Investigation System (PRÉCIS). With this system, a risk assessor can calculate the doses and risks associated with multiple environmental and exposure pathways, for both chemicals and radioactive contaminants. Exposure assessment models in the system account for transport of contaminants to receptor points from a source zone

---

Senior Research Scientist, INTERA Inc., 1650 University Blvd NE; Suite 300; Albuquerque, New Mexico 87102

Project Leader, Sandia National Laboratories; P.O. Box 5800; MS 0720; Albuquerque, New Mexico 87185

originating in unsaturated soils above the water table. In addition to performing calculations of dose and risk based on initial concentrations, PRÉCIS can also be used in an inverse manner to compute soil concentrations in the source area that must not be exceeded if prescribed limits on dose or risk are to be met. Such soil contaminant levels, referred to as soil guidelines, are computed for both single contaminants and chemical mixtures and can be used as action levels or cleanup levels. Probabilistic estimates of risk, dose and soil guidelines are derived using Monte Carlo techniques.

KEYWORDS: dose, inverse procedure, Latin Hypercube Sampling, Monte Carlo method, risk, sensitivity analysis, soil guideline

---

During the last few years, several software packages have been developed to assist environmental scientists in conducting risk assessments (Block 1995; Renner 1995). These packages vary widely in terms of scope, complexity, approach to estimating risks, methodology for evaluating risk uncertainty, and ancillary features for entering data and analyzing computed risks. Many of the software tools focus on the use of the Monte Carlo method for directly quantifying risk uncertainty. Others have incorporated extensive databases that contain such information as climate statistics or fate and toxicity data for a large number of chemicals. Still others emphasize multimedia mass balance fate models, wherein conservation of mass for the contaminants of concern is maintained throughout the risk calculations (Renner, 1995). This latter feature is particularly important at sites where transport of a contaminant away from a source area by one pathway reduces the level of contamination and resulting exposure that can occur in an alternative pathway. Consequently, balancing mass within a multi-media system reduces the potential for overestimating risk due to the inclusion of contaminant levels that are no longer present. Regardless of the methods applied in the software packages, each is potentially useful in that it can be used to assess risk efficiently at a given site or at many sites.

Sandia National Laboratories (SNL), Albuquerque, New Mexico, has developed a software system for conducting human health risk assessments that is particularly suited to the evaluation of numerous sites that contain a variety of contaminants. The package, referred to as the Probabilistic Risk Evaluation and Characterization Investigation System, or PRÉCIS, contains several individual features as well as combinations of features that distinguishes it from previously-developed software tools. With this system, a risk assessor can calculate the risks and hazard indices associated with chemicals at hazardous waste sites and the doses resulting from exposure to environmental contamination from radioactive wastes. PRÉCIS can be used for single deterministic estimates of risk as well as in a probabilistic manner using the Monte Carlo method (e.g. Thompson et al. 1992; Zimmerman et al. 1990). All probabilistic calculations are performed internally within the package, as there is no dependence on a separate piece of software to conduct the sampling of parameters for Monte Carlo simulations. PRÉCIS can be used to conduct both the exposure assessment and risk characterization phases of a risk assessment. The fate, transport, and exposure analysis methods in the package conserve contaminant mass as it is distributed through a variety of pathways. In addition to providing defensible estimates of risk, the system is designed to aid operable unit leaders, responsible parties, stakeholders, and regulators in establishing concentration thresholds for contaminants in source areas, as well as prioritizing site characterization needs. Source concentration thresholds computed by PRÉCIS, which are called soil guidelines, can be determined for both single contaminants or contaminant mixtures. Site characterization needs can be prioritized using sensitivity analysis techniques in the package that identify which risk assessment parameters have the greatest effect on computed risk.

CURRENT FEATURES AND APPLICATIONS OF PRÉCIS

PRÉCIS contains two separate models to evaluate risk at a site. Exposure assessment methods in both models account for mass-conservative transport of contaminants to receptor points from a source zone originating in unsaturated soils above the water table. The first model, known as RISKRAD, is designed to compute equivalent doses resulting from radioactive contaminants. As many as nine environmental pathways operating simultaneously and three general forms of exposure pathways can be evaluated in this model. The second model, RISKCHEM, is a hazardous chemical version of RISKRAD. In addition to calculating chemical intakes, RISKCHEM computes incidences of cancer risk and the hazard indices resulting from exposure to toxic constituents.

Computation of soil guidelines is accomplished in PRÉCIS using "inverse methods" built into the system. The techniques employed are referred to as inverse procedures because they perform the opposite of the risk calculations, i.e. they permit the calculation of allowable source area concentrations so that specified levels of risk will not be exceeded. In addition to determining single-source guidelines, PRÉCIS is designed to compute soil guidelines on the basis of contaminant mixtures. The mixture guidelines take into account what are assumed to be the additive effects of multiple contaminants on dose, risk and toxicity. The assumption of risk additivity, which is recommended in the Risk Assessment Guidance for Superfund (RAGS) (EPA 1989), obviously ignores any synergistic or antagonistic effects that may occur between co-contaminants. The soil guidelines computed in PRÉCIS are useful in the sense that they can be employed as action levels during initial site investigations or, in some cases, as site-specific cleanup levels.

Sampling of uncertain parameters, when applying PRÉCIS in a probabilistic manner, is accomplished using Latin Hypercube Sampling (Iman and Shortencarrier 1984), a procedure that allows risk uncertainty to be examined with fewer Monte Carlo simulations than would be required using pure random sampling. Input parameter values, including values describing the probability density functions (PDFs) of uncertain parameters, are entered into the system through a graphical user interface. All input parameters to the risk models in PRÉCIS can be treated as uncertain variables. Alternatively, a variable can be assigned a fixed constant value. For each uncertain parameter, the PRÉCIS user can select any of sixteen PDFs to represent its distribution.

Performing assessments in a probabilistic manner allows the PRÉCIS user to quantitatively account for the transfer of parameter uncertainty to uncertainty in risk. Consequently, a risk assessor can compute a realistic range of risks associated with a site rather than a single risk estimate based on traditionally conservative assumptions that lead to both compounding and additive error. During the past several years, numerous investigators (e.g. Burmaster and Lehr 1991; Thompson et al. 1992) have pointed out the inherent limitations of the conservative Reasonable Maximum Exposure (RME) concept, as published in RAGS (EPA 1989) and traditionally applied to risk assessment, and discussed the benefits of probabilistic risk analysis. Probabilistic results from PRÉCIS for computed risk measures and soil guidelines can be examined in both report and graphical form. Graphical output from probabilistic assessments consists of complementary cumulative distribution functions (CCDFs) of dose, intake, risk, hazard index, and soil guidelines.

PRÉCIS is currently being employed by SNL to assess risk at more than eighty separate sites. The numerous features of the software system allow SNL personnel to evaluate risk at each site relatively quickly, and to prioritize, or rank, the sites on the basis of their relative risks. Probabilistic assessment of the risk at each site makes it possible to observe quantitatively the effects of parameter uncertainty on computed risk. Accordingly, parameter sensitivity analyses conducted in PRÉCIS are being used to identify which parameters have the greatest effect on computed risk and should, therefore, be focused on during future site characterization activities.

RADIATION PATHWAYS ANALYSIS

The model used in PRÉCIS to assess human health risk at a

radioactive waste site, RISKRAD, is designed to compute radiation doses to members of a population group residing at or near the site after it has been designated for uses other than waste disposal. RISKRAD consists of a variation of the dose estimation code in RESRAD (Gilbert et al. 1989; Yu et al. 1993), developed at Argonne National Laboratory for the U.S. Department of Energy (DOE). In the model, exposures of humans to radionuclides are assumed to occur from wastes originally occurring in soil above the water table. Exposure can be direct from soil constituents, or indirect as a result of releases from the contaminated soil zone and subsequent environmental transport to receptor points away from the waste source.

Exposure to ionizing radiation due to waste releases from landfills and other waste depositories can occur as a result of transport through a variety of pathways. Figure 1 summarizes the radiation pathways that are included in RISKRAD. As this schematic indicates, there are three main exposure pathways corresponding to the three mechanisms by which radionuclides can enter the body: (1) external radiation from radionuclides in the contaminated zone; (2) internal radiation from inhaled radionuclides; and (3) internal radiation from ingested radionuclides. In addition, there are nine environmental pathways that are taken into account in RISKRAD: (1) direct gamma radiation from radionuclides in the soil; (2) inhalation of resuspended dust (if the contaminated area is exposed at the ground surface); (3) ingestion of food from crops or other plants growing in the contaminated soil; (4) ingestion of milk from livestock raised in the contaminated area; (5) ingestion of meat from livestock raised in the contaminated area; (6) ingestion of fish from a nearby pond contaminated by water percolating through the contaminated zone; (7) ingestion of

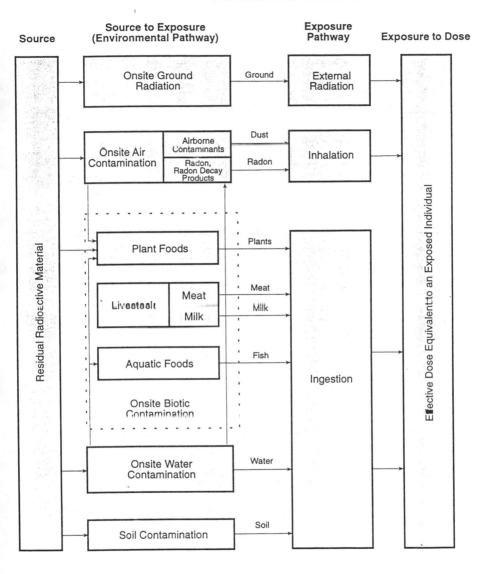

FIG. 1--Exposure pathway diagram for calculating the dose to an onsite resident from residual radioactive material (Source: Modified from Yu et al. 1993, Figure 2.2)

water from a well contaminated by water percolating through the contaminated zone; (8) inhalation of radon gas diffusing from the contaminated soil or dissolved in water; and (9) ingestion of contaminated soil. Many of the environmental pathways can occur as segments in other pathways. For example, contaminated groundwater can contribute to both the food pathways and the drinking water pathway if contaminated well water is used for irrigation and livestock watering in addition to human consumption.

The pathways analysis employed in RISKRAD for deriving doses from surface or buried radioactive wastes has three parts: (1) source analysis; (2) environmental transport analysis; and (3) dose/exposure analysis. Source analysis involves the derivation of source terms that determine the rate at which radionuclides are released into the environment. Environmental transport analysis consists of (a) identifying environmental pathways by which contaminants can migrate from the source to a human exposure location and (b) determining the rate of migration along these pathways. Dose/exposure analysis addresses the problem of deriving and applying dose conversion factors for the radiation dose that will be incurred by exposure to ionizing radiation. RISKRAD contains algorithms that affect all three pathways analysis components.

Waste Source in RISKRAD

The source term in RISKRAD is defined by a subsurface contaminated zone in unsaturated soils in which constituents exist at above-background concentrations. All pathways originate at the source area, which is assumed by default to be a cylindrically-shaped contaminated zone wherein contaminants are "uniformly" distributed. Uniform contamination implies that radionuclide concentrations are exactly the same at every point, which rarely occurs at actual sites. Such an idealized source shape and contaminant distribution is necessary to accomodate analytical solutions used in RISKRAD to estimate contaminant concentrations in various media. To account for nonideal conditions, the PRÉCIS user may elect to treat both the source shape and initial source concentrations of relevant contaminants as uncertain parameters. Accordingly, these parameters will vary with each Monte Carlo simulation in conformance with user-specified parameter ranges and distributions.

The schematic in Figure 2 illustrates an idealized contaminated zone, as used in RISKRAD, of source thickness T. Overlying this zone is a cover layer of depth C_d, which corresponds to the distance from the ground surface to the uppermost contaminated soil sample. The cover depth plus the contaminated zone thickness $(C_d + T)$ corresponds to the distance to the lowest contaminated soil sample. Radioactive doses computed in RISKRAD are largely affected by three rate-limited processes occurring in these two layers: (1) the rate of ingrowth and decay of the radionuclides; (2) the rate at which radionuclides are leached from the contaminated zone; and (3) the rate of erosion of the cover and contaminated zones.

Contaminant leaching from the waste source is assumed in the current version of RISKRAD to be sorption-controlled. This means that the dissolved concentration of a radionuclide in infiltrating soil water leaving the base of the contaminated zone (i.e. leachate concentration) is directly affected by a user-specified soil/water distribution coefficient for that radionuclide. It also means that, if infiltration

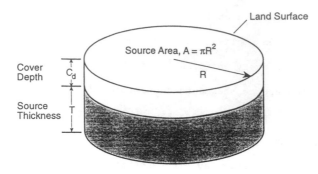

FIG. 2--Geometry of idealized contaminated zone

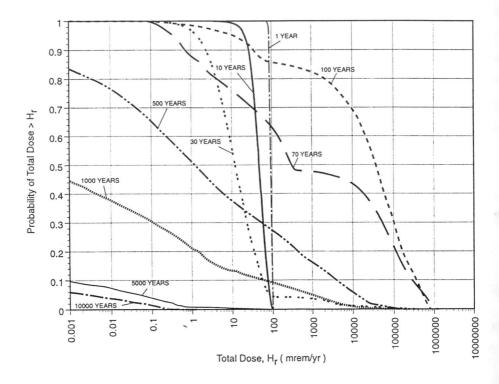

FIG. 3--Complementary cumulative distribution function curves for
total dose from all pathways.

at the ground surface is sufficient to cause leaching and the calculated
dissolved concentration of a radionuclide is not greater than its
solubility, the leachate concentration is constantly decreasing with
time. Currently, RISKRAD does not contain a solubility constraint on the
the radionuclide concentration of the leachate; a version of the model
now under development does include such a constraint.

Environmental Transport in RISKRAD

For all radiation pathways but the radon pathway, RISKRAD
calculates two separate types of quantities, known as exposure
parameters: (1) unit intakes of radionuclides in the case of internal
radiation (inhalation and ingestion), and (2) unit concentrations of
radionuclides in the environment at the point of exposure in the case of
external radiation. For all pathways other than the radon pathway, an
exposure parameter for a single radionuclide transported through a

single pathway is computed as the product of three quantities (Gilbert et al. 1989; Yu et al. 1993)

$$E_r(t) = ETF_r(t) \cdot SF_r(t) \cdot S_r(0) \qquad (1)$$

where

$E_r(t)$	=	exposure parameter, in the form of the annual intake of the radionuclide (pCi/yr) for internal radiation, and concentration of the radionuclide in the contaminated zone (pCi/cm^3) for external radiation,
$ETF_r(t)$	=	environmental transport factor [(g/yr) for internal radiation, (g/cm^3) for external radiation],
$SF_r(t)$	=	$S_r(t)/S_r(0)$ = source factor (dimensionless),
$S_r(t)$	=	time-dependent radionuclide concentration at the waste source (pCi/g),
$S_r(0)$	=	initial radionuclide concentration at the waste source (pCi/g),
t	=	time (years), and
r	=	index for radioactive contamination.

The environmental transport factor $ETF_r(t)$ represents the time-varying ratio of the exposure parameter to the source concentration. Values of $ETF_r(t)$ are pathway- and radionuclide-dependent. Detailed formulations of the models used to calculate the environmental transport factors for each pathway are presented in Gilbert et al. (1989) and Yu et al. (1993). The radon pathway does not depend on the calculation of an environmental transport factor. The source factor $SF_r(t)$ is the ratio of time-dependent source concentration of a radionuclide $S_r(t)$ to its initial concentration $S_r(0)$ (Yu et al. 1993). It represents the time-dependent ratio of the activity of a radionuclide remaining in the contaminated zone after contributions from ingrowth and removal by leaching and decay of the radionuclide. Equation **(1)** is presented in terms of initial source concentration and a source factor rather than time-dependent source concentration to help facilitate the description of soil guidelines, as discussed in later sections.

The radon pathway in RISKRAD considers exposure from inhalation of both radon-222 and radon-220. Both outdoor exhalation of radon from the ground surface and indoor radon exposure from a house built onsite are modeled. The radon flux is attributed to molecular diffusion from soil sources to the ground surface and/or the foundation of a building. Flow of radon-contaminated soil air in response to air pressure gradients is not considered.

Radiation Dose

The exposure factors computed as a result of environmental transport analysis must be translated into radioactive doses to the human body so that the potential risks posed by the radionuclides can be assessed. The computation of doses from intakes and concentrations is accomplished using dose conversion factors. A dose conversion factor accounts for the overall biological effectiveness of a radioactive dose, which depends on the type of radiation, the location of the radionuclides emitting the radiation (i.e. internal or external to the body), and the body organs receiving the radiation. RISKRAD takes these factors into consideration by presenting doses in the form of an effective dose equivalent (ICRP 1979-1982). For internal exposure to radiation, acute intakes of radionuclides commit an individual to receiving doses over future times (even with no further intake) until activity is removed from the body by biological elimination or radioactive decay. Taking this into consideration, doses of internal radiation are analyzed in terms of committed effective dose equivalent. In RISKRAD, committed doses are determined assuming 50 years of internal exposure following acute intake by inhalation or ingestion. The model reports radioactive doses in the form of annual effective dose equivalent, in units of millirems per year (mrem/yr).

For all pathways other than the radon pathway, dose from a single principal radionuclide transported through an individual pathway is computed as (Gilbert et al. 1989; Yu et al. 1993)

$$H_r(t) = DCF_r \cdot E_r(t) \tag{2}$$

where

$H_r(t)$ = annual effective dose equivalent (mrem/yr), and

DCF_r = dose conversion factor [(mrem/pCi) for internal radiation from inhalation or ingestion, $(mrem/yr)/(pCi/cm^3)$ for external gamma radiation].

RISKRAD contains default values of dose conversion factors for each pathway and radionuclide incorporated in the model. These values are derived from years of study and compilation by individual researchers and agencies such as the International Commission on Radiological Protection (ICRP) and DOE.

Radiation dose from radon and its decay products is calculated by using the accumulated exposure in terms of Working Level Month (WLM). The WLM is a cumulative exposure unit historically applied to uranium miners. Because exposure for the general population is continuous and the breathing rate is lower and shallower than for miners, the use of WLM for estimating doses in RISKRAD has to be adjusted for the general population. This is accomplished by employing proportional factors published by the National Research Council (1988).

One of the objectives of a radiation risk assessment is to determine the total dose to which an individual may be exposed. RISKRAD determines total dose (in mrem/yr) by summing the doses from all relevant radionuclides for all active pathways. To further assess the importance of individual pathways and radionuclides, it also calculates the total dose for a given active pathway for all relevant radionuclides, and the total dose from a given radionuclide for all active pathways.

Dose-to-Source Ratio

Substitution of (1) into (2) leads to a new equation for radiation dose that is expressed in terms of a mathematical construct known as the dose-to-source ratio

$$H_r(t) = DSR(t) \cdot S_r(0) \tag{3}$$

where

DSR(t)   =   dose-to-source ratio [(mrem/yr)/(pCi/g)]

= $DCF_r \cdot ETF_r(t) \cdot SF_r(t)$.

The dose-to-source ratio allows the RISKRAD user to observe how doses change with time in reference to the initial concentration (at time zero) of a radionuclide. In addition, the DSR(t) quantity facilitates a simplified description of the methods used to calculate soil guidelines, as discussed in subsequent sections. In the same manner that total doses from relevant radionuclides and active pathways are calculated, dose-to-source ratios are also totaled.

CHEMICAL PATHWAYS ANALYSIS

The chemical risk assessment model RISKCHEM computes chemical intakes and the associated cancer risks and/or hazard indices resulting from exposure to carcinogenic and toxic chemicals at a hazardous waste site. RISKCHEM is a hazardous chemical version of RISKRAD developed at SNL. The current version of the model includes the chemical equivalent of the environmental pathways in RISKRAD, with the exception of the external radiation and radon pathways. Thus, RISKCHEM currently handles only seven environmental pathways, all of them dealing with internal exposure: (1) dust inhalation, (2) plant ingestion, (3) milk ingestion, (4) meat ingestion, (5) aquatic food ingestion, (6) water ingestion, and (7) soil ingestion. A version of the model currently being developed will include a dermal uptake pathway and a pathway for inhalation of volatile chemicals. RISKCHEM is designed to calculate intakes of hazardous chemicals in units of milligrams per kilogram per day (mg/kg/day). The chemical intakes are in turn used to compute incidences of cancer risk and the hazard indices resulting from ingestion and dust inhalation of toxic constituents.

The pathways analysis for deriving cancer risks and hazard indices from surface or buried chemical waste has four parts: (1) source analysis; (2) environmental transport analysis; (3) intake/exposure analysis; and (4) risk/intake analysis. The first two components accomplish the same risk assessment steps as their counterparts in RISKRAD. Intake/exposure analysis, which is analogous to RISKRAD's dose/exposure analysis, consists of determining and employing intake conversion factors to transform annual intake quantities into chemical intake rates that are normalized with regard to exposure duration, exposure averaging time, and body weight. Risk/intake analysis is applied to convert the normalized intakes into incidences of excess cancer as well as any hazard quotients and indices resulting from exposure to toxic chemicals.

Waste Source in RISKCHEM

The source term in RISKCHEM is developed using most of the same techniques employed in RISKRAD. The contaminated source area is assumed to be cylindrically-shaped (Figure 2), located in unsaturated soils, and uniformly contaminated. Unlike RISKRAD, however, the current version of RISKCHEM does not account for chemical decay and ingrowth. Thus, processes affecting the concentration of a chemical in the waste source are limited to those that control leaching of the chemical by infiltrating water and erosion of the cover and contaminated zones. Leaching of the chemical source area is sorption-controlled.

Chemical Intake and Environmental Transport

In developing RISKCHEM, it has been assumed that chemical intake, as normalized by exposure duration, body weight, and exposure averaging time, is the hazardous chemical equivalent of annual effective dose equivalent for a radioactive contaminant. As a consequence, as indicated by **(2)**, chemical intake can also be viewed as the product of an exposure parameter and a conversion factor, i.e.

$$H_c(t) = ICF_c \cdot E_c(t)$$

(4)

where

$H_c(t)$ =   normalized chemical intake (mg/kg/day),

$E_c(t)$ =   chemical exposure parameter, or annual mass intake of a chemical (mg/yr),

ICF_c = $ED/(BW \cdot AT)$ = intake conversion factor (yr/kg/day),

ED =   exposure duration (years),

BW =   body weight (kg),

AT =   averaging time (days), and

c =   index for chemical contamination.

As shown in **(4)**, chemical intake in RISKCHEM is calculated with relatively basic parameters that are largely identical to the parameters used in RAGS (EPA 1989). Accordingly, the current version of RISKCHEM does not incorporate explicit methods to account for such factors as chemical bioavailibility or the ability of humans to detoxify some chemicals.

The version of RISKCHEM currently in PRÉCIS allows the user to specify three separate intake conversion factors for each relevant chemical: (1) a factor for all ingestion pathways other than the soil ingestion pathway; (2) a soil ingestion factor; and (3) a dust inhalation factor.

The chemical exposure parameter $E_c(t)$ (i.e., non-normalized annual intake) is computed for active pathways in RISKCHEM using the chemical equivalent of **(1)**

$$E_c(t) - ETF_c(t) \cdot SF_c(t) \cdot S_c(0) \tag{5}$$

where

$$ETF_c(t) \quad = \quad \text{environmental transport factor for a chemical (g/yr),}$$

$$SF_c(t) \quad = \quad S_c(t)/S_c(0) = \text{source factor for a chemical, as affected by leaching and erosion (dimensionless),}$$

$$S_c(t) \quad = \quad \text{time-dependent chemical concentration at the waste source (mg/g), and}$$

$$S_c(0) \quad = \quad \text{initial chemical concentration at the waste source (mg/g).}$$

The chemical environmental transport factor for a specific pathway and chemical is calculated using the same equations employed in the computation of the analogous radionuclide environmental transport factor $ETF_r(t)$. Thus, the methods and parameters presented in RESRAD documentation (Gilbert et al. 1989; Yu et al. 1993) for calculating transport factors apply to RISKCHEM as well. Similar to Equation (1), Equation (5) is presented in terms of initial source concentration and a source factor rather than a time-dependent source concentration to facilitate discussion of chemical guidelines, as presented later. As in the case of radioactive waste, a risk assessor is also interested in deriving the total hazardous chemical intake to which an individual may be subjected. Total intakes are presented in RISKCHEM in both report and graphical form.

Risk/Intake Analysis

Excess cancer incidence, or cancer risk, for a single chemical and pathway is computed with the equation

$$R_c(t) = SLF_c \cdot H_c(t)$$

(6)

where

$R_c(t)$ = chemical cancer risk (dimensionless),

SLF_c = cancer slope factor $(mg/kg/day)^{-1}$, and

$H_c(t)$ = chemical intake $(mg/kg/day)$.

RISKCHEM utilizes two types of slope factors: oral and inhalation. The values for these factors are taken largely from EPA's

1994 IRIS database (EPA 1994). As in the case of intakes, site-specific cancer risks for all relevant chemicals and active pathways are also totaled and reported in RISKCHEM.

Hazard quotients for a single chemical and a single pathway are computed in RISKCHEM using the equation

$$HQ_c(t) = \frac{H_c(t)}{RfD_c} \tag{7}$$

where

$HQ_c(t)$ =   hazard quotient (dimensionless), and

RfD_c =   reference dose for the chemical (mg/kg/day)

Following methodology presented in the Risk Characterization chapter of the Risk Assessment Guidelines for Superfund (EPA 1989), hazard indices are computed by summing hazard quotients from individual contaminants and individual pathways. As in the case of cancer slope factors, the RISKCHEM user utilizes both oral and inhalation reference doses, which are also taken largely from EPA's 1994 IRIS database (EPA 1994).

Intake-, Risk-, and Hazard Index-to-Source Ratios

Hazardous chemical equivalents to the dose-to-source ratio defined in (3) for radiation pathway analysis are computed in RISKCHEM. These time-dependent quantities describe, respectively, the ratio of chemical intake, cancer risk, and hazard index to initial chemical concentration in the contaminated source area. Inspection of (4) and (5) indicates that, in the current version of RISKCHEM, an intake-to-source-ratio [ISR(t)] is defined by the product of an intake conversion factor, a chemical environmental transport factor, and a chemical source factor. Similarly, **(6)** and **(7)** show that a risk-to-source ratio [RSR(t)] is formed by the product of an intake-to-source ratio and a slope factor, and a hazard index-to-source ratio [HSR(t)] is the quotient of an intake-to-source ratio and a reference dose. The ratios [ISR(t), RSR(t), and HSR(t)] may be used to calculate soil guidelies, as described below, based on prescribed limits on total intake, total cancer risk, and total hazard index, respectively.

SOIL GUIDELINES

In addition to performing calculations for the estimation of various risk measures based on initial contaminant concentrations, PRÉCIS performs inverse calculations for estimates of acceptable contaminant soil concentrations given prescribed limits on the risk measures. Such concentrations are referred to as soil concentration guidelines, or simply soil guidelines. They can be used as action levels in RCRA investigations or as cleanup levels in assessing remedial alternatives. Soil guidelines calculated with PRÉCIS can also be used to: (a) guide the adequacy of field-screening equipment; (b) allow an early determination of whether a site is safe (perhaps resulting in a No Further Action proposal); and (c) determine which constituents are of concern.

Soil guidelines are computed assuming that individual chemicals are either (a) the only source of contamination or (b) part of a mixture comprising several chemicals. The calculation of single-source guidelines is accomplished without any foreknowledge of or assumptions about the contaminant mixtures at a site. In contrast, to calculate mixture guidelines, PRÉCIS requires that estimates be given for the soil concentrations of all contaminants in the source area.

Single-Source Radiation Soil Guidelines

A radionuclide soil guideline is the level of radioactivity (activity concentration) in contaminated zone soil that must be achieved and maintained so that a prescribed dose limit is not exceeded. The time-dependent soil guideline for an individual radionuclide transported over multiple pathways is calculated in RISKRAD as

$$G_r(t) = \frac{RDL}{\sum_{p} DSR_{p,r}(t)} \tag{8}$$

where

$G_r(t)$ = single-source soil guideline in the contaminated zone (pCi/g),

RDL = basic radiation dose limit (mrem/year), and

$DSR_{p,r}(t)$ = dose-to-source concentration ratio for pth environmental pathway at time t [(mrem/yr)/(pCi/g)].

Additional Features of RISKRAD

In addition to calculating guidelines at designated output times, RISKRAD also computes the minimum guideline for each chemical during the entire time that doses are calculated. This corresponds to the guideline resulting from **(8)** at the time of maximum dose for a radionuclide, which is determined using search algorithms built into RISKRAD.

An additional feature built into RISKRAD permits the user to determine minimum guidelines at a time following waste emplacement. This feature is provided so that the risk assessor can develop action levels for a site on the basis of exposures that are potentially occurring today, perhaps numerous years after the wastes at a site were first placed there. In other words, if the calculated maximum dose occurs at some point in the past, the associated guideline may be irrelevant to current decisions regarding corrective measures at a site.

Guidelines for Radionuclide Mixtures

The general equation employed in RISKRAD for calculating a time-dependent mixture guideline for an individual radionuclide is

$$RDL = \sum_{i=1}^{n} \left[\sum_{P} DSR_{ip,r}(t) \right] \cdot G_{i,rm}(t) \tag{9}$$

where

$DSR_{ip,r}(t)$ =   dose-to-source ratio for the ith radionuclide

and the pth environmental pathway at time t
[(mrem/yr)/(pCi/g)],

$G_{i,rm}(t)$ =   mixture guideline for the ith radionuclide at
time t (pCi/g), and

n   =   number of initially-existent radionuclides.

Equation (9) can be applied to any of the output times specified in a RISKRAD run. Doing so in conjunction with a scheme that apportions dose between the n radionuclides results in soil guidelines that produce a combined dose for that time that is equal to the dose limit. However, utilization of the guidelines from a specific time does not assure that the dose limit will not be exceeded at other times. Moreover, using the minimum computed guideline for a contaminant over all times does not guarantee that the computed total dose will always be less than the basic radiation dose limit. Thus a more conservative form of (9), that makes use of the maximum dose-to-source ratio for a radionuclide, is actually employed in RISKRAD.

Equation (9) contains n unknowns corresponding to the n initially existent radionuclides in the contaminated zone. Therefore, the unknowns must be defined in relative terms. Although there are many ways that this can be done, the current version of RISKRAD applies two different methods that are referred to as weighting schemes. The first scheme assumes that the radionuclides comprising the mixture will exist in the same proportion as specified by the initial concentrations used in the RISKRAD simulation. This scheme is referred to as "weighting by initial concentration." The second approach assumes that the guideline for a radionuclide will be inversely proportional to the relative dose contributed by this radionuclide. This latter scheme is referred to as "weighting by total dose."

Chemical Soil Guidelines

Single-source soil guidelines are computed in RISKCHEM using the hazardous chemical equivalents of (8). In lieu of a radiation dose limit, three different sets of chemical guidelines are derived on the basis of a basic chemical intake limit (CIL), a cancer risk limit (CRL), and a hazard index limit (HIL). The respective sets of guidelines make use of previously described intake-to-source ratios, risk-to-source ratios, and hazard index-to-source ratios. These ratios are also employed in the calculation of related mixture guidelines using hazardous chemical equivalents of (9). By comparing the guidelines resulting from the respective risk measure limits, a risk assessor can discern which limit produces the most restrictive action or cleanup levels.

As in RISKRAD, a feature in RISKCHEM permits the user to determine minimum guidelines at a time following waste emplacement. As previously stated, this feature allows the risk assessor to develop action levels for a site on the basis of exposures that are potentially occurring today, perhaps numerous years after the wastes at a site were first placed there.

SENSITIVITY ANALYSIS

Sensitivity analysis techniques built into PRÉCIS are conducive to rapid assessment of model results. One of the benefits derived from sensitivity analysis is the identification of parameters that most strongly affect risk and would, therefore, benefit from further field characterization. The current version of PRÉCIS contains tools for conducting two types of sensitivity analysis. Both techniques are considered to be "local" sensitivity methods in that they can only be employed with single model simulations taken from the full ensemble of simulations that comprise the Monte Carlo analysis.

The first local sensitivity tool is analogous to the dose-versus-time graphs included with the RESRAD model (Yu et al. 1993). Graphing tools currently in PRÉCIS allow the user to plot doses with time from a RISKRAD run, and normalized intakes with time from a RISKCHEM run. The graphical sensitivity technique allows the PRÉCIS user to view these plots for simulations based on both original and perturbed parameter values. Parameter values are perturbed by a user-specified percentage. The second local sensitivity analysis tool built into PRÉCIS also examines the effects of parameter perturbation, but is more objective than the first tool in that it also allows the user to compare the relative importance of each parameter through the calculation of normalized sensitivity coefficients (Cheng et al. 1989). Parameters producing the largest coefficients have the greatest influence on computed risk. Thus this approach quantifies the relative importance of each parameter so that site characterization needs can be more rigorously identified.

MODEL OUTPUT

RISKRAD and RISKCHEM input and results are tabulated for each

Monte Carlo run in a variety of ASCII-formatted reports. In addition to echoing all input parameters, the reports list time-dependent risk measures by pathway and contaminant, summarize dose-to-source ratios and analogous ratios, and list single-source and mixture guidelines.

Graphical output of the probabilistic results from Monte Carlo analysis consists of complementary cumulative distribution functions (CCDFs) (Zimmerman et al. 1990). In the current version of RISKRAD, CCDFs can be requested for computed doses and guidelines. Figure 3 illustrates examples of CCDFs developed for total radiation dose at different simulation times. The current version of RISKCHEM produces CCDF plots for chemical intake and intake-limited guidelines.

PRÉCIS ENHANCEMENTS

An enhanced version of PRÉCIS that incorporates a variety of pathway model changes is currently being developed. Most of the changes are focused on RISKCHEM and include the following: (1) a dermal absorption pathway; (2) inhalation of volatile organic chemicals; and (3) improved groundwater pathway estimates using a model of multi-dimensional advective-dispersive transport in the saturated zone. The last of these enhancements will enable simulation of additional fate and transport processes such as dispersion, retardation, and biodegradation. This will in turn enable the calculation of attenuated groundwater concentrations and associated exposures at a receptor located considerable distances downgradient of a waste site. Similar groundwater pathway improvements are being applied to the radioactive waste model. CCDFs for cancer risk and hazard index are also being included as standard output from RISKCHEM.   A more global approach to sensitivity analysis is currently being added to PRÉCIS in the form stepwise multiple regression analysis (Zimmerman et al. 1990), using original variables, standardized variables, or rank-transformed data.   This method will facilitate the identification of parameters that significantly impact risk estimates over the full probability space examined in a Monte Carlo analysis.

SUMMARY

A series of computer tools known as the Probabilistic Risk Evaluation and Characterization Investigation System, or PRÉCIS, has been developed to conduct human health risk assessments at sites containining either chemical or radioactive contaminants.   In addition to the fact that PRÉCIS can be used to assess risks from either chemical exposure or radiation, several features of this software system distinguish from many other software packages currently employed for risk assessment.   PRÉCIS can be used for single deterministic estimates of risk as well as in a probabilistic manner using the Monte Carlo method.   Performing assessments in a probabilistic manner allows the PRÉCIS user to quantitatively account for the transfer of parameter uncertainty to uncertainty in risk.   All probabilistic calculations are performed internally within the system, as there is no dependence on a separate piece of software to conduct the sampling of parameters for Monte Carlo simulations.   Exposure assessment models in the system account for multimedia transport of contaminants from a source zone originating in unsaturated soils above the water table.   The fate, transport, and exposure analysis methods in the package conserve contaminant mass as it is distributed through a variety of pathways. In addition to providing defensible estimates of risk at a site, the system can compute site-specific source concentration thresholds, or soil guidelines, that correspond to levels of soil contamination that cannot be exceeded if specified risk limits are to be met. Soil guidelines can be determined for both single contaminants and contaminant mixtures, which can in turn be used as action levels or possibly cleanup levels. Site characterization needs can be prioritized using sensitivity analysis techniques in PRÉCIS that identify the risk assessment parameters having the greatest effect on computed risk.

PRÉCIS, like many software packages designed to aid risk assessment, can be employed to efficiently evaluate risk at numerous sites. Sandia National Laboratories (SNL) is currently applying PRÉCIS at more than eighty of its sites for both site ranking purposes and to identify the risk parameters that would benefit most from further site characterization. Probabilistic calculations with the system allow SNL personnel to quantitatively and objectively examine the effects of parameter uncertainty on computed risk uncertainty, rather than using subjective means to evaluate risk uncertainty.

ACKNOWLEDGMENTS

This system was developed with funding from the U.S. Department of Energy's Office of Environmental Restoration, and the work performed by Sandia National Laboratories and its contractors under contract DE-AC04-94AL85000.

REFERENCES

Block, R.M., 1995, "Software Packages Ease Risk Assessment Tasks," Environmental Solutions, March, pp. 55-60.

Cheng, J.-J., C. Yu, and A.J. Zielen, 1991, "RESRAD Parameter Sensitivity Analysis," Argonne National Laboratory, Environmental Assessment and Information Sciences Division, ANL/EAIS-3.

Gilbert, T.L., C. Yu, Y.C. Yuan, A.J. Zielen, M.J. Jusko, and A. Wallo III, 1989, "A Manual for Implementing Residual Radioactive Material Guidelines," Argonne National Laboratory, Energy and Environmental Systems Division, ANL/ES--160, DOE/CH/8901 (draft revised, 1991).

Iman, R.L. and M.J. Shortencarrier, 1984, "A FORTRAN 77 Program and User's Guide for the Generation of Latin Hypercube and Random Samples for Use with Computer Models," Sandia National Laboratories, NUREG/CR-3624, SAND83-2362.

International Commission on Radiological Protection (ICRP), 1979-1982, "Limits for Intakes of Radionuclides by Workers," A Report of Committee 2 of the International Commission on Radiological Protection, adopted by the Commission in July 1978, ICRP Publication 30, Annals of the ICRP.

Burmaster, D.E. and J.H. Lehr, 1991, "It's Time to Make Risk Assessment a Science," Ground Water Monitoring Review, Summer 1991, pp. 5-15.

National Research Council, 1988, "Health Risks of Radon and Other Internally Deposited Alpha Emitters, BEIR IV," Committee on the Biological Effects of Ionizing Radiation, National Academy Press, Washington, D.C.

Renner, R., 1995, "Predicting Chemical Risks with Multimedia Fate Models," Environmental Science and Technology, Vol. 29, No. 12, pp. 556A-559A.

Thompson, K.M., D.E. Burmaster, and E.A.C. Crouch, "Monte Carlo Techniques for Quantitative Uncertainty Analysis in Public Health Risk Assessments," Risk Analysis, Vol. 12, No. 1, 1992, pp. 53-63.

U.S. Environmental Protection Agency (EPA), 1989, "Risk Assessment Guidance for Superfund: Volume I, Human Health Evaluation Manual (Part A)," Office of Emergency and Remedial Response, Washington, D.C. 20460.

U.S. Environmental Protection Agency (EPA), 1994, "IRIS, Integrated Risk Information System (data base)," Office of Research and Development.

Yu, C., A.J. Zielen, J.-J. Cheng, Y.C. Yuan, L.G. Jones, D.J. LePoire, Y.Y. Wang, C.O. Loureiro, E. Gnanapragasam, E. Faillace, A. Wallo III, W.A. Williams, and H. Peterson, 1993, "Manual for Implementing Residual Radioactive Material Guidelines Using RESRAD, Version 5.0," Argonne National Laboratory, Environmental Assessment Division, ANL/EAD/LD-2.

Zimmerman, D.A., R.T. Hanson and P.A. Davis, 1990, "A Comparison of Parameter Estimation and Sensitivity Analysis Techniques and Their

Impact on the Uncertainty in Ground Water Flow Model Predictions,"
Prepared for U.S. Nuclear Regulatory Commission by Sandia National
Laboratories, NUREG/CR-5522, SAND90-0128.

Laura A. Mahoney[1], Douglas M. Petroff[2], and John C. Batey[3]

THE RISK IMPLICATIONS OF THE DISTRIBUTION OF CHROMIUM FORMS IN ENVIRONMENTAL MEDIA

REFERENCE: Mahoney, L. A., Petroff, D. M., and Batey, J. C., "The Risk Implications of the Distribution of Chromium Forms in Environmental Media," *Environmental Toxicology and Risk Assessment: Biomarkers and Risk Assessment—Fifth Volume, ASTM STP 1306,* David A. Bengtson and Diane S. Henshel, Eds., American Society for Testing and Materials, 1996.

ABSTRACT: Chromium exhibits multiple oxidation (valence) states, ranging from (-II) to (+VI). Under natural conditions, however, chromium typically exists in the Cr(III) (trivalent) and/or Cr(VI) (hexavalent) form, with the hexavalent form exhibiting higher solubility and much greater toxicity than the trivalent form. Due to the large differences in toxicity, the distribution of chromium oxidation states (Cr(III) and Cr(VI)) in site media is potentially of great importance to the calculation of site risk levels, and thus ultimately to cleanup activities. Despite its importance, chromium oxidation states are often not available for media samples collected at waste sites.

Typical assumptions regarding the chromium distribution in site media are presented. Actual chromium distribution data from media from baseline investigations of several waste sites are also presented for groundwater, surface water, and soil and compared in terms of background chromium levels and the nature of site wastes. The differences in toxicity of Cr(III) and Cr(VI) are briefly discussed. Risk estimates and risk-based cleanup levels generated using different assumptions for the distribution of chromium in site media for a selected example site are then given. These risk-based cleanup levels are compared to various state regulatory limits, MCLs, and Practical Quantitation Limits (PQLs) for chromium.

---

[1]Senior Manager, Risk Assessment Services, ECKENFELDER INC., 227 French Landing Drive, Nashville, TN 37228
[2]Project Engineer, ECKENFELDER INC., 227 French Landing Drive, Nashville, TN 37228
[3]Scientist III, ECKENFELDER INC., 227 French Landing Drive, Nashville, TN 37228

KEYWORDS: Chromium; valence; oxidation states; trivalent; hexavalent; risk assessment

---

INTRODUCTION

Chromium (Cr) is one of the most commonly occurring constituents at waste sites. Although Cr is an essential micronutrient for humans and other organisms, at high concentrations, some forms can be highly toxic (ATSDR, 1992). Chromium exhibits multiple oxidation states, ranging from (-II) to (+VI) (Bodek, 1988). Under natural conditions, however, Cr typically exists in the Cr(III) (trivalent) and/or Cr(VI) (hexavalent) form, with the hexavalent form exhibiting higher solubility and much greater toxicity than the trivalent form (ATSDR, 1988). Due to the large differences in toxicity, the distribution of Cr oxidation states (Cr(III) and Cr(VI)) in site media is potentially of great importance to the calculation of site risk levels and the comparison to other standards, and thus, ultimately to cleanup activities. Despite its importance, chromium oxidation states are often not available for media samples collected at waste sites.

Chromium occurs naturally in ores, with a reported concentration range in soil of 1.0 to 2,000 mg/kg in the conterminous U.S., with a mean of 54 mg/kg (Dragun, 1991). Hem (1985) reported that concentrations of Cr in natural waters (unaffected by anthropogenic sources) are commonly less than 10 μg/L. Chromium is important commercially; chromite ore is used in the metallurgical and chemical industries for the manufacture of stainless steels, alloy cast irons, pigments, wood preservatives, and also in metal finishing, electroplating, and leather tanning (ATSDR, 1992).

Although very stable, elemental Cr (Cr°) is not usually found pure in nature (Eisler, 1986). In most soils, Cr will be present predominately as Cr(III) (ATSDR, 1992). Chromium speciation (between III and VI) in groundwater depends on the pH and redox conditions, which are primarily controlled by the amount of dissolved oxygen in the aquifer. Generally, oxidizing conditions, which favor the predomination of Cr(VI) over Cr(III), are found in shallow (typically higher dissolved oxygen) aquifers; reducing conditions, which favor the predomination of Cr(III) over Cr(VI), typically exist in deeper (typically, lower dissolved oxygen) groundwaters (ATSDR, 1992).

Anthropogenic Cr impacts to groundwater, surface water, or soil may result in very different Cr speciation than that expected in these media under natural conditions. Even under oxidizing conditions, depending upon the source, a release of Cr(VI) to the environment might be transformed to less mobile and less toxic Cr(III) in the presence of the appropriate minerals. Conversely, strongly oxidizing chemicals associated with released wastes may maintain significant amounts of Cr in the Cr (VI) state, or even oxidize Cr (III) to the Cr (VI) state.

The differences in toxicity associated with Cr(III) and Cr(VI) compounds are well documented in the literature. The known harmful effects of Cr to humans are primarily attributable to the hexavalent form. The difference between the toxicity of Cr(VI) and Cr(III) compounds is thought to be due to the ability of hexavalent compounds to penetrate biological membranes and bind to intracellular proteins, whereas trivalent compounds typically do not (ATSDR, 1992). For quantitative risk assessment applications, the USEPA currently recommends the use of an oral noncarcinogenic reference dose (RfD) of 1.0 mg/kg-day for Cr(III) and an oral RfD of 5×10^{-3} mg/kg-day for Cr(VI) (IRIS, 1995).

Laboratory analysis of Cr(VI) has historically not been performed during site investigations. Hexavalent chromium analyses for water samples are often omitted from sampling programs because of the difficulty in meeting the rigorous holding time limit of 24 hours (Method 7196 A; USEPA, 1990). In addition, until very recently (Vitale, et al, 1995), there has been no USEPA-approved method for the analysis of Cr(VI) in soil (USEPA, 1990). Another common problem with respect to measurements of Cr in water is the difference in results between filtered (soluble) and unfiltered (total) samples. Analyses of unfiltered samples often include significant concentrations of Cr associated with suspended solids.

The objective of this paper is to illustrate how the distribution of the oxidation states of Cr can affect the interpretation of environmental data in several media, as well as the risk estimates performed using the data. To accomplish this, the paper is divided into three components: (1) the presentation of examples of Cr distribution data in media including groundwater, surface water, and soil from four waste sites in the U.S.; (2) the presentation of several variations in Cr risk estimates using the environmental data collected from one of the four waste sites; and (3) the comparison of risk-based concentrations to other state and federal criteria which may be evaluated for use as target cleanup levels in the three media of interest.

EXAMPLES OF CHROMIUM DISTRIBUTION IN ENVIRONMENTAL MEDIA

As a part of different types of baseline site characterizations (e.g., remedial investigation for a Superfund site), chromium (as well as other constituents) data were collected at four waste sites being investigated for environmental impacts. Groundwater samples were analyzed for Cr at three of these sites; surface water samples were analyzed for Cr at one of the sites; and soil was analyzed for Cr at one of the sites. Table 1 lists the operations involving Cr at each of these sites, the maximum Cr concentrations, the ranges of Cr (VI) distributions in each medium (i.e., the percent

TABLE 1--Ranges of hexavalent chromium distributions for the sites evaluated

Site Number	Operations at Site	Maximum Cr Concentration	Range of Cr(VI) (% of Total)	Dominant Oxidation State
1	Cr ore processed for manufacture of pigments	Groundwater (unfiltered): 131,000 μg/L (CrVI)	Unfiltered: <0.04-151 (groundwater) Filtered: 0.1-380 (groundwater)	Cr(VI), but variable
2	No known uses of Cr-containing materials	Groundwater (unfiltered): 59.8 μg/L (total) 0.03 μg/L (CrVI)	Unfiltered: <0.002-0.18 (groundwater)	Cr(III)
3	Cr-bearing metal parts finishing (grinding and polishing)	Soil: 820 mg/kg (total) 1.9 mg/kg (CrVI) 15-100 mg/kg (Background)	<0.16-0.39 (soil)	Cr(III) Cr°(?)
4	Electroplating	Groundwater (unfiltered): 58,800 μg/L (total) 51,000 μg/L (CrVI)	Unfiltered: 12.0-89.6 (groundwater) Filtered: 88-106 (groundwater)	Cr(VI)
		Surface Water (unfiltered): 169 μg/L (total) 129 μg/L (CrVI) 3.0 μg/L (Background)	Unfiltered: 18.9-108 (surface water)	Cr(VI)

of total Cr concentration accounted for by Cr(VI)), and the dominant Cr oxidation state present. It should be noted that the chromium measurements made at these sites were for site characterization, not for the express evaluation of the oxidation states of chromium. Therefore, it is acknowledged that other key parameters (e.g., dissolved oxygen), may have provided additional information regarding the oxidation states of chromium, but were not measured at the time of the site investigations. Each site is further discussed below.

Site 1 (Groundwater)

As shown in Table 1, based upon the availability of soluble Cr(VI) sources at this site, a preponderance of Cr(VI) in groundwater would be expected relative to Cr(III). In fact, concentrations of Cr(VI) (unfiltered) were significant in a number of the 104 groundwater samples collected, ranging as high as 131,000 μg/L. However, the proportion of total Cr (unfiltered) in each sample accounted for by Cr(VI) ranged from less than 0.04 to 151 percent, indicating that a simple generalization as to the speciation of Cr in groundwater at the site would be seriously in error (values greater than 100 percent reflect normal variation in analytical precision). Sampling technique (not filtering) may have biased the results in favor of high concentrations of Cr(III) in the groundwater samples.

Site 2 (Groundwater)

Impacts at this site have primarily been related to organic constituents, and there are no known uses of Cr-containing materials at Site 2; however, groundwater samples were analyzed for Cr in response to regulatory requirements. Since there are no known sources of Cr at the site, downgradient groundwater Cr concentrations would be expected to be similar to those upgradient and representative of natural background conditions in the aquifer.

Of the 45 downgradient groundwater samples (unfiltered) evaluated, two had anomalously high concentrations, 320 μg/L and 634 μg/L, respectively. Neglecting these samples, total Cr concentrations (unfiltered) ranged only as high as 59.8 μg/L. Hexavalent Cr (unfiltered) was below the detection limit of 0.013 μg/L in all but four samples, with the highest concentration at 0.03 μg/L. The distribution of Cr(VI) in all samples was consequently very low, ranging from less than 0.002 to 0.18 percent, implying that the Cr present in groundwater was primarily in the trivalent form. Analyses were not conducted on filtered samples at this site; therefore, the effect of suspended solids on the total Cr concentrations can not be evaluated.

Site 3 (Soil)

Chromium analyses of six soil samples were performed at Site 3. Total Cr concentrations ranged from 460 mg/kg to 820 mg/kg, and hexavalent concentrations ranged from less than 1.0 mg/kg to 1.9 mg/kg. Unlike the water analyses presented for Sites 1 and 2, a significant portion of the total Cr concentrations in soil at Site 3 may be attributable to elemental Cr, because of the nature of the source at Site 3.

Background Cr concentrations for soil in this area would be expected to be within the ranges of 15 mg/kg to 100 mg/kg (Dragun, 1991). Although hexavalent Cr was detected in four of the six samples, the proportion of total Cr in each sample accounted for by Cr(VI) was very low, ranging from less than 0.16 to 0.39 percent.

Site 4 (Groundwater, Surface Water, Soil)

Eight groundwater samples at Site 4 were analyzed for total Cr (unfiltered), hexavalent Cr (unfiltered), and total Cr (filtered). Concentrations of trivalent Cr (unfiltered) were obtained by subtracting the measured Cr(VI) from the total Cr measurements (both unfiltered). The distribution of Cr (VI) in the unfiltered data was expressed as a percent of the total unfiltered Cr data, and is given in Table 2.

As shown in Table 2, concentrations of Cr in some of the unfiltered groundwater samples at Site 4 were notable, ranging as high as 58,800 μg/L for total Cr and 51,000 μg/L for Cr(VI). Based on the potential sources at the site noted in Table 1, a significant variation in the distribution of Cr(VI) in the site groundwater may be expected. Indeed, based on these data, the percent of Cr(VI) of the total unfiltered total Cr measurements spans a wide range, varying from 12.0 to 89.6 percent.

Figure 1 presents two different representations of the Site 4 Cr groundwater data. The darkly shaded bars represent the soluble fractions of Cr in the total Cr measurements for each sample as a percent, by the ratio: Concentration Total Cr (filtered)/Concentration Total Cr (unfiltered) x 100.

The lighter bars represent the hexavalent Cr fractions (unfiltered) in each sample as a percent, by the ratio: Concentration Cr(VI) (unfiltered)/Concentration Total Cr (unfiltered) x 100.

It can be assumed that the difference between 100 percent and the height of the darkly shaded bars represents the portion of a given sample which was insoluble, and that the difference between 100 percent and the height of the lighter bars represents the portion of a given sample which is trivalent. Theoretically, if all of the Cr(VI) is soluble, the height of the bars should be equal; the difference between the heights of the two bars essentially shows how good the soluble fraction is at predicting the Cr(VI) concentrations in the unfiltered samples. As would be expected, the sets of bars for each of the samples are very similar, indicating that the soluble fraction is a good indicator of the measured Cr(VI) concentrations.

TABLE 2--<u>Percent distribution of hexavalent chromium in groundwater and surface water at site 4</u>[a]

Sample ID	Chromium Concentration (Unfiltered) (µg/L)			Percent Hexavalent Chromium (Unfiltered) (%)	Total (III and VI) Chromium (Filtered) (µg/L)	Percent Soluble Total Chromium[c] (%)
	Total (III and VI)	Trivalent (Total-VI)[b]	Hexavalent (VI)			
Groundwater						
1	343	293	50	14.6	--d	--
2	251	221	30	12.0	--	--
3	1,230	1,020	210	17.1	200	16.3
4	95	35	60	63.2	68	71.6
5	90	30	60	66.7	62	68.9
6	20,100	2,100	18,000	89.6	17,000	84.6
7	58,800	7,800	51,000	86.7	54,800	93.2
8	1,180	901	279	23.6	293	24.8
UCL[e]:	58,800	7,800	51,000	**Range:** 12.0 - 89.6		**Range:** 16.3 - 93.2
Stream						
1	169	137	32	18.9	--	--
2	84	49	35	41.7	--	--
3	83	57	26	31.3	--	--
4	166	130	36	21.7	--	--
5	119	0	129	108	--	--
6	126	11	115	91.3	--	--
7	130	14	116	89.2	--	--
UCL[e]:	161	137	129	**Range:** 18.9 - 108		

[a]Only samples with detections of <u>both</u> chromium (total) and hexavalent chromium are presented.

[b]Trivalent Cr was not measured, it was derived by Total Cr-Cr(VI) measurements.

[c]Percentage derived from following ratio: total Cr (filtered)/total Cr (unfiltered).

[d]Dashes (--) indicate that filtered chromium analysis was not performed for this sample.

[e]UCL is the log-transformed 95th percent upper confidence limit of the arithmetic mean, or the maximum concentration, whichever is smaller.

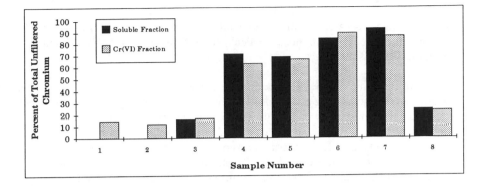

FIGURE 1. THE DISTRIBUTION OF CHROMIUM IN GROUNDWATER AT SITE 4

The heights of the sets of bars relative to one another and to 100 percent are also an indication of how much of the Cr in the groundwater, based on these samples, is present as Cr (III) and how much is Cr(VI). As shown in Figure 1, groundwater at Site 4 appears to be predominantly in the Cr(VI) state, with the exception of samples 3 and 8 (no filtered measurements were obtained for samples 1 and 2). It is likely that the variation in the unfiltered Cr(VI) data (12.0 to 89.6 percent) can be attributed to suspended solids in the samples.

The distribution of Cr(VI) in surface water was also evaluated for Site 4. Sources of Cr in the stream adjacent to the site may have included treated wastewater discharges and the discharge of impacted groundwater. As shown in Table 2, the concentrations of Cr in surface water were significantly lower than the concentrations detected in site groundwater, ranging only as high as 169 μg/L for total Cr (unfiltered) and 129 μg/L for Cr(VI) (unfiltered); however, the concentrations are significantly higher than the background concentration of 3.0 μg/L detected upstream. The distribution of Cr(VI) in each of these seven (unfiltered) samples spans a considerable range, 18.9 to 108 percent.

VARIATIONS IN RISK ESTIMATES USING CHROMIUM DISTRIBUTIONS

As mentioned previously, due to the lack of oxidation state-specific environmental data for many sites, and the differences in toxicity of the two oxidation states, assumptions concerning the distribution of Cr(III) and Cr(VI) must often be made during the risk assessment process. Many times, it is conservatively assumed that the total Cr data represent either 100 percent Cr(III) compounds or 100 percent Cr(VI) compounds, and a wide range of risks is presented. Even if oxidation state-specific data are obtained, there are variations in how these data can be used to estimate risks from exposure to Cr because there are separate toxicity factors for Cr(III) and Cr(VI). Because there are separate toxicity factors, this leads to two separate estimates of Cr risk (and risk-based concentrations, if calculated), effectively treating Cr(III) and Cr(VI) as different chemicals.

To illustrate the variations in risk estimates which may result from using different Cr distributions, actual data and exposure scenarios from Site 4 (previously discussed) were used. For consistency in this illustration, only the ingestion routes were evaluated for a potential future residential or recreational population who may encounter Cr as measured in samples of site groundwater, surface water from a nearby stream, or surficial soil under baseline conditions. The intake calculations and risk estimates were performed using the methods given in the current federal Superfund guidance (USEPA, 1989), and the noncarcinogenic toxicity factors, called reference doses (RfDs) for Cr(III) and Cr(VI) from IRIS (1.0 and 0.005 mg/kg-day, respectively). Consistent with federal guidance, the concentration term used was the log-transformed 95th percent upper confidence limit (UCL) of the arithmetic mean, or the maximum, whichever was smaller. Carcinogenic risk estimates are not given for this illustration since carcinogenicity was only relevant for the inhalation route (i.e., no oral slope factors are currently available from IRIS for Cr(III) or Cr(VI)).

Noncarcinogenic risk estimates (called "hazard quotients") for Cr were generated by calculating ratios of the oxidation state-specific intake factor (resulting from a combination of exposure parameter values for both Cr(III) and Cr(VI)) divided by the oxidation state-specific RfD (USEPA, 1989). Values which exceed one (1.0) are of potential concern. Hazard quotients (HQs) for Cr were calculated using unfiltered groundwater and surface water data for the following variations of Cr(III)/(VI) distributions: assuming 100 percent of the measured total Cr (unfiltered) concentration was Cr(III) to calculate a UCL and use of the Cr(III) RfD; assuming 100 percent of the measured total Cr concentration was Cr(VI) to calculate a UCL and use of the Cr(VI) RfD; using an estimated Cr(III) concentration (subtracting the measured hexavalent data from the total Cr data and calculating a UCL) and the Cr(III) RfD; and using the measured Cr(VI) data to calculate a UCL and the Cr(VI) RfD. For surficial soil, only the first two variations were performed because only total Cr data (no hexavalent) were available. The range of HQs for Cr generated using these variations are presented in Table 3. Also presented are the concentration terms (UCLs or maximums) used to calculate the HQs.

As shown in Table 3, for groundwater, the HQs ranged from 0.27 to 400. The minimum value was obtained by use of the measured distribution data for Cr(III), and the maximum was obtained assuming 100 percent of the total Cr was as Cr(VI). In reviewing the assumption (not measured) data for Cr(III) and Cr(VI), a range of 2 to 400 for the HQ is evident. Because the groundwater concentration (58.8 mg/L total Cr) used to calculate both HQs and the exposure parameters were all the same, this range simply represents the range in toxicity of Cr(III) and Cr(VI). This wide range in

TABLE 3--Variations in noncarcinogenic risk estimates resulting from different chromium distributions

Exposure Route and Cr Distributions	95th UCL[a] (ppm)	Noncarcinogenic Hazard Quotient (HQ)
INGESTION OF GROUNDWATER		
-Assumed 100% Cr(III)	58.8 *	2.0
-Assumed 100% Cr(VI)	58.8 *	400
-Measured Cr(III)[b]	7.8 *	0.27
-Measured Cr(VI)	51.0 *	360
INGESTION OF SURFACE WATER		
-Assumed 100% Cr(III)	0.161	3.9E-05
-Assumed 100% Cr(VI)	0.161	7.8E-03
-Measured Cr(III)[b]	0.137 *	3.4E-05
-Measured Cr(VI)	0.129 *	6.4E-03
INGESTION OF SURFICIAL SOIL		
-Assumed 100% Cr(III)	153	3.7E-05
-Assumed 100% Cr(VI)	153	7.4E-03

[a]Unfiltered data are presented for both groundwater and surface water; units for soil are in mg/kg. If an asterisk (*) noted, UCL exceeded maximum, so the maximum concentration was used to estimate HQs.
[b]"Measured" Cr(III) value determined by subtracting measured Cr(VI) concentration from measured total Cr concentration.

risk estimates indicates that, if oxidation state-specific data were not available and assumptions about Cr oxidation states were used instead, and predominately Cr(III) was present in groundwater, the risks would be greatly overestimated. However, if Cr(VI) was the predominant oxidation state, risks on the upper end of the range would be expected to be more representative.

Using the actual measured distributions of Cr(III) and Cr(VI) in groundwater (7.8 and 51.0 mg/L, respectively) from Site 4, a range of HQs of 0.27 to 360 is obtained. This range is very similar to the range obtained from just assuming 100 percent of either Cr(III) or Cr(VI). The similarity is due to the fact that most of the Cr present in groundwater was demonstrated to be hexavalent. More specifically, the UCL used to estimate Cr(VI) risks (51.0 mg/L) is approximately 87 percent of the total Cr measurement (58.8 mg/L). The minimum HQ value (0.27) is lower than the minimum HQ obtained assuming 100 percent Cr(III) (2.0) because the UCL used is smaller.

For surface water, the HQs were much lower than those for groundwater (reflecting much lower measured concentrations of Cr), ranging from 3.4×10^{-5} to 7.8×10^{-3}. The differences in groundwater and surface water concentrations may reflect differences in site sources, or proximity to sources, or a higher percentage of Cr(III) in surface water, which is likely bound to sediment. As was the case with groundwater, the minimum value was also obtained by use of the measured distribution and using measured distribution data for Cr(III), and the maximum value was obtained from assuming 100 percent of the total Cr was Cr(VI). The HQs obtained assuming a 100 percent distribution and using measured distribution data reflect differences similar to groundwater (i.e., 3.9×10^{-5} compared to 3.4×10^{-5}, and 7.8×10^{-3} compared to 6.4×10^{-3}).

Only two HQs were generated for the surficial soil ingestion route because no hexavalent data were measured for soils. Although the HQ values for soil are relatively low, they still represent a large range, from 3.7×10^{-5} to 7.4×10^{-3}. The distribution of Cr(III) and Cr(VI) in soil cannot be predicted by the percentages observed in water samples, and would be expected to be very different. Although the HQs are below the "acceptable" limit of 1.0, the range of HQ values points to the importance of having hexavalent Cr measurements. It should be noted that there are sources of uncertainty in the risk estimates inherent in the process other than the assumptions about Cr distribution. Also, the distribution of oxidation states of Cr left at sites may change through natural processes over time.

RISK-BASED AND OTHER CLEANUP LEVELS

For the purposes of comparison to regulatory criteria for Cr, risk-based preliminary remediation goals (PRGs) were calculated using the same methods, exposure scenarios, and parameters from Site 4 used in the risk estimates (HQs) previously presented in Table 3. PRGs are chemical-specific concentrations, generated by "back-calculating" from an HQ value of 1.0 to arrive at an "acceptable" Cr concentration in each relevant medium. Figure 2 provides a summary of the most and least conservative PRGs for Cr (i.e., assuming total Cr is 100 percent Cr(VI) or 100 percent Cr(III), respectively) for each medium, groundwater, surface water, and soil, along with selected state and federal regulatory limits for comparison. As shown in Figure 2, some of the criteria are for specific valence of Cr (III or VI), and some are for total Cr.

Groundwater

The groundwater risk-based PRGs calculated for Cr ranged from 0.14 mg/L (assuming 100 percent Cr(VI)) to 29 mg/L (assuming 100 percent Cr(III)). Both of the risk-based PRGs are greater than the Practical Quantitation Limit (PQL) of 10 μg/L for Cr. The federal MCL (or Maximum Contaminant Level) for total Cr, the Massachusetts Cr(VI) standard, and the Wisconsin groundwater standard for total Cr are all 0.1 mg/L, just below the risk-based PRG based on 100 percent Cr(VI). The Massachusetts (Cr(III) groundwater standard is 2 mg/L, an order of magnitude below the risk-based PRG based on 100 percent Cr(III).

Surface Water

The surface water risk-based PRGs calculated for Cr ranged from 19 mg/L (assuming 100 percent Cr(VI)) to 3,700 mg/L (assuming 100 percent Cr(III)). Both of the risk-based PRGs are greater than the PQL of 10 μg/L for Cr. The federal freshwater chronic ambient water quality criteria for Cr(III) and Cr(VI) are 0.21 mg/L and 0.011 mg/L, respectively. The Wisconsin chronic surface water standards for Cr(III) and Cr(VI) are 0.055 mg/L and 0.0097 mg/L, respectively. The New Jersey surface water standard (based on total Cr) is 0.16 mg/L. As shown in Figure 2, all of these regulatory levels are orders of magnitude below both risk-based PRGs presented. This is presumably because the regulatory levels are based upon toxicity to aquatic organisms rather than humans.

Soil

The soil risk-based PRGs calculated for Cr ranged from 1,300 mg/kg (assuming 100 percent Cr(VI)) to 270,000 mg/kg (assuming 100 percent Cr(III)). Both of the risk-based PRGs are greater than the PQL of 0.5 mg/kg for Cr. The draft federal soil screening level for Cr(VI) (390 mg/kg), the Massachusetts Cr(VI) soil standard (200 mg/kg), and the Wisconsin Cr(VI) soil standard (135 mg/kg) are all well below the Cr(VI) risk-based PRG. The Massachusetts Cr(III) soil standard (1,000 mg/kg) and the Wisconsin Cr(III) standard (50,000 mg/kg) are also well below the Cr(III) risk-based PRG.

FIGURE 2. SUMMARY OF CHROMIUM RISK-BASED PRELIMINARY REMEDIATION GOALS AND REGULATORY LEVELS BY MEDIUM

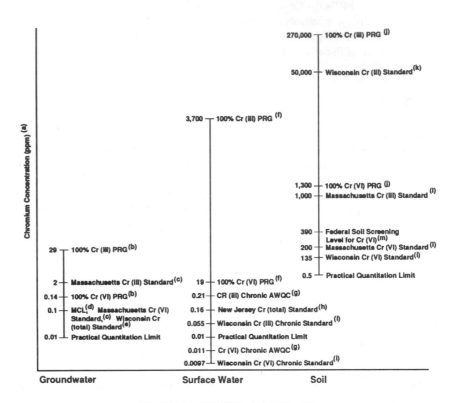

ENVIRONMENTAL MEDIA OF INTEREST

Footnotes:

(a) Due to the large range of chromium concentrations presented in this figure, the levels indicated are not to scale.

(b) PRG based on the ingestion exposure route for a residential child/adult population.

(c) Based on groundwater category GW-3 (category of groundwater at all disposal sites) (ASTM, 1995).

(d) "Maximum Contaminent Levels" Title 40 Code of Federal Regulations Pt.142.

(e) Source: ASTM, 1995.

(f) PRG based on the dermal contact, incidental ingestion, and inhalation exposure routes for a recreational child/adult population.

(g) AWQC = Ambient Water Quality Criteria (USEPA, 1984).

(h) Criteria for FW2 surface waters (New Jersey Administrative Code).

(i) Assumes hardness of 100 ppm (Wisconsin Administrative Code).

(j) PRG based on the dermal contact, incidental ingestion, and inhalation exposure routes for a residential child/adult population.

(k) Nonindustrial level (ASTM, 1995).

(l) Source: ASTM, 1995.

(m) Based on ingestion exposure route from draft USEPA Soil Screening Guidance (USEPA, 1994).

As shown in Figure 2, there can be a great deal of variation in the criteria which may be used at a site as target cleanup levels. This variation is likely due to differences in the assumptions made concerning what constitutes an acceptable exposure. For the risk-based PRG levels calculated for Cr, the assumptions used (or the actual distributions) of Cr(III)/Cr(VI) within the associated media have an enormous effect on the level calculated. Thus, the Cr distribution may determine whether or not a cleanup level exceeds an associated regulatory level, and potentially whether, and how much, remediation at a site is necessary.

CONCLUSIONS

It has been demonstrated that the distribution of Cr oxidation states varies widely throughout waste sites and environmental media, and there is no apparent or consistent trend in the proportions of the Cr oxidation states observed. The distributions observed at the four waste sites evaluated are most likely due more to the oxidation states and concentrations in site sources as compared to the environmental transformation reactions which may be taking place in the media. It was also shown that the filtering of water samples can have a profound effect on the determination of the predominant oxidation states present.

Risk estimates (HQs) calculated using data from one of the waste sites evaluated also showed a wide range. Because the risk estimates are directly related to concentrations in site media as well as toxicity, and the toxicity value for Cr(III) is much lower than that for Cr(VI), this variability is not unexpected.

In addition, an evaluation of risk-based PRGs and selected state and federal criteria showed a wide range in acceptable levels of Cr in site media; this range is also a function of the oxidation state of Cr assumed/measured. Although oxidation state-specific measurements of Cr are not routinely performed at all waste sites, this paper illustrates the importance that the distribution of Cr(III) and Cr(VI) in environmental media has on the characterization of data, the evaluation of potential risks associated with the media, and also possibly the level of cleanup required at a site.

REFERENCES

Agency for Toxic Substances and Disease Registry, 1992, Draft Toxicological Profile for Chromium. U.S. Department of Health and Human Services, October 1991.

ASTM, 1995, *Cleanup Criteria for Contaminated Soil and Groundwater*, DS 64, American Society for Testing and Materials, Philadelphia, PA.

Bodek, Itamar, 1988, *Environmental Inorganic Chemistry Properties, Processes, and Estimation Methods*. Pergamon Press Inc.

Dragun, James, 1991, *Elements in North American Soils*. Hazardous Materials Control Resources Institute, Greenbelt, Maryland.

Eisler, R., 1986, Chromium Hazards to Fish, Wildlife, and Invertebrates: A Synoptic Review. U.S. Fish Wildl. Serv. Biol. Rep. 85(1.6) Contaminant Hazard Reviews Report No. 6., January 1986.

Hem, John D., 1985, "Study and Interpretation of the Chemical Characteristic of Natural Water". U.S. Geological Survey Water-Supply Paper 2254, third Edition.

Integrated Risk Information System, 1995, U.S. Environmental Protection Agency, Office of Health and Environmental Assessment, March 17, 1995.

New Jersey Administrative Code 7:9 B-1.14, "Criteria for FW2 Surface Waters".

U.S. Environmental Protection Agency, 1994, *Draft Soil Screening Guidance*, EPA/540/R-94/101, December 1994.

U.S. Environmental Protection Agency, 1990, *Test Methods for Evaluating Solid Wastes, Physical/Chemical Methods, SW-846, 3rd ed.* Office of Solid Waste and Emergency Response, Washington, DC.

U.S. Environmental Protection Agency, 1989, *Risk Assessment Guidance for Superfund - Human Health Evaluation Manual, (Part A)*, Interim Final, EPA/540/1-89/002, Office of Emergency and Remedial Response, December 1989.

U.S. Environmental Protection Agency, 1984, *Ambient Water Quality Criteria for Chromium*, EPA/440/5-84/029.

Vitale, et al., "Hexavalent Chromium Quantification in Soils: An Effective and Reliable Procedure". American Environmental Laboratory, April, 1995.

Wisconsin Administrative Code Chapter NR 105.06, "Wisconsin Water Quality Standards".

Hui-Tsung Hsu[1] and Albert T. Yeung[2]

DEVELOPMENT OF A MATHEMATICAL MODEL FOR DESIGN OF MULTIPLE-WELL SOIL VAPOR EXTRACTION SYSTEMS

REFERENCE: Hsu, H.-T. and Yeung, A. T., "Development of A Mathematical Model for Design of Multiple-Well Soil Vapor Extraction Systems," *Environmental Toxicology and Risk Assessment: Biomarkers and Risk Assessment—Fifth Volume, ASTM STP 1306,* David A. Bengtson and Diane S. Henshel, Eds., American Society for Testing and Materials, 1996.

ABSTRACT: Soil vapor extraction (SVE) is a proven technology that can remove volatile organic compounds (VOCs) from the subsurface effectively if the conditions are favorable. However, most systems are designed by empirical methods or engineering judgement based on results of pilot tests. An attempt is made to develop a mathematical model for the technology so that optimal operating parameters can be obtained. The pressure distributions induced by multiple-well extractions are obtained by superimposing an existing analytical solution. Concentrations of VOCs as a function of time and space are obtained by numerical simulation of the migration and fate of VOC. The effectiveness of SVE systems using different operating parameters is evaluated on the basis of the quantity of contaminant removed. The developed mathematical model provides the necessary engineering design tools to evaluate different operation scenarios.

KEYWORDS: volatile organic compound, soil vapor extraction, numerical simulation, multiple-well operation, site remediation, subsurface contamination, soil venting, mathematical model

INTRODUCTION

Soil vapor extraction (SVE) or soil venting is an *in-situ* process developed to remove VOCs, liquid-phase hydrocarbons, and semi-volatile compounds from the subsurface. It has been used to remove VOCs from numerous contaminated sites successfully (Crow et al. 1986; Knieper 1988; Malot 1989). The fundamental phenomena governing the performance of SVE can be understood easily. The vapor flow through an unsaturated soil is induced by applying a vacuum through an

---

[1]Graduate Research Assistant, Department of Civil Engineering, Texas A&M University, College Station, Texas 77843-3136.
[2]Assistant Professor of Civil Engineering, Texas A&M University, College Station, Texas 77843-3136.

extraction well. A pressure gradient is thus created to drive gas flow through the contaminated zone to the extraction well. Contaminated vapor so collected can be either discharged directly to the atmosphere or treated by a vapor treatment device. Commonly used vapor treatment devices include: granular activated carbon, catalytic combustion, and vapor incinerator. A typical SVE system is presented in Fig. 1.

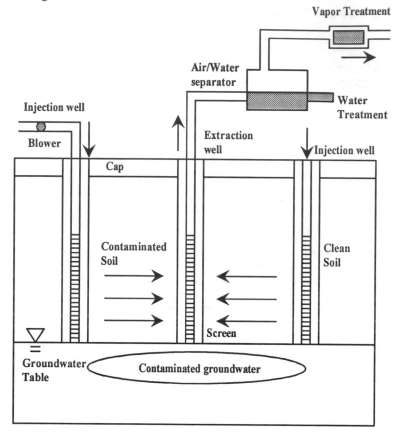

FIG. 1 -- Schematic of a typical soil vapor extraction system

At present, SVE systems are often designed by empirical methods. Many designs are based on engineering judgment and experience gained from expensive and time-consuming pilot tests (Massmann 1989; Johnson et al. 1990). Hence, there is a need to develop rational design methods. Much effort has been devoted to develop a mathematical simulation method to describe the performance of the SVE system. Theoretically, the performance of a SVE system can be assessed by a two step approach: (1) determination of the pressure distribution in the domain of interest; and (2) simulation of contaminant transport and contaminant interactions between different phases.

While many earlier studies have provided a deeper insight into the design and operation of the SVE system, their uses to simulate more complex and practical configurations of SVE systems are quite limited. For example, there is still no systematic study of the effectiveness and efficiency of using multiple-well extraction (Johnson et al. 1990). Most studies to date use only one extraction well installed at the center of the contaminated zone. Therefore, studies on (1) advantages and disadvantages of using multiple wells; and (2) optimization of multiple-well operation are yet to be performed.

In this paper, an approach to address these problems is presented. The Baehr and Hult (1991) analytical approach is adopted to determine the pressure distribution in the subsurface during a multiple-well extraction. The transport of VOCs to the extraction wells is simulated by the advection-dispersion equation. The distribution of VOCs in different phases is determined by equilibrium relationships between concentrations of VOCs in various phases. Solutions obtained from these numerical simulations are used to assess the performance of SVE systems using different operating parameters.

ASSUMPTIONS

Though the concept of a SVE operation can be understood easily, successful application of the technology depends on these factors:

(1)   favorable chemical properties of contaminant (high Henry's constant or high vapor pressure and low aqueous phase partition coefficient);

(2)   favorable characteristics of the soil environment (high porosity, low water content, and high air permeability); and

(3)   optimal operating parameters, such as number of wells, well configuration, pumping rate, screen length, etc., of the SVE system.

These factors must be considered carefully in the development of a mathematical model for the simulation of SVE operations. However, certain simplifications are necessary so that the mathematical model is able to represent the SVE process adequately and the resulting equations can be solved efficiently. The assumptions made in the formulation of the mathematical model are summarized in Table 1.

DETERMINATION OF PRESSURE DISTRIBUTION

Using Darcy's law, continuity equation, and ideal gas laws, the steady state pressure distribution in the scenario depicted in Fig. 2 is described by (Baehr and Hult 1991)

$$k_r \left(\frac{\partial^2 \phi}{\partial r^2} + \frac{1}{r} \frac{\partial \phi}{\partial r} \right) + k_z \frac{\partial^2 \phi}{\partial z^2} - \frac{k_c}{b b_c} \left(\phi - P_{atm}^2 \right) = 0 \qquad (1)$$

where $\phi = P^2$ and P = pressure [g/cm-s^2]; k_r = intrinsic air permeability of soil in the radial direction [cm^2]; k_z = intrinsic air permeability of soil in the vertical direction [cm^2]; k_c = intrinsic air permeability of cover material in the vertical direction [cm^2]; b = depth of unsaturated zone [cm]; b_c = thickness of the cover [cm]; and P_{atm} = atmospheric pressure [g/cm-s^2]. The last term on the left

TABLE 1 -- Assumptions made in the formulation of the mathematical model

Classifications	Assumptions
Subsurface environment	(a) the soil is homogeneous and isothermal (b) source of contamination has been removed (c) Darcy's law is valid for gas flow
Contaminant properties	(a) the VOC vapor is an ideal gas and a Newtonian fluid (b) slip flow and Klinkenberg effect are negligible (c) water and immiscible fluid phases are immobile (d) chemical equilibrium between phases can be reached instantaneously (e) sorption of contaminant on soil particle surface can be described by a linear isotherm (f) the rate of biodegradation and chemical reactions are negligible
SVE system	(a) the upper soil surface is covered by an impermeable material (b) the pressure field in the subsurface is at steady state

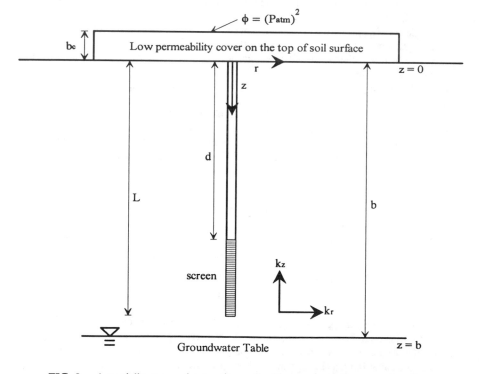

FIG. 2 -- A partially screened extraction well with a cover on the ground surface

hand side accounts for the air leakage through the cover. For the boundary conditions given by

$$\frac{\partial \phi}{\partial z}(r, 0) = \frac{\partial \phi}{\partial z}(r, b) = 0 \tag{2}$$

$$\lim_{r \to \infty} \phi(r, z) = P_{atm}^2 \tag{3}$$

and at $r = r_w$

$$\frac{\partial \phi}{\partial r} = 0 \qquad\qquad 0 < z < d \tag{4}$$

$$\frac{\partial \phi}{\partial r} = \frac{-Q_c}{\pi k_r(L - d)r_w} \qquad\qquad d < z < L \tag{5}$$

$$\frac{\partial \phi}{\partial r} = 0 \qquad\qquad L < z < b \tag{6}$$

where r_w = radius of the well [cm]; $Q_c = (Q \mu RT)/M_{air}$; Q = mass pumping rate [g/s]; μ = dynamic viscosity of air [g/cm-s]; M_{air} = molecular weight of air [g/mole]; R = universal gas constant [8.3145×10^7 erg/mole-K]; T = temperature [K]; L = distance from the lower surface of cover to the bottom of well screen; d = distance from the lower surface of cover to the top of well screen; and $(L-d)$ = length of screened portion of the extraction well; the analytical solution to Eq. (1) is given by (Baehr and Hult 1991)

$$\phi = P_{atm}^2 + \frac{aQ_c}{\pi k_r r_w} \left\{ \frac{K_0\left(\dfrac{M_0 r}{a}\right)}{b M_0 K_1\left(\dfrac{M_0 r_w}{a}\right)} + \frac{2}{\pi(L-d)} \sum_{n-1}^{\infty} \left(\sin\left(\frac{n\pi L}{b}\right) - \sin\left(\frac{n\pi d}{h}\right) \right) \right.$$

$$\left. \times \frac{K_0\left(\dfrac{M_n r}{a}\right)}{n M_n K_1\left(\dfrac{M_n r_w}{a}\right)} \cos\left(\frac{n\pi z}{b}\right) \right\} \tag{7}$$

where $a = \sqrt{k_r / k_z}$; K_0 = the zeroth order modified Bessel function of the second kind; K_1 = the first order modified Bessel function of the second kind; and $M_n = \sqrt{(n\pi/b)^2 + k_o/(b b_c k_z)}$.

As Eq. (1) is linear in ϕ, the value of ϕ at any location due to a multiple-well extraction can be obtained by superimposing the solution given in Eq. (7). Thus, the pressure induced at any location A by m extraction wells is given by

$$P_A = \sqrt{\sum_{i-1}^{m} \phi(r_i, z) - (m-1)P_{atm}^2} \tag{8}$$

where P_A = pressure at point A [g/cm^2-s]; and r_i = distance between extraction well i and point A [cm].

SIMULATION OF VOC TRANSPORT AND INTER-PHASE PARTITIONING

The vapor flux through an unsaturated zone is described by the advection-dispersion equation

$$J_a = q_a C_a - D\nabla C_a \tag{9}$$

where J_a = vapor flux [g/cm^2-s]; $q_a = -k\nabla P/(n\mu)$ = average linear velocity of air through the porous medium; C_a = concentration of VOC in the gaseous phase [g/cm^3]; and D = hydrodynamic dispersion tensor [cm^2/s]. Neglecting dispersion in the transverse direction, the hydrodynamic dispersion coefficient in the i-direction D_i is given by

$$D_i = \alpha_L |q_{a,i}| + D_f^e \tag{10}$$

where α_L = longitudinal dispersivity [cm]; $q_{a,i}$ = component of the average linear velocity of air in the i-direction; and D_f^e = effective molecular diffusion coefficient of gas in soil [cm^2/s]. Millington (1959) defined the effective molecular diffusion of gas phase as

$$D_f^e = \frac{(nS_a)^{10/3}}{n^2} D_f \tag{11}$$

where D_f = free-air diffusion coefficient [cm^2/s]. The mass balance equation of VOC is thus given by

$$R_T \frac{\partial C_a}{\partial t} + \nabla \cdot J_a = 0 \tag{12}$$

where $R_T = nS_w/K_h + nS_a + \rho_b K_{sa}$ = retardation factor; S_w and S_a = degrees of water and air saturation, respectively; $K_h = C_a/C_w$ = Henry's constant; C_w = concentration of VOC in the aqueous phase [g/cm^3]; ρ_b = dry density of the porous medium [g/cm^3]; $K_{sa} = C_s/C_a$ = soil-gas partition coefficient [cm^3/g]; and C_s = concentration of VOC in the sorbed phase [g/g]. Solutions to Eq. (12) give the concentration of VOC as a function of time and space.

The soil-gas partition coefficient K_{sa} is estimated by (Ong and Lion 1991)

$$K_{sa} = \frac{K_{sw}}{K_h} + \frac{\theta}{K_h \rho_w} \tag{13}$$

where K_{sw} = soil-water partition coefficient [cm^3/g]; θ = water content by mass in decimal; and ρ_w = density of water [g/cm^3]. The soil-water partition coefficient K_{sw} is related to the carbon content of the soil by (Hamaker and Thompson 1972; Rao and Davidson 1980; Jury et al. 1983)

$$K_{sw} = f_{oc}K_{oc} \tag{14}$$

where f_{oc} = fraction of organic carbon in the soil [dimensionless]; and K_{oc} = organic carbon normalized partition coefficient [cm^3/g].

The pressure distribution in the subsurface is determined by Eqs. (7) and (8), and the vapor flux is then calculated using Eq. (9). Then solutions to Eq. (12) give the concentration of VOC in the gaseous phase as a function of time and space. The numerical scheme used to solve Eq. (12) is the discretization method developed by Patankar (1981). The domain of simulation is divided into continuous non-overlapping control volumes. A grid point is located at the geometric center of each control volume and the partial differential equation is integrated over each control volume and over the time interval from t to t+Δt. The concentration at the grid point is thus representative of that of the control volume. The profile of flux over each face of the control volume is assumed to be uniform. The technique of implicit finite difference is used for time marching. Applying the power law scheme to interpolate the concentration at the surface of the control volume, the two-dimensional discretization equation for VOC concentration can be expressed as

$$a_P C_P = a_W C_W + a_E C_E + a_S C_S + a_N C_N + b \tag{15}$$

where a_i = discretization coefficients; and C_i = concentration of VOC of grid point i at t+Δt [g/cm^3]. W, E, S, and N are the grid points surrounding grid point P. The discretization coefficients are calculated by

$$a_E = G_e A(|P_e|) + [[F_e, 0]] \tag{16}$$

$$a_W = G_w A(|P_w|) + [[-F_w, 0]] \tag{17}$$

$$a_N = G_n A(|P_n|) + [[F_n, 0]] \tag{18}$$

$$a_S = G_s A(|P_s|) + [[-F_s, 0]] \tag{19}$$

$$a_P = R_T \frac{\Delta x \Delta y}{\Delta t} \tag{20}$$

$$b = a_P C_P^0 \tag{21}$$

where the operator [[a,b]] denotes the greater of a and b; Δx and Δy = dimensions of control volume in the x and y directions, respectively; F_e, F_w, F_s, and F_n = mass flow rates through the respective control-volume interfaces; P_e, P_w, P_s, and P_n = Peclet numbers of the flows at interfaces e, w, s, and n, respectively; C_P^0 = concentration of VOC at grid point P at time t; and the interpolation function $A(|P|)$ is given as

$$A(|P|) = [[0, (1 - 0.1|P|)^5]] \tag{22}$$

The coefficients G_e, G_w, G_s, and G_n are defined as

$$G_e = \frac{D_e \Delta y}{I_e} \tag{23}$$

$$G_w = \frac{D_w \Delta y}{I_w} \tag{24}$$

$$G_s = \frac{D_e \Delta x}{I_s} \tag{25}$$

$$G_n = \frac{D_n \Delta x}{I_n} \tag{26}$$

where D_e, D_w, D_s, and D_n are the hydrodynamic dispersion tensors; and I_e, I_w, I_s, and I_n are the grid spacings between grid point P and its neighboring grid points E, W, S, and N, respectively.

The discretization equation, i.e. Eq. (15), can be solved numerically by the line-by-line iteration technique for the given initial and boundary conditions (Patankar 1981). The method uses the Thomas algorithm or the tridiagonal matrix algorithm as the basic operator. The discretization equations along a chosen line of grid points can be solved when the concentrations of VOC at grid points on neighboring lines are given the best estimates. The solving process is continued iteratively in all directions until the concentrations of VOC at all the grid points converge. Interested readers should refer to Hsu (1995) for details of the algorithm.

RESULTS AND DISCUSSIONS

A hypothetical benzene (C_6H_6) contaminated site 16 m long by 16 m wide is used to demonstrate the capability of the developed mathematical model. The soil properties of the site and chemical properties of benzene are tabulated in Tables 2 and 3, respectively. The surface of the contaminated site is covered by a material of very low air permeability to enhance removal efficiency. The performance of three different SVE systems is evaluated. One, three, and five extraction wells are installed at the center of the contaminated zone in Cases A, B, and C, respectively. The well configurations are depicted in Figs. 3a, 4a, and 5a. The operating parameters are tabulated in Table 4. The total mass pumping rate for all three cases is chosen to be 18 g/s to evaluate the effects of number of wells on VOC removal efficiency.

As all three cases being studied are axisymmetric, only one-quarter of the contaminated zone is simulated. The pressure distributions in a horizontal soil layer at the middle of the well screen for one, three, and five extraction wells are presented in Figs. 3b, 4b, and 5b, respectively. In general, there is a cone of pressure depression adjacent to each extraction well. Theoretically, the extent of the reduced pressure zone determines the effectiveness of the extraction well in generating a pressure gradient to drive gas flow. For Case A as presented in Fig. 3b, the extent of the reduced pressure zone appears to be quite limited to the close vicinity of the extraction well. The pressure gradient diminishes rapidly with increase in distance from the extraction well. Thus, increasing mass pumping

TABLE 2 -- Soil Properties of the hypothetical benzene contaminated site

Soil properties	Values
Porosity n	0.4
Intrinsic air permeability in r-direction k_r	1.28×10^{-7} cm^2
Intrinsic air permeability in z-direction k_z	4.92×10^{-8} cm^2
Longitudinal dispersivity α_L	0.004 cm
Temperature T	20°C
Degree of air saturation S_a	0.8
Degree of water saturation S_w	0.2
Dry density of soil ρ_b	1.73 g/cm^3
Fraction of organic carbon in the soil f_{oc}	5%
Depth of unsaturated zone b	500 cm

TABLE 3 -- Chemical properties of benzene

Chemical properties	Values [a]
Molecular weight MW	78.1 g/mole
Vapor pressure P_v	0.1 atm [b]
Solubility in water S	1,780 mg/l [b]
Organic carbon normalized partition coefficient K_{oc}	85 cm^3/g [b]
Henry's constant K_h	0.186 [c]
Free-air diffusion coefficient D_f	0.088 cm^2/s

[a] All the parameters are measured at 20°C.
[b] Values adapted from Krishnayya et al. (1994).
[c] Values adapted from Rathfelder et al. (1991).

TABLE 4 -- Operating parameters of SVE systems evaluated

Operating parameters	Case A	Case B	Case C
Number of extraction wells	1	3	5
Mass pumping rate per well Q [g/s]	18	6	3.6
Dist. from bottom of cover to bottom of well screen L [cm]	500	500	500
Dist. from bottom of cover to top of well screen d [cm]	300	300	300
Thickness of cover b_c [cm]	20	20	20
Intrinsic air permeability of cover k_c [cm^2]	1.9×10^{-9}	1.9×10^{-9}	1.9×10^{-9}

rate does not necessarily improve the performance of a SVE system when the contaminated zone is relatively large. Even when the total mass pumping rate is identical, Cases B and C generate much larger reduced pressure zones as depicted in Figs. 4b and 5b, respectively. Therefore, it is more advantageous to install multiple extraction wells at a reduced mass pumping rate when the contaminated zone is relatively large.

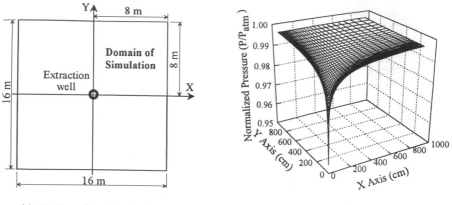

(a) Well configuration in plan   (b) Pressure distribution

FIG. 3 -- Case A: Single extraction well

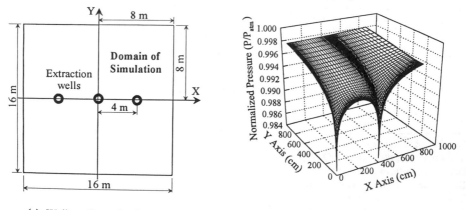

(a) Well configuration in plan   (b) Pressure distribution

FIG. 4 -- Case B: Three extraction wells

Contours of benzene vapor concentration after 40 and 110 hours of continuous pumping at constant rates for the three cases are presented in Figs. 6, 7, and 8. These figures indicate that benzene vapor in the contaminated soil is driven toward the extraction wells and the mass of benzene in the soil is decreasing with duration of soil vapor extraction. Moreover, it can be observed that the pattern of the contours is dependent on the well configuration. Removal of benzene vapor at the corner of the contaminated zone is the most difficult as the flow path is the longest in that direction. It is another good indication that multiple-well extraction should be used in a relatively large contaminated zone so as to shorten the flow path for the VOC to reach the extraction well.

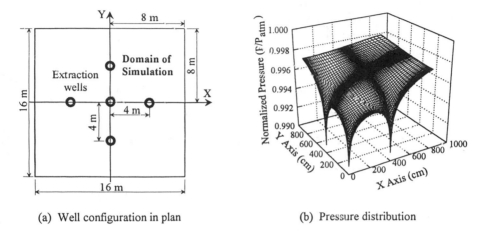

(a) Well configuration in plan   (b) Pressure distribution

FIG. 5 -- Case C: Five extraction wells

The benzene vapor removal efficiencies of the three different well configurations as a function of time is plotted in Fig. 9. Initially, the removal efficiency increases with the number of wells even though the total mass pumping rates are equal in all three well configurations. However, the inward migration of contaminant with time makes the single-well extraction system progressively more efficient. When the contaminated zone is relatively large at the onset of the cleanup operation, a multiple-well extraction system can create a larger reduced pressure zone at a lower pressure gradient than a single-well extraction system. Thus, the zone of influence of a multiple-well extraction system is much larger than that of a single-well extraction system. Though the extraction rate of a single-well extraction system in the close vicinity of the well is higher, more contaminant can be removed by a multiple-well extraction system because of its larger zone of influence. As the zone of contamination decreases with time, the multiple-well extraction system starts to lose its advantage. The higher extraction rate of a single-well extraction system begins to dominate the rate of contaminant removal. An optimization strategy can be formulated on the basis of these observations. Initially, a multiple-well extraction system should be operated with the maximum available power. The number of extraction wells is then reduced progressively while the power supplied to each pump is increased

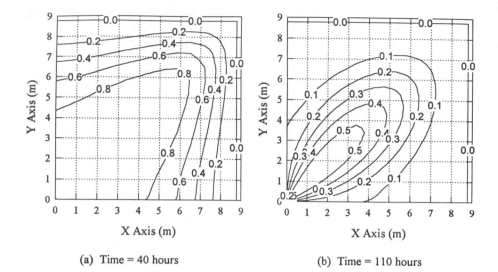

(a) Time = 40 hours   (b) Time = 110 hours

FIG. 6 -- Normalized concentration distribution of benzene in Case A

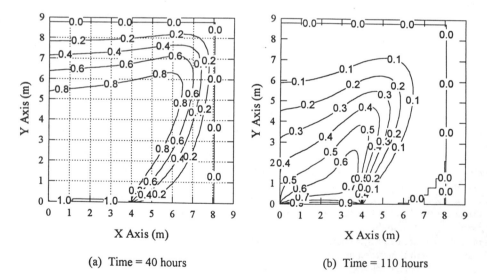

(a) Time = 40 hours   (b) Time = 110 hours

FIG. 7 -- Normalized concentration distribution of benzene in Case B

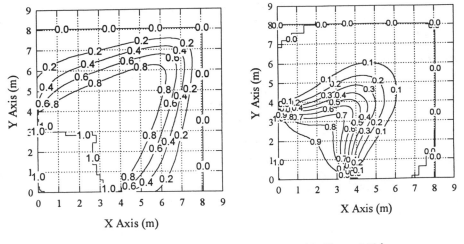

(a) Time = 40 hours   (a) Time = 110 hours

FIG. 8 -- Normalized concentration distribution of benzene in Case C

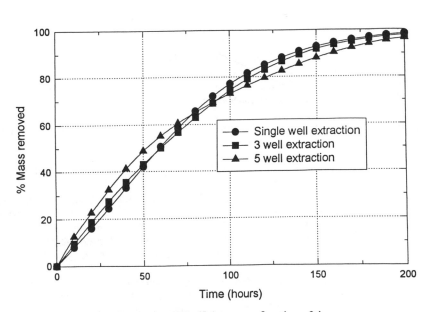

FIG. 9 -- Removal efficiency as a function of time

accordingly. The performance of the SVE system can thus be kept at its best throughout the operation.

CONCLUSIONS

Soil vapor extraction has been proven to be an efficient technology to remove VOC from the subsurface. However, the lack of proper engineering design tools makes it very difficult to design an optimal operating system. A mathematical model describing the pressure distribution generated by vacuum extraction wells and the transport and fate of VOC in the unsaturated zone has been developed in this study. The pressure distribution generated by a multiple-well extraction system is obtained by superposition of an analytical solution for a single-well extraction system. The approach is extremely useful in the simulation of complex and practical system configurations where there are multiple extraction wells installed in the contaminated zone. The equation describing the transport and fate of VOC is solved iteratively by the discretization method. The developed mathematical model can be applied to simulate field-scale operations.

A hypothetical case is presented to demonstrate the capability of the developed mathematical model to predict the performance of the SVE system, and to evaluate the efficiency of a single-well versus that of a multiple-well extraction. The results indicate that the performance of a SVE system can be optimized by the use of proper combination of single well and multiple wells at different stages of the cleanup operation.

REFERENCES

Baehr, A. L. and Hult, M. F., 1991, "Evaluation of Unsaturated Zone Air Permeability through Pneumatic Tests," Water Resources Research, Vol. 29, No. 10, 2605-2617.

Crow, W. L., Anderson, E. P., and Minugh, E. M., 1986, "Subsurface Venting of Vapors Emanating from Hydrocarbon Product on Groundwater," Ground Water Monitoring Review, Vol. 7, No. 1, pp. 51-57.

Hamaker, J. W. and Thompson, J. M., 1972, "Adsorption," Organic Chemicals in the Soil Environment, C. A. I. Goring and J. W. Hamaker, Eds., Marcel Dekker, Inc., New York, pp. 49-144.

Hsu, H.-T., 1995, "Three Dimensional Semi-Analytical Simulation of Multiple Well Soil Vapor Extraction," Ph.D. dissertation, Texas A&M University, College Station.

Johnson, P. C., Stanley, C. C., Kemblowski, M. W., Byers, D. L., and Colthart, J. D., 1990, "A Practical Approach to the Design, Operation, and Monitoring of in-Situ Soil-Venting Systems," Ground Water Monitoring Review, Vol. 10, No. 2, pp. 159-178.

Jury, W. A., Spencer, W. F., and Farmer, W. J., 1983, "Behavior Assessment Model for Trace Organics in Soil: I. Model Description," Journal of Environmental Quality, Vol. 12, No. 4, pp. 558-564.

Knieper, L. H., 1988, "VES Cleans up Gasoline Leak," Pollution Engineering, 20(8), p. 56.

Krishnayya, A. V., Williams, D. R., Agar, J. G., and O'Connor, M. J., 1994, "Significance of Organic Chemical Adsorption in Soil and Groundwater Remediation," Journal of Soil Contamination, Vol. 3, No. 2, pp. 191-202.

Malot, J. J., 1989, "Vacuum Extraction Technology," Forum on Innovative Hazardous Waste Treatment Technologies: Domestic and International, U S. EPA Report No. EPA/540/2-89/056, U.S. EPA, Cincinnati, OH, pp. 77-91.

Massmann, J. W., 1989, "Applying Groundwater Flow Models in Vapor Extraction System Design," Journal of Environmental Engineering, ASCE, Vol. 115, No. 1, pp. 129-149.

Millington, R. J., 1959, "Gas Diffusion in Porous Media," Science, Vol. 130, No. 3267, 100-103.

Ong, S. K. and Lion, L. W., 1991, "Mechanisms for Trichloroethylene Vapor Sorption onto Soil Minerals," Journal of Environmental Quality, Vol. 20, No. 1, pp.180-188.

Patankar, S. V., 1981, "A Calculation Procedure for Two-dimensional Elliptic Situations," Numerical Heat Transfer, Vol. 4, No. 4, pp. 409-425.

Rao, P. S. C. and Davidson, J. M., 1980, "Estimation of Pesticide Retention and Transformation Parameters Required in Nonpoint Source Pollution Models," Environmental Impact of Nonpoint Source Pollution, M. R. Overcsh, Ed , Ann Arbor Sci. Publ. Inc., Ann Arbor, pp. 23-67.

Rathfelder, K., Yeh, W. G., and Mackay, D., 1991, "Mathematical Simulation of Soil Vapor Extraction Systems: Model Development and Numerical Examples," Journal of Contaminant Hydrology, Vol. 8, No. 3/4, pp. 263-297.

Bai-Lian Li[1] and Albert T. Yeung[2]

A WAVELET-BASED METHOD TO ANALYZE CPT DATA FOR GEOTECHNICAL AND GEO-ENVIRONMENTAL SITE CHARACTERIZATION

REFERENCE: Li, B.-L. and Yeung, A. T., "A Wavelet-Based Method to Analyze CPT Data for Geotechnical and Geo-Environmental Site Characterization," *Environmental Toxicology and Risk Assessment: Biomarkers and Risk Assessment—Fifth Volume, ASTM STP 1306,* David A. Bengtson and Diane S. Henshel, Eds., American Society for Testing and Materials, 1996.

ABSTRACT: The applications of cone penetration technology (CPT) in geotechnical and geo-environmental engineering are increasing due to recent advances in electronics and sensors that can be installed on the cone. However, interpretation of CPT data is a complex process and most existing methods are either empirical or semi-empirical. In order to fully utilize the capability of CPT, issues of local feature identification, uncertainty quantification, and scale effects on the interpretation of collected data have to be addressed properly. In this paper, wavelet transform and wavelet variance are used to characterize the essential scales of CPT data, and wavelet transform modulus maxima and phases are used to detect instantaneous frequency change. The scale effects of site stratigraphy determination using CPT data are demonstrated. The results indicate that this wavelet-based approach can provide a promising tool to reduce uncertainties in CPT data interpretation.

KEYWORDS: wavelet analysis, site characterization, cone penetrometer test, CPT, scale effects, site stratigraphy, subsurface contamination, spatial data analysis, feature extraction

INTRODUCTION

Accurate characterization of the subsurface is an integral part of successful design and implementation of waste management/environmental remediation strategies for contaminated sites. Reliable modeling of the chemical, biological, and mechanical processes affecting

---

[1]Assistant Research Scientist, Center for Biosystems Modelling, Department of Industrial Engineering, Texas A&M University, College Station, Texas 77843-3131.

[2]Assistant Professor of Civil Engineering, Texas A&M University, College Station, Texas 77843-3136.

subsurface transport and fate of the contaminant are needed for risk assessment. The subsurface has to be characterized and important parameters have to be identified before any model can be developed. The model will gain credibility only if it can identify and verify critical processes and their interactions in the modeling processes (Li et al. 1996). Localized processes in the subsurface and multi-scale effects in geologic sampling data have to be addressed during site characterization as the characterization may change with scale of subsurface processes, e.g., ground-water recharge is significantly affected by soil depth and small scale topography (Seyfried and Wilcox 1995) and transport processes significant at small scales may not be relevant at large scales. New emerging processes are identified as a result of the increase in scale. However, methods used to represent these processes in a model may depend on the assumed model structure (Carrera 1993). From the analytical perspective, the process of localization introduces important aspects, such as scale dependence of localization zone and evolution of an affined structure within the region, that may violate conventional assumptions made for continua. From the computational standpoint, issues associated with localization include the role of adaptivity and mesh objectivity in the development of unique patterns of localization and stability of such numerical schemes. These unresolved issues are addressed in terms of their relevance to applications in geotechnical engineering, geo-environmental engineering, constitutive parameter identification, error analysis, and risk assessment in this paper.

The need for accurate subsurface information is ever-increasing. Increases in data requirements demand more rapid and economical analyses of collected data. The current trends in dynamic geo-environmental engineering are focused on a better understanding of the dynamic properties of geologic media used in engineering practice. *In-situ* measurements are often preferred to laboratory testing because they eliminate possible sample disturbance during retrieval, and handling and transport of samples. Accurate subsurface strata identification and delineation are prerequisites for both geotechnical and geo-environmental engineering applications. In most geo-environmental engineering projects, chemical data and hydraulic properties of the subsurface strata are typically the focus. The cone penetration technology (CPT) has gained widespread popularity for these purposes due to recent advances in electronics and sensors that can be installed on the cone (Bowders and Daniel 1994; Akhtar 1995). It offers numerous advantages that are being capitalized in the geo-environmental arena. Some of these advantages are: (1) the technique can provide a rapid and inexpensive means to study the subsurface physical and chemical characteristics of a hazardous waste site (data are collected at the standard penetration rate of 2 cm/s); (2) continuous subsurface profile information can be obtained; (3) the data collected can be processed in real time on site so that field decisions can be made; (4) *in-situ* measurements can be made and there is no time lag between collection and chemical analyses of samples; (5) there is no direct contact between workers and contaminated materials; (6) the results obtained are almost operator independent; (7) no contaminated cuttings have to be handled; and (8) impact to the surrounding environment is kept at a minimum. However, some of these advantages can also be disadvantages of the CPT, e.g., not having a soil sample (cutting) can make strata identification more challenging (Bowders and Daniel 1994; Olsen 1994). In general, current criticisms on the cone penetration technology include: resolution, sensitivity, accuracy and confidence of the information obtained. Interpretation of CPT data is a complex process due to the presence of localized and multi-scale features in th subsurface. Most existing interpretation methods are either empirical or semi-empirical. These methods are thus soil specific.

Geostatistical methods are widely accepted tools used to integrate static data for subsurface characterization. However, their uses in the processing of dynamic data are very limited. Moreover, they cannot address critical issues such as data sensitivity and scale, and are inadequate in evaluating different data types. Data integration is a non-trivial task because different data types span different length scales of heterogeneity. In the analysis of any given data set, the length scale of heterogeneity that can be resolved and the associated uncertainties have to be quantified. More promising tools to address these issues are needed for the analyses of CPT data.

Wavelet analysis is a newly developed mathematical theory and computational technique for the separation and sorting of structures on different time scales at different times, or on different spatial scales at different locations (Brewer and Wheatcraft 1994; Pike 1994; Li 1995; Loehle and Li 1996). In wavelet representation, a geophysical signal is decomposed into a sum of elementary building blocks describing its local frequency contents. It is also very useful in the investigation of energy contents of different components of geologic signals within subbands or subspectra and their relationships among different rated processes in the subsurface. In this paper, the limitations of current geostatistical approach to process data are discussed. Wavelet analysis is used as an innovative method to identify and characterize the subsurface at different scales using CPT data. It is demonstrated that wavelet analysis can provide a natural way of sorting multiple scales and localized processes, and determining spatial scale features and site stratigraphy hidden in CPT data.

LIMITATIONS OF CURRENT GEOSTATISTICAL APPROACHES

Multi-scale and localized structures in CPT data are difficult to identify and analyze using current geostatistical methods as the principal frequencies and scales of geotechnical and geo-environmental properties of the subsurface change very rapidly over space. Current geostatistical methods such as semi-variance analyses or kriging have four major limitations: (1) Semi-variance is a global statistic as it compares all data points at a given lag over the entire data set. Local spatial features that produce anomalous results cannot thus be detected. For example, if there are alternating soil types along a drilled core, the semi-variance plot of the data is wavy and difficult to interpret. Moreover, a semi-variance plot does not provide sufficient information to back-calculate details of specific structures, such as strata, that generate the correlations. (2) Current geostatistical methods do not provide stratigraphic description. While data collected from a detailed site investigation can be used to construct a 3-d picture of stratigraphic features, current geostatistical methods do not allow quantitative description of such a spatially explicit data set. Therefore, it is not possible to compare stratigraphic structures of different sites, such as degree of blockiness or degree of interbedding, quantitatively. However, these properties have significant influence on the hydrology and characteristics of contaminant transport at the site. (3) Current geostatistical methods do not capture discontinuities. These methods cannot describe such features and they fail to deal with discontinuities such as those at stratigraphic boundaries. However, information on fractures and discontinuities is crucial for contaminant or microbial transport studies. (4) Geostatistical methods do not allow detection or description of multi-resolution structures that are extremely important in relating phenomena across scales. In summary, current geostatistical methods work best within homogeneous strata or in randomly heterogeneous unstructured media. New methods are thus needed to describe heterogeneous spatial structures and patterns.

Kriging is a collection of generalized linear regression techniques used to minimize the variance of an estimate defined by a chosen covariance model and it is the dominant method used to interpolate geologic data. Kriging techniques include ordinary kriging (point, site, and block), universal kriging, disjunctive kriging, indicator kriging, and cokriging (Deutsch and Journel 1992). When kriging techniques are applied to perform statistical interpolation, the data are assumed to be: (1) intrinsic-stationarity or second-order (weak) stationarity; (2) ergodicity or partial ergodicity; and (3) existence of distribution-based estimation (Li et al. 1992). However, the distributions of data are skewed in many applications (especially in CPT data) rendering accurate estimation very difficult to make. When data are multi-variate normally distributed and variogram is known and well behaved, ordinary kriging is known to be statistically optimal. Similarly, multi-variate lognormal kriging is optimal if data are lognormally distributed. However, it is very difficult to guess the correct distribution for nonlinear and spatially distributed data. The user of geostatistics is therefore faced with the formidable task of choosing the most appropriate stationary model for his data. It is very difficult to make the proper choice as the only given information is from a single realization (set of samples). Since the kriging estimator depends only on the semi-variogram (or the covariance function) and the configuration of observation points (Haining 1990), it also has the disadvantages of semi-variogram. Different types of kriging require different assumptions. Nonetheless, these assumptions are at best only approximately satisfied in practice. For a strongly structured subsurface, the soil and rock parameters that control contaminant flow often change abruptly over short distances. Thus, the assumptions made by kriging cannot even be satisfied approximately. Therefore, new spatial statistical methods are needed to interpolate between unsampled areas for many types of non-stationary, singular, and discontinuous subsurface data.

Singularities and irregular structures often carry the most important information in heterogeneous subsurface systems. Until recently, Fourier transformation has been the most accepted mathematical tool used to analyze singularities. It is a global technique that provides a description of the overall regularity of signals, but it is not well adapted to find the locations and spatial distribution of singularities. Fourier transforms are localized in frequency but not in time (or space). Therefore, they contain information on the frequencies of the signal at all times (or depths) but do not indicate how the frequency vary with time (or space).

WAVELET ANALYSIS

Wavelet analysis is a new computational method developed for signal processing. Because of its capability to perform time (or space) - frequency localization and multi-resolution analysis, the wavelet transform of a signal can provide detailed information on the underlying processes as a function of time or spatial scale. It provides a new technique to analyze geophysical signals at various scales. In wavelet representation, a geophysical signal is decomposed into a sum of elementary building blocks describing its local frequency content. The algorithm is fast and very easy to implement.

Wavelet transforms are integral transforms using integration kernels called wavelets. These transforms enable the study of non-stationary processes (signals) that have good localization properties both in time (or space) and frequency (Chui 1992; Gao and Li 1993; Meyer 1993). Locations of rapid changes in a signal can be detected easily as illustrated in Fig. 1. The signal consists of parts of frequencies 5 Hz and 20 Hz. Its wavelet transform contour map clearly identifies the time when the activity shifts from low frequency to high frequency. The shape of the basic wavelet function in the time (or space) domain varies with frequency to provide an improved fitting to nonlinear and irregular geophysical data. The wavelet analysis provides both scale and time (or space) information and allows separation and sorting of different structures on different time (or space) scales at different times (or locations). The integral wavelet transform of a function f is defined by

$$(W_\psi f)(a,b) \quad = \quad \frac{1}{\sqrt{|a|}} \int f(t)\, \psi\left(\frac{t-b}{a}\right) dt \tag{1}$$

where the function $\psi\left((t-b)/a\right)/\sqrt{|a|}$ is called the "basic" or "mother wavelet". The parameters $a(\neq 0)$ and b are used to adjust the shape and location of the wavelets, respectively. The $1/\sqrt{|a|}$ term keeps the energy of the scaled wavelet equal to the energy of the original mother wavelet. As a changes, the shape of the wavelet is compressed or stretched to cover different frequency ranges. Changing b allows the time (or space) localization center to move and translate wavelets through all data points as shown in Fig. 2. Thus, wavelet transform provides a time (or space) - frequency description of a geophysical signal f. In comparison to the windowed Fourier transformation, wavelet transformation possesses an improved ability to "zoom in" and "zoom out" structures at different scales (Chui 1992; Meyer 1993).

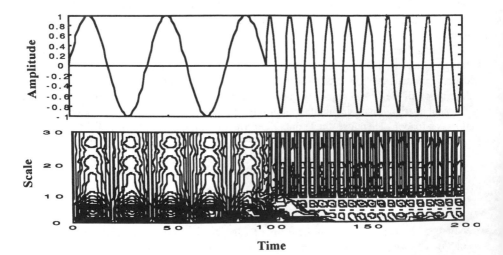

FIG. 1 -- A signal consists of parts of different frequencies and its wavelet transform contour map

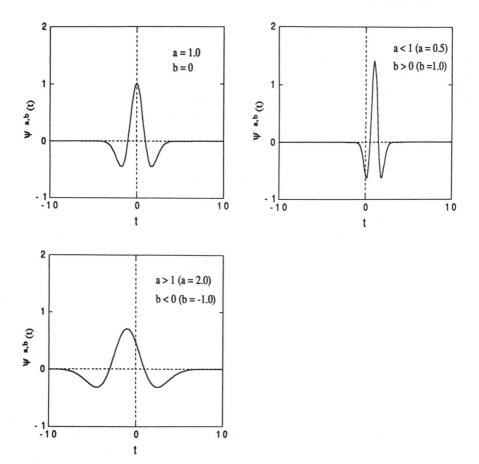

FIG. 2 -- Changes in shape of the "mother wavelet" defined by the "Mexican hat" function with different values of a and b

Let f be a given experimental geophysical signal with energy content $E_f = <f, f>$. For the analysis of wavelet ψ, the wavelet variance WV_f of f is defined as the integral sum of the squares of transform coefficients at different scales of all data points as follows,

$$WV_f(a) = \frac{1}{T_2(a) - T_1(a)} \int_{T_1(a)}^{T_2(a)} [(W_\psi f)(a,b)]^2 \, db \qquad (2)$$

where $T_1(a)$ and $T_2(a)$ are the lower and upper bounds of the spatial range where transform coefficients are computed for a given scale a. The wavelet variance is simply the average of the squares of the wavelet coefficients at every point along the transection for a given scale. As energy is conserved in wavelet transformation, the area under a wavelet variance is proportional to the energy content of the signal. Its relative magnitudes can thus be used to measure the scale dependence of the relative strengths of different structures. Moreover, a dominant structure or correlation length is usually characterized by a large local WV_f (a) value. The scale at the peak of WV_f (a) (dWV_f (a)/da = 0) can be used as an objective estimate of the scale of the dominant structure (Li 1995; Gao and Li 1993; Collineau and Brunet 1993; Li and Loehle 1995). Thus, wavelet variance can be used to capture appropriate correlation scales of spatial heterogeneity of CPT data. Phase change and local wavelet transform modulus maxima (Delprat et al. 1992; Muzy et al. 1994) can be used to characterize scale effects and to extract local features and site stratigraphy from the collected CPT data.

Recent research indicates that Fourier analysis and classical box-counting methods cannot reveal the multi-fractal structure of a signal easily and that wavelet analysis can provide an immediate access to information that is obscured by time (or space) - frequency methods (Meyer 1993). The wavelet-based method provides a natural generalization of the classical box-counting techniques for fractal objects as the wavelets actually play the role of "generalized boxes" (Muzy et al. 1994). The method thus provides a more generalized tool to analyze non-stationary, nonlinear, and multi-scale geophysical signals. Beyond statistical characterization of the scaling properties of fractal objects, the advantages of the wavelet transform microscope can also be taken to address the fundamental issue of solving the inverse fractal problem. In many cases, the self-similarity properties of fractals can be expressed in terms of a dynamic system that leaves the object invariant. The inverse fractal problem consists of recovering the dynamical system or its main characteristics from the data.

APPLICATION OF WAVELETS TO CPT DATA ANALYSIS

Data interpretation and accuracy in determining stratigraphy by CPT technology are complex processes due to the presence of localized and multi-scale features in the subsurface. Most current interpretation methods are empirical or semi-empirical. Each of these methods is often applicable only to limited types of soils. In order to develop a rapid, reliable, safe and cost effective technique for *in-situ* and real-time characterization of subsurface contamination, CPT data processing techniques need to be improved. In this preliminary study, wavelet transform and wavelet variance are used to characterize multi-scale features of CPT data, and wavelet transform modulus maxima and phases are used to evaluate scale effects and site stratigraphy. The "Mexican hat" mother wavelet function $\psi(t') = (1-16t'^2)\exp(-8t'^2)$, the second-order derivative of the Gaussian function defined within $-1 \leq t' \leq 1$, is used in the analyses. The radius of the window mother wavelet function is 1. This "Mexican hat" function is well localized in both time (or space) and frequency as shown in Fig. 2. When the wavelet function is applied to Eq. (1), t' is replaced by $(t - b)/a$. A wavelet variance, defined by integrating the wavelet coefficient fluctuations as presented in Eq. (2), is used to detect the characteristic scales of non-periodically spaced spatial structures. Results indicate that this method can provide a basis for the quantification and characterization of the subsurface.

The CPT data used for the analyses include pore pressure, sleeve friction, and tip resistance as a function of depth. The characteristic scales of spatially correlated heterogeneity of pore pressure, sleeve friction, and tip resistance in the CPT data are presented in Fig.

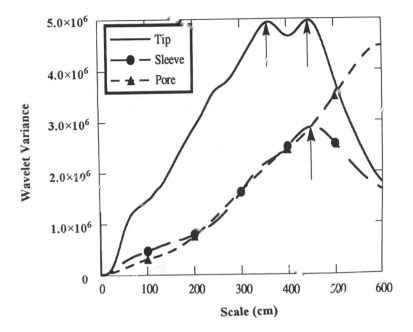

FIG. 3 -- Characteristic multi-scales of spatially correlated heterogeneity of pore pressure, sleeve friction, and tip resistance measured by CPT. (Curves indicate magnitude of variability as a function of scale, and arrows indicate scale of local maximum variance.)

3. When all the data are included in the evaluation of Eq. (2), two peaks can be observed in the tip resistance data at 3.63 m and 4.47 m. A single dominant scale is observed in the sleeve friction data at 4.54 m. However, no dominant scale under 6 m is observed in the pore pressure data. It is very interesting to observe that the single dominant scale of the sleeve friction data is very close to one of the dominant scales of the tip resistance data. From the scaling and resolution standpoints, this observation provides support for the validity of current CPT data interpretation methods that use tip resistance and sleeve friction information to characterize the subsurface. However, extreme care must be exercised to handle different CPT variables with different scales. These scaling results will improve our current data interpretation, especially in the integration of different scale data in CPT measurement. These scaling information may also help to detect different contaminants in the subsurface as different materials have their specific physical and chemical features in time (or space) and/or frequency domain. The results of phase changes of CPT data, e.g., pore pressure, sleeve friction and tip resistance, at scales from 0 to 0.5 m, 0 to 1 m, and 0 to 1.5 m are presented in Fig. 4. The curves give the scales at which the wavelet transform modulus maxima occur within the limits as a function of depth. It is obvious that these scales depend on the upper

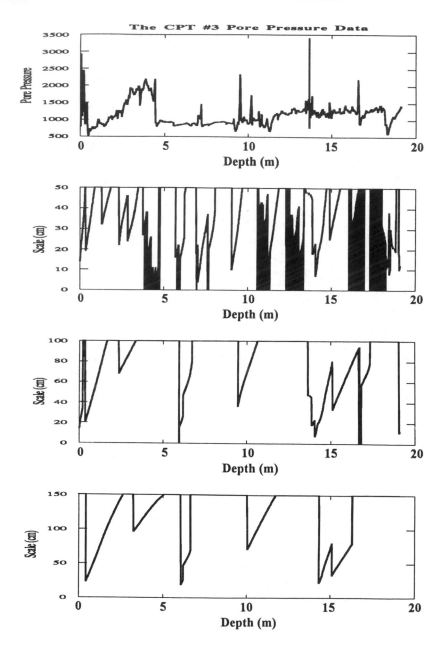

FIG. 4a -- Scaling effects on the determination of site stratigraphy by pore pressure
    measured by CPT

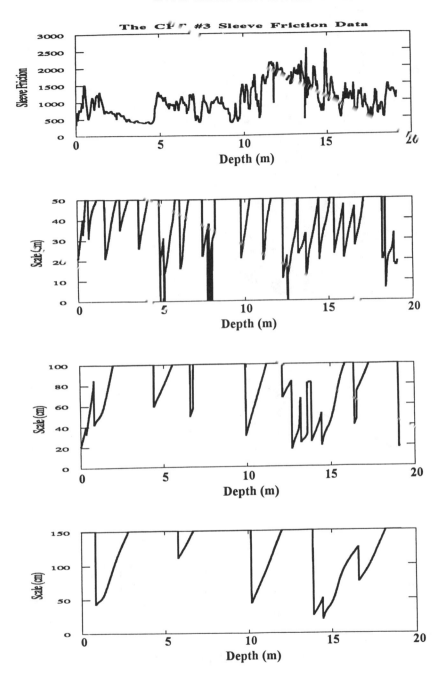

FIG. 4b -- Scaling effects on the determination of site stratigraphy by sleeve friction
measured by CPT

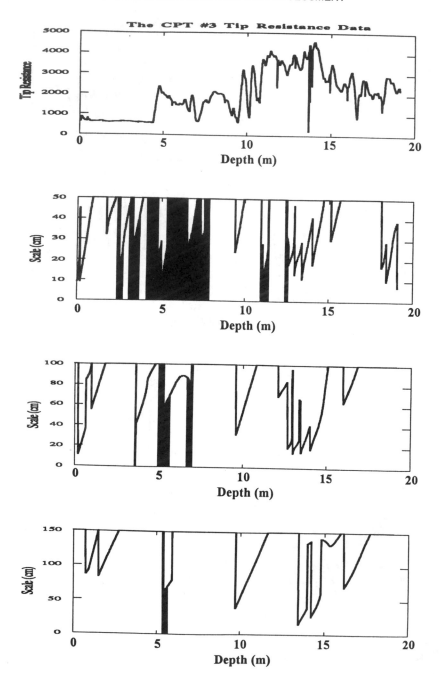

FIG. 4c -- Scaling effects on the determination of site stratigraphy by tip resistance measured by CPT

bound of the scale. When a scale is chosen, the curves give the depths at which the data change phase as the locations of wavelet transform modulus maxima give the depths where the data change phase. Thus, the space between any two wavelet transform modulus maxima at a given scale can be interpreted statistically as a phase. Physically, the subsurface layer between any two wavelet transform modulus maxima can be interpreted as a stratum. The interpreted site stratigraphy agree well with the observations made in confirmatory boreholes. These information can also be used to determine soil structures, and type/concentration/ location of subsurface contaminants. As the scale changes, one can "zoom in" and "zoom out" the detailed structures at different scales.

DISCUSSIONS AND CONCLUSIONS

In the analysis and interpretation of signals such as the CPT data and seismic signals, the ability of the technique used to extract relevant features from the data is of vital importance. The important features of the signals, such as edges, spikes, or transients, are often characterized by localized information either in the time (or space) domain, the frequency (or wave number) domain, or both. In this preliminary research, wavelet transformation and wavelet transform modulus maxima are used to filter CPT data. The technique may provide a new approach for the analysis and interpretation of CPT data. These information can be used as a basis to quantify and characterize any subsurface properties relevant to contamination. Current wavelet transform methods (1-d, 2-d and 3-d) require evenly spaced data. However, this requirement does not impose any restriction on the interpretation of CPT data as they are collected at regular intervals in depth.

Many decision processes in CPT data analysis and interpretation involve several variables or dimensions. Therefore, the acceptability of an alternative interpretation method depends on how well it addresses the characteristics of the problem in concern with respect to these variables or dimensions. Combining this approach and an adaptive fuzzy modeling technique (Li and Yeung 1994) will provide great potential for rapid assessment and prioritization of many contaminated sites across the country.

Characterization of the subsurface needs to integrate data from a variety of sources such as cores, logs, seismic traces, pressure transients, tracer tests, cone penetrometer measurements, borehole flowmeter measurements, etc. Such data integration is computing intensive and non-trivial since different data types span different length scales of heterogeneities. Wavelet analysis will surpass current geostatistical methods by using techniques from geophysical inverse theory along with high resolution numerical modeling to identify dominant patterns in subsurface heterogeneities and examine their impact on environmental remediation and other subsurface processes.

ACKNOWLEDGEMENTS

This research is supported in part by the U. S. Department of Energy Subsurface Science Program under Contract No. W-31-109-ENG-38 through the Argonne National Laboratory at Chicago, Illinois, and the National Science Foundation under Grant No. CMS

9211336. The support is gratefully acknowledged. The authors also wish to thank Craig Loehle, Andrew Chan, Charles Chui, Weigang Gao, Akhil Datta-Gupta, and Ching Wu for many helpful discussions. The CPT data used in the analyses are provided by the Argonne National Laboratory.

REFERENCES

Akhtar, A. S., 1995, "Development of a Cone and an Apparatus for the Measurement of Electrical Properties of Contaminated Soils," M.Eng. Report, Department of Civil Engineering, Texas A&M University, College Station.

Bowders, J. J. and Daniel, D. E., 1994, "Cone Penetration Technology for Subsurface Characterization," Geotechnical News, Vol. 12, No. 3, pp. 24-29.

Brewer, K. E. and Wheatcraft, S. W., 1994, "Including Multi-scale Information in the Characterization of Hydraulic Conductivity Distributions," Wavelets in Geophysics, E. Foufoula-Georgiou and P. Kumar, Eds., Academic Press, San Diego, pp. 213-248.

Carrera, J., 1993, "An Overview of Uncertainties in Modelling Groundwater Solute Transport," Journal of Contaminant Hydrology, Vol. 13, No. 1, pp. 23-48.

Chui, C. K., 1992, An Introduction to Wavelets, Academic Press, Inc., Boston.

Collineau, S. and Brunet, Y., 1993, "Detection of Turbulent Coherent Motions in a Forest Canopy. Part I: Wavelet Analysis," Boundary-Layer Meteorology, Vol. 65, pp. 357-379.

Delprat, N., Escudie, B., Guillemain, P., Kronland-Martinet, R., Tchamitchian, P., and Torresani, B., 1992, "Asymptotic Wavelet and Gabor Analysis: Extraction of Instantaneous Frequencies," IEEE Transaction on Information Theory, Vol. 38, No. 3, pp. 644-664.

Deutsch, C. V. and Journel, A. G., 1992, GSLIB: Geostatistical Software Library and User's Guide. Oxford University Press, New York.

Gao, W. and Li, B. L., 1993, "Wavelet Analysis of Coherent Structures at the Atmosphere-Forest Interface," Journal of Applied Meteorology, Vol. 32, No. 11, pp. 1717-1725.

Haining, R., 1990, Spatial Data Analysis in the Social and Environmental Sciences. Cambridge University Press, Cambridge.

Kumar, P. and Foufoula-Georgiou, E., 1994, "Wavelet Analysis in Geophysics: An Introduction," Wavelets in Geophysics, E. Foufoula-Georgiou and P. Kumar, Eds., Academic Press, San Diego, pp. 1-43.

Li, B. L., 1995, "Wavelet Analysis for Characterizing Spatial Heterogeneity in the Subsurface," Wavelet Applications in Signal and Image Processing III, A. F. Laine, M. A. Unser, and M. V. Wickerhauser, Eds., Vol. 2569, SPIE Press, Bellingham.

Li, B. L. and Loehle, C., 1995, "Wavelet Analysis of Multiscale Permeabilities in the Subsurface," Geophysical Research Letters, Vol. 22, No. 23, pp. 3123-3126.

Li, B. L., Loehle, C., and Malon, D., 1996, "Microbial Transport through Heterogeneous Porous Media: Random Walk, Fractal, and Percolation Approaches," International Journal of Ecological Modelling, in press.

Li, B. L., Wu, Y., and Wu, J., 1992, "Patchiness and Patch Dynamics: II. Description and Analysis," Chinese Journal of Ecology, Vol. 11, No. 5, pp. 28-37.

Li, B. L. and Yeung, A. T., 1994, "An Adaptive Fuzzy Modeling Framework for Character-ization of Subsurface Contamination," Proceedings of the 1st International Joint Conference of the North American Fuzzy Information Processing Society Biannual Conference, the Industrial Fuzzy Control and Intelligent Systems Conference, and the NASA Joint Technology Workshop on Neural Network and Fuzzy Logic, San Antonio, Texas, L. Hall, H. Ying, R. Langari, and J. Yen, Eds., IEEE Press, pp. 194-195.

Loehle, C. and Li, B. L., 1996, "Statistical Properties of Ecological and Geologic Fractals," International Journal of Ecological Modelling, in press.

Meyer, Y., 1993, Wavelets: Algorithms and Applications, SIAM, Philadelphia.

Muzy, J. F., Bacry, E., and Arneodo, A., 1994, "The Multifractal Formalism Revisited with Wavelets," International Journal of Bifurcation and Chaos, Vol. 4, No. 2, pp. 245-302.

Olsen, R. S., August 1994 "Normalization and Prediction of Geotechnical Properties Using the Cone Penetrometer Test (CPT)," Technical Report GL-94-29, Waterways Experiment Station, US Army Corps of Engineers, Vicksburg, Mississippi.

Pike, C. J., 1994, "Analysis of High Resolution Marine Seismic Data Using the Wavelet Transform," Wavelets in Geophysics, E. Foufoula-Georgiou and P. Kumar, Eds., Academic Press, San Diego, pp. 183-211.

Seyfried, M. S. and Wilcox, B. P., 1995, "Scale and the nature of spatial variability: field examples having implications for hydrologic modeling," Water Resource Research.

Author Index

Subject Index

A

Acid volatile sulfides, 53
Alcohol exposure, 79
Ammonia, 285
Amphibian toxicity, 188
Amphipods, 53, 285
Aquatic species, 285, 301, 323
   amphipods, 53, 285
   crayfish, 344
   estrogen tests, 23
   fish, 37, 79, 310
   invertebrates, 323
   mosquitofish, 117
   mysids, 257
   oyster larvae, 53
   plants, 163, 270
   test quality procedures, 349,
     374
ASTM standards
   E 1191, 257
   E 1367, 285
Atrazine, 270

B

Benthic invertebrates, 323
Benzo(a)pyrene, 138
Biphenyls, polychlorinated, 53,
   219, 230
Birds, 95
Brain, 219
   gross rain asymmetry, 230

C

Cadmium, 344
Carbon, total organic, 53
Chicken embryo method, 204,
   219
Chlorophyll content, 163
Chromium, 426
Chromosone, 109
Cladoceran, 79, 177
Clastogenic exposure, 109
Cleanup levels, 426

Coal tar, 138
Competition, aquatic
   invertebrates, 323
Computer tomography, 230
Cone penetrometer test, 456
Copepod, 79
Copper, 177, 188
Cotinine, 149
Cover-seeking behavior,
   crayfish, 344
Creosote, 163
Crustaceans, 323
Cytochrome P450, 53, 95

D

Daphnia, 177
Daphnia magna, 79
di-4-ANEPPS, 177
Diazinon, 177
Dibenzofuran, 219
Dioxin, 204
DNA adducts, quantifying, 117
DNA damage, translocations,
   109
Dose, risk assessment, 392
Duckweed, 163

E

Earthworm, 79
Ecological significance, 310
Effluent testing, 374, 349
Egg injection method, 204, 219
Electroretinogram, 239
ELISA tests, 23, 149
Embryonic exposure, 204, 219,
   230
Enzyme-linked immunosorbant
   assay (ELISA), 23, 149
Estrogen, 3, 23
Estuarine variables, 270
Ethyoxyresorufin-O-deethylase
   (EROD) induction, 204
Eurytemora affinis, 79

473